T0271934

Spatio-Temporal Methods in Environmental Epidemiology with R

Spatio-Temporal Methods in Environmental Epidemiology with R, like its First Edition, explores the interface between environmental epidemiology and spatio-temporal modeling. It links recent developments in spatio-temporal theory with epidemiological applications. Drawing on real-life problems, it shows how recent advances in methodology can assess the health risks associated with environmental hazards. The book's clear guidelines enable the implementation of the methodology and estimation of risks in practice.

New additions to the Second Edition include: a thorough exploration of the underlying concepts behind knowledge discovery through data; a new chapter on extracting information from data using R and the tidyverse; additional material on methods for Bayesian computation, including the use of NIMBLE and Stan; new methods for performing spatio-temporal analysis and an updated chapter containing further topics. Throughout the book there are new examples, and the presentation of R code for examples has been extended. Along with these additions, the book now has a GitHub site (https://spacetime-environ.github.io/stepi2) that contains data, code and further worked examples.

Features:
- Explores the interface between environmental epidemiology and spatio-temporal modeling
- Incorporates examples that show how spatio-temporal methodology can inform societal concerns about the effects of environmental hazards on health
- Uses a Bayesian foundation on which to build an integrated approach to spatio-temporal modeling and environmental epidemiology
- Discusses data analysis and topics such as data visualization, mapping, wrangling and analysis
- Shows how to design networks for monitoring hazardous environmental processes and the ill effects of preferential sampling
- Through the listing and application of code, shows the power of R, tidyverse, NIMBLE and Stan and other modern tools in performing complex data analysis and modeling

Representing a continuing important direction in environmental epidemiology, this book – in full color throughout – underscores the increasing need to consider dependencies in both space and time when modeling epidemiological data. Readers will learn how to identify and model patterns in spatio-temporal data and how to exploit dependencies over space and time to reduce bias and inefficiency when estimating risks to health.

CHAPMAN & HALL/CRC

Texts in Statistical Science Series

Joseph K. Blitzstein, *Harvard University, USA*
Julian J. Faraway, *University of Bath, UK*
Martin Tanner, *Northwestern University, USA*
Jim Zidek, *University of British Columbia, Canada*

Recently Published Titles

Bayes Rules!
An Introduction to Applied Bayesian Modeling
Alicia Johnson, Miles Ott and Mine Dogucu

Stochastic Processes with R
An Introduction
Olga Korosteleva

Design and Analysis of Experiments and Observational Studies using R
Nathan Taback

Time Series for Data Science: Analysis and Forecasting
Wayne A. Woodward, Bivin Philip Sadler and Stephen Robertson

Statistical Theory
A Concise Introduction, Second Edition
Felix Abramovich and Ya'acov Ritov

Applied Linear Regression for Longitudinal Data
With an Emphasis on Missing Observations
Frans E.S. Tan and Shahab Jolani

Fundamentals of Mathematical Statistics
Steffen Lauritzen

Modelling Survival Data in Medical Research, Fourth Edition
David Collett

Applied Categorical and Count Data Analysis, Second Edition
Wan Tang, Hua He and Xin M. Tu

Geographic Data Science with Python
Sergio Rey, Dani Arribas-Bel and Levi John Wolf

Models for Multi-State Survival Data
Rates, Risks, and Pseudo-Values
Per Kragh Andersen and Henrik Ravn

Spatio–Temporal Methods in Environmental Epidemiology with R, Second Edition
Gavin Shaddick, James V. Zidek, and Alex Schmidt

A Course in the Large Sample Theory of Statistical Inference
W. Jackson Hall and David Oakes

For more information about this series, please visit: https://www.routledge.com/
Chapman--HallCRC-Texts-in-Statistical-Science/book-series/CHTEXSTASCI

Spatio-Temporal Methods in Environmental Epidemiology with R

Second Edition

Gavin Shaddick
James V. Zidek
Alexandra M. Schmidt

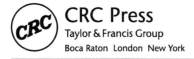

CRC Press
Taylor & Francis Group
Boca Raton London New York

CRC Press is an imprint of the
Taylor & Francis Group, an **informa** business

A CHAPMAN & HALL BOOK

Second edition published 2024
by CRC Press
2385 NW Executive Center Drive, Suite 320, Boca Raton FL 33431

and by CRC Press
4 Park Square, Milton Park, Abingdon, Oxon, OX14 4RN

CRC Press is an imprint of Taylor & Francis Group, LLC

© 2024 Gavin Shaddick, James V. Zidek, and Alexandra M. Schmidt

First edition published by Taylor and Francis Group, LLC 2021

ISBN: 978-1-032-39781-8 (hbk)
ISBN: 978-1-032-40351-9 (pbk)
ISBN: 978-1-003-35265-5 (ebk)

DOI: 10.1201/9781003352655

Typeset in Nimbus font
by KnowledgeWorks Global Ltd.

Publisher's note: This book has been prepared from camera-ready copy provided by the authors.

Dedications:

Gavin to Jo and Cynthia;

Jim to Lynne;

Alex to Lourdes, Artur and Marco

Contents

List of Figures

List of Tables

Preface

Motivated by increased societal concerns about environmental hazards, this book explores the interface between environmental epidemiology (EE) and spatio-temporal (ST) modeling. Its aim is to promote the interface between statisticians and practitioners in order to allow the rapid advances in the field of spatio-temporal statistics to be fully exploited in assessing risks to health. The aim of EE is to understand the adverse health effects of environmental hazards and to estimate the risks associated with those hazards. Such risks have traditionally been assessed either over time at a fixed point in space or over space at a fixed point in time. ST modeling characterizes the distribution of those hazards and associated risks over both geographical locations and time. Understanding variation and exploiting dependencies over both space and time greatly increases the power to assess those relationships.

Motivated by real-life problems, this book aims to provide both a link between recent advances in ST methodology and epidemiological applications and to provide a means to implement these methods in practice. The book recognizes the increasing number of statistical researchers who are collaborating with environmental epidemiologists. Many excellent books on spatial statistics and spatial epidemiology were available when this book was written, including: Banerjee, Carlin, and Gelfand (2015), N. Cressie (1993), N. Cressie and Wikle (2011), P. J. Diggle and Ribeiro (2007), Le and Zidek (2006), Schabenberger and Gotway (2000), Stein (1999), Waller and Gotway (2004), Lawson (2013) and Elliott, Wakefield, Best, and Briggs (2000). This selection provides an excellent resource; however, none specifically addresses the interface between environmental epidemiology and spatio-temporal modeling. This is the central theme of this book and we believe it promotes a major new direction in environmental epidemiology where there is an increasing need to consider spatio-temporal patterns in data that can be used to borrow strength over space and time and to reduce bias and inefficiency.

The genesis of the book was a thematic year at the Statistical and Applied Mathematical Sciences Institute (SAMSI) on 'Space–time Analysis for Environmental Mapping, Epidemiology and Climate Change'. It was the basis of a course in spatio-temporal epidemiology and was successfully used in a 13-week graduate statistics course at the University of British Columbia. A key feature of the book is the coverage of a wide range of topics from an introduction to spatio-temporal and epidemiological principles along with the foundations of ST modeling, with specific focus on their application, to new directions for research. This includes both traditional and Bayesian approaches, the latter providing an important unifying framework for the integration of ST modeling into EE and which is key to many of the approaches presented within the book. Coverage of current research topics includes visualization and mapping; the analysis of high-dimensional data; dealing with stationary fields; the combination of deterministic and statistical models; the design of monitoring networks and the effects of preferential sampling.

Throughout the book, the theory of spatial, temporal and ST modeling is presented in the context of its application to EE and examples are given throughout. These examples are provided together with embedded R code and details of the use of specific R packages and other software, including Win-BUGS/OpenBUGS and modern computational methods such as integrated nested Laplace approximations (INLA). Additional code, data and examples are provided in the online resources associated with the book. A link can be found at http://www.crcpress.com/product/isbn/9781482237030.

As a text, this book is intended for students in both epidemiology and statistics. The original course at the University of British Columbia (UBC) was intended for graduate-level students in statistics and epidemiology and lasted for 13 weeks, with two 90-minute lectures and a two-hour lab session each week.

The main topics covered included:

- Types of epidemiological studies: cohort, case–control, ecological.

- Measures of risk: relative risks, odds ratios, absolute risk, sources of bias, assessing uncertainty.

- Bayesian statistics and computational techniques: Markov Chain Monte Carlo (MCMC) and Integrated nested Laplace approximations (INLA).

- Regression models in epidemiology: Logistic and Poisson generalized linear models, generalized additive models, hierarchical models, measurement error models.

- Temporal models: time series models, temporal auto-correlation, smoothing splines.

- Spatial models: point processes, area and point referenced methods, mapping, geostatistical methods, spatial regression, non-stationary models, preferential sampling.

- Spatial-temporal models: separable models, non-separable models, modeling exposures in space and time, correction for ecological bias.

In addition to the material covered in this course, the book contains details of many other topics, several of which are covered in greater technical depth.

Many universities operate a 15-week schedule, and this book was initially designed for such courses. Three examples include: (i) a course for epidemiologists with the emphasis on the application of ST models in EE; (ii) a course for biostatisticians, covering underlying principles of modeling and application and (iii) an advanced course on more theoretical aspects of spatio-temporal statistics and its application in EE. Further information on possible course structures, together with exercises, lab projects and other material, can be found in the online resources.

To conclude, we would like to express our deepest gratitude to all of those who have contributed to this book, both in terms of specific assistance in its creation and also in a much wider sense. This includes our many co-authors and past and present students. In regard to the latter, special thanks goes out to the Class of 2013 at UBC, who provided invaluable feedback when the material in the book was first presented. A huge 'Thank You' goes to Song Cai, whose work as a lab instructor was instrumental in developing the exercises and projects. Thank you also to those who attended the short courses on this topic at Telford (RSS), Toronto (SSC) and Cancun (ISBA).

The book was written jointly in the Department of Mathematical Sciences at the University of Bath and the Department of Statistics at the University of British Columbia, both as home institutions but also as hosts of visits by the two authors. We thank the staff and faculty of these two departments for their support and guidance. We would like to thank Yang 'Seagle' Liu (UBC), Yiping Dou (UBC) and Yi Liu (Bath) for allowing us to include their code and other material in the book and in the online resources. Similarly, thanks go to Ali Hauschilt (UBC), Kathryn Morrison and Roni English for proofreading and Millie Jobling (Bath) for comments and help in preparing the text. Many thanks also to Duncan Lee for providing data and code for some of the examples. The Peter Wall Institute for Advanced Studies (PWIAS, UBC) generously supported an opportunity for both authors to work together at PWIAS and to finalize the book.

We appreciate the support of CRC/Chapman and Hall and particularly Rob Calver, Senior Acquisitions Editor for the Taylor and Francis Group, who played a key role in encouraging and supporting this work throughout its production. Many thanks also to Suzanne Lassandro. Special thanks go to the anonymous reviewers of the book, who provided extremely helpful and insightful comments on early drafts.

The first author would like to give special thanks to Paul Elliott and Jon Wakefield for stimulating and maintaining his interest in the subject, and to Jon for continued statistical enlightenment. Finally, he would like to give special thanks to his mum (Cynthia) for everything, from beginning to end, and to Jo for encouragement, patience, support and continued good nature during a period in which plenty was required. From both authors, very special thanks go to Lynne for continual encouragement, support and providing essential sustenance. Above all, she took on the virtually impossible role of ensuring that this transatlantic co-authorship actually resulted in a book!

Bath, UK   *Gavin Shaddick*
Vancouver, Canada   *James V. Zidek*
February 2015

Preface to Second Edition

The overall aims and academic level of the revision remain the same as those of the first edition. Briefly, it aims to explore the interface between environmental epidemiology (EE) and spatio-temporal (ST) modeling. Its intended audience: graduate students in epidemiology with an intermediate-level background in statistics, and graduate students in statistics. The original steered a course between a cut-and-paste style cookbook and a scholarly work on underlying theory.

The field of spatio-temporal statistics has continued to evolve rapidly since the original version was published in 2015, and thanks especially to the addition of Professor Alex Schmidt as a third author, we have been able to include a broader range of theoretical methods, methods for computational implementation and more applications. New ways of implementing theory and methods in applications have been added, replacing some of the now lesser used approaches that were in the first edition. As a result of these changes, the book has grown from 368 to almost 500 pages. This gives instructors more topics to choose from when planning their courses, depending on the educational backgrounds of their students. This book will also assist practitioners to take advantage of these changes, as these advances in statistical science have led to the possibility of more sophisticated models for evaluating the health risks of exposures, which vary over space and time. In summary, motivated by real-life problems, this book will continue to aim at providing a link between recent advances in spatial-temporal methodology and epidemiological applications, together with the means to implement these methods in practice. Compared to the first edition, some of the chapter titles have been changed to better reflect the story the book is trying to tell.

The book's foundation has three general components, which together will lead to an understanding of processes associated with spatio-temporal environmental epidemiology, and hence lead to a reduction in the uncertainty associated with them:

(i) The first component is represented by a process model, which incorporates direct and indirect prior knowledge about the natural process of interest, for example a pollution field.

(ii) Together with the form of the underlying process model we require prior knowledge to inform the parameters of the model, that may change dynamically over space and/or time.

(iii) The third, empirical component of the investigation, leads to the data model that is measurement model. This third route to understanding has seen an explosion of interest in data science, and has lead to an entire chapter being devoted to it in this book.

The book now has a GitHub site (https://spacetime-environ.github.io/stepi2) that contains a toolbox of R-packages that has grown to enhance the value of the new methods now available for spatio-temporal modeling and make a wider array of applications feasible. That GitHub site *provides R code, data and links to data files, together with solutions to selected exercises, on a chapter-by-chapter basis. It also contains material from the first edition of the book.* The authors intend to keep the site updated and will add errata, additional data, code, reviews and so on.

The authors remain indebted to all those individuals and institutions named above in the Preface to the first edition. To this list we now add, acknowledge, and warmly thank, individuals who helped put this revision together:

- Ms. Mariana Carmona Baez inspired the creation of the Bookdown format for the examples on the GitHub site associated with the second edition;

- Dr. Sara Zapata-Marin together with Mariana provided the code and analyses for the worked examples using Bookdown and helped develop the GitHub site they can be accessed;

- Mr. Paritosh Kumar Roy provided the code for the forward-filtering-backward-sampling algorithm discussed in Chapter 11;

- Mr. Johnny Li assisted with a number of software issues and assembled solutions for selected exercises;

- Dr. Laís P. Freitas, for her inspired graphic on the front cover, of spatio-temporal processes combined with their epidemiological impacts;

- Dr. Joe Watson, for help in assembling his preferential sampling software for modeling the effect.

- Dr. Matthew L. Thomas, for providing code, models, data and ideas related to the examples based on the WHO air quality database and modeling air pollutants in Europe.

A big thanks also to Mr. Rob Calver, Senior Publisher-Mathematics, Statistics, and Physics, Chapman and Hall/CRC Press, Taylor and Francis Group, for his advice and encouragement. Also, to Shashi Kumar, for assistance with the LaTeX file. Finally, thank you, Lynne Zidek, for an enormous amount of help in coordinating and managing the revision.

In the second edition, R code is now fully listed in the examples where it is used. These examples are provided as in the first edition, along with embedded R code and details on the use of specific R packages and other software.

Additional code, data and examples are provided on the book's GitHub site, along with other online resources associated with the book. These can be found on the GitHub site for the book.

Updates from the first edition include:

- Dramatic new advances in spatio-temporal modeling, especially R packages for implementing those models, notably with NIMBLE and STAN, which replace the WinBugs used in the first edition;

- A new chapter on data science that includes such things as data wrangling, along with a clear description of the complimentary roles of data modeling, process modeling and parameter modeling;

- Listed code for software used in examples;

- Modern computational methods, including INLA, together with code for implementation are provided;

- A new section on causality showing how the comparison of the impact of Covid in China and Italy are completely reversed when Simpson decomposition is applied:

- The R code for the examples is now fully listed in the text and available, with addition examples and code, on the book's GitHub site;

- Solutions to selected problems appear in the GitHub site;

- How to wrap a deterministic model in a stochastic shell by a unified approach to physical and statistical modeling;

- New sections on causality and confounders, including the relationship of Simpson's paradox with process models.

London, UK   *Gavin Shaddick*
Vancouver, Canada   *James V. Zidek*
Montreal, Canada   *Alexandra M. Schmidt*
May 2023

Abbreviations

ACF	Autocorrelation function
AIC	Akaike information criterion
AR	Autoregressive process
ARIMA	Autoregressive regressive integrated moving average
ARMA	Autoregressive regressive moving average
Be–Ne–Lux	Belgium, Netherlands, Luxembourg region
BIC	Bayesian information criteria
BLUP	Best linear unbiased predictor
BSP	Bayesian spatial predictor
CapMon	Canadian Acid Precipitation Monitoring Network
CAR	Conditional autoregressive approach
CAR	Conditional autoregressive
CDF	Cumulative distribution function
CI	Confidence interval or in Bayesian analysis, credible interval
CMAQ	Community multi–scale air quality model
CMT	Chemical transport models
CO	Carbon monoxide
CRF	Concentration response function
CSD	Census subdivision
CV	Cross validation
DIC	Deviance information criterion
DLM	Dynamic linear model
DT	Delauney triangle
ERF	Exposure response function
EU	European union
GCV	Generalised cross validation
GEV	Generalized extreme value distribution
GF	Gaussian field
GMRF	Gaussian Markov random field
GPD	Generalized Pareto distribution
Hg	Mercury
ICD	International Classification Codes for Diseases
IRLS	Interactively re–weighted least squares
KKF	Kriged Kalman filter
LHS	Latin hybercube sampling
MAR	Multivariate autoregressive process

MCAR	Multivariate CAR
MESA	Multi–ethnic study of atherosclerosis
mg/kg or mg^{-1}	Micrograms per kilogram
μgm^{-3}	Micrograms per meter cubed
MRF	Markov random field
MSE	Mean squared error
NADP	National Atmospheric Deposition Program
NCS	Natural cubic splines
NO$_2$	Nitrogen dioxide
NUSAP	Numerical–Units–Spread–Assessment–Pedigree
O$_3$	Ozone
PACF	Partial autocorrelation function
Pb	Chemical symbol for lead
PDF	Probability density function
PMF	Probability mass function
PM$_{10}$	Airborne particulates of diameter less than 10 μgm^{-3}
PM$_{2.5}$	Airborne particulates of diameter less than 2.5 μgm^{-3}
POT	Peak over threshold
ppb	Particles per billion
ppm	Particles per million
PYR	Person year at risk
RR	Relative risk
RS	Relative sensitivity
SAR	Simultaneous autoregressive
SIR	Susceptible–infective–recovered model for infectious diseases
SMR	Standard mortality ratio
SO$_2$	Sulphite or sulphur dioxide
SPDE	Stochastic partial differential equations
UTM	Universal Transverse Mercator (coordinate system)
VAR	Vector autoregressive process
VOC	Volatile organic compounds
WHO	World Health Organization

The Authors

Professor Gavin Shaddick is the Executive Dean of the School of Engineering, Mathematical and Physical Sciences and a Professor of Data Science and Statistics at Royal Holloway, University of London and a Turing Fellow at The Alan Turing Institute. His research interests lie at the interface of statistics, AI, epidemiology and environmental science. He is a member of the UK government's Committee on the Medical Effects of Air Pollutants (COMEAP) and the sub-group on Quantification of Air Pollution Risk (QUARK). He leads the World Health Organization's Data Integration Taskforce for Global Air Quality and led the development of the Data Integration Model for Air Quality (DIMAQ) that is used to calculate a number of air pollution related to United Nations Sustainable Development Goals indicators.

Professor James V. Zidek is a Professor Emeritus at the University of British Columbia. He received his M.Sc. and Ph.D. from the University of Alberta and Stanford University, both in Statistics. His research interests include the foundations of environmetrics, notably on the design of environmental monitoring networks and spatio-temporal modeling of environmental processes. His contributions to statistics have been recognized by a number of awards including Fellowships of the ASA and IMI, the Gold Medal of the Statistical Society of Canada and Fellowship in the Royal Society of Canada, one of that country's highest honors for a scientist.

Professor Alexandra M. Schmidt has joined the Shaddick-Zidek team of co-authors. She is a Professor of Biostatistics at McGill University. She is distinguished for her work in the theory of spatio-temporal modeling and more recently for that in biostatistics as well as epidemiology. In recognition of that work, she received awards from The International Environmetrics Society (TIES) and the American Statistical Association's Section on Statistics and the Environment (ENVR-ASA). She was the 2015 President of the International Society for Bayesian Analysis and Chair of the Local Organizing Committee for the 2022 ISBA meeting. Her current topics of research include nonnormal models for spatio-temporal processes and the analysis of joint epidemics of dengue, Zika and chikungunya in Latin America.

Chapter 1

An overview of spatio-temporal epidemiology and knowledge discovery

1.1 Overview

Spatial epidemiology is the description and analysis of geographical data, specifically health data, in the form of counts of mortality or morbidity, and factors that may explain variations in those counts over space. These may include demographic and environmental factors together with genetic and infectious risk factors (Elliott and Wartenberg, 2004). It have a long history dating back to the mid-1800s when John Snow's map of cholera cases in London in 1854 provided an early example of geographical health analyzes that aimed to identify possible causes of outbreaks of infectious diseases (Hempel, 2014). Since then, advances in statistical methodology together with the increasing availability of data recorded at very high spatial and temporal resolution have led to great advances in spatial and, more recently, spatio-temporal epidemiology.

There are a number of reasons for considering measurements over both space and time in epidemiological studies, including an increase in power when processes evolve over both the spatial and temporal domains, gaining additional information on risks when we have contrasting levels over the two domains and when spatial fields are temporally independent, replicates of the spatial field become available and spatial dependence is easier to model. However, in the latter case, the likely presence of temporal dependence leads to a need to build complex dependence structures. At the cost of increased complexity, such models may use the full benefit of the information contained in the spatio-temporal field. This means that dependencies across both space and time can be exploited in terms of 'borrowing strength'. For example, values could be predicted at unmonitored spatial locations or at future times to help protect against predicted overexposure.

Advances in spatio-temporal methodology that address the challenges of modeling with increasingly complex data have been driven in part by increased awareness of the potential effects of environmental hazards and potential increases in the hazards themselves. In order to assess and manage the risks associated with environmental hazards, there is a need for monitoring and modeling the associated environmental processes that will lead to an increase in a wide variety of adverse health outcomes. Recent advances in methodology that allows complex patterns of dependencies over space and time to be exploited in producing predictions of environmental hazards play an important role in monitoring progress towards the United Nations' 2030 Agenda for Sustainable Development. This calls for a plan of action for people, planet and prosperity. It aims to take the bold and transformative steps that are urgently needed to shift the world onto a sustainable and resilient path. Quality, accessible, timely and reliable disaggregated data are essential for understanding the scale of the challenges and in measuring progress to ensure that no one is left behind. However, the United Nations Environmental Programme estimates that of the 93 environment-related Sustainable Development Goals (SDGs) indicators, there is insufficient data to assess progress for 68% of them.

Example 1.1. *Global modeling of fine particulate air pollution*

An example of the need for modeling over space and time is in the global assessments of air quality and health require comprehensive estimates of the exposures to air pollution experienced by populations in every country. However, there are many countries in which measurements from ground-based monitoring are sparse, or non-existent, with quality-control and representativeness providing additional challenges. While ground-based monitoring provides a far from complete picture of global air quality, there are other sources of information that provide comprehensive coverage across the globe. The Data Integration Model for Air Quality (DIMAQ; (Shaddick et al., 2018)) was developed to combine information from ground measurements with that from other sources such as atmospheric chemical transport models and estimates from remote sensing satellites to produce the information required for health burden assessment and the calculation of air pollution-related Sustainable Development Goals indicators, including indicator 11.6.2 (Annual mean levels of fine particulate matter (e.g. $PM_{2.5}$ and PM_{10}) in cities). The result can be seen in Figure 1.1 that shows the locations of monitoring sites in the World Health Organization's air quality database. Whilst there are extensive measurements in Northern America, Western Europe and increasingly in China and India, there are large parts of the world where monitoring is sparse, or even non-existent. DIMAQ is a Bayesian spatio-temporal model with inference performed using integrated nested Laplace approximations (see Chapters 6 and 12 for further details) that provides predictions of $PM_{2.5}$ on a high-resolution grid covering the world and thus provides estimates of exposures for each country that, when matched to population estimates, are used to calculate country-level estimates of exposures for the SDG indicators.

Models such as DIMAQ are now possible due to advances in methodology, computational ability and an explosion in the availability of large and complex data sets from diverse sources (e.g. environmental monitoring, remote sensing, numerical modeling) and the ability to integrate data from multiple sources provides a fantastic opportunity to produce high-resolution estimates of exposures to environmental hazards, over both space and time, that can be linked to health data to estimate risks.

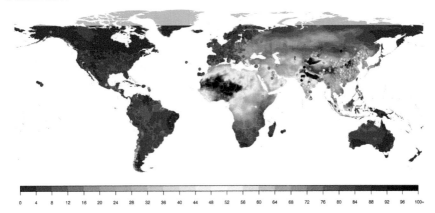

Figure 1.1: Estimated annual average concentrations of $PM_{2.5}$ μgm^{-3} for 2016. Estimates are the medians of the posterior distributions from a Bayesian spatio-temporal model (DIMAQ), shown together with the locations (and concentrations) of monitoring sites within the WHO Air Quality Database

Increasingly, as in this example, data is used to answer questions and form the basis of decision-making outside the sphere of its intended use. The differences between using routinely available data and data that has been collected as part of a carefully designed experiment requires a fundamental change in approach, acknowledging all aspects of data, including interactions between collection (including potential biases), governance, analysis, interpretation, communication and the future use of resulting composite datasets in other fields. This requires the ability to use information from data within the context of knowledge of the quality and provenance of the data. It also highlights the importance of uncertainty associated with data and the need to fully integrate it into decision making processes.

The importance of uncertainty has increased dramatically as the twentieth century ushered in the era of post-normal science, as articulated by Funtowicz and Ravetz (1993). Gone were the days of the solitary scientist running carefully controlled bench-level experiments with assured reproducibility, the hallmark of good classical science. Then came a science characterized by great risks and high levels of uncertainty, an example being climate science with its associated environmental health risks. Funtowicz–Ravetz post-normality has two major dimensions (Aven, 2013): (i) decision stakes or the value dimension (cost–benefit) and (ii) system uncertainties. Dimension (i) tends to increase with (ii); just where certainty is needed the most, uncertainty is reaching its peak.

Post-normal science called for a search for new approaches to dealing with uncertainty, ones that recognized the diversity of stakeholders and evaluators needed to deal with these challenges. That search led to the recognition that characterizing uncertainty required a dialogue amongst this extended set of peer reviewers through workshops and panels of experts. Such panels are convened by the US Environmental

Protection Agency (EPA) who may be required to debate the issues in a public forum with participation of outside experts (consultants) employed by interest groups, for example the American Lung Association and the American Petroleum Producers Association in the case of air pollution.

In this chapter we start by describing the underlying concepts behind investigations into the effects of environmental hazards and, in particular, the importance of considering diseases and exposures over both space and time in epidemiological analyzes. Throughout the book we advocate a Bayesian approach to modeling, and later in this chapter, we consider a general framework for how data is used to update knowledge and the important role of uncertainty. Throughout this chapter, concepts and theory are presented together with examples.

1.2   Health-exposure models

An analysis of the health risks associated with an environmental hazard will require a model which links exposures to the chosen health outcome. There are several potential sources of uncertainty in linking environmental exposures to health, especially when the data might be at different levels of aggregation. For example, in studies of the effects of air pollution, data often consists of health counts for entire cities with comparisons being made over space (with other cities experiencing different levels of pollution) or time (within the same city) whereas exposure information is often obtained from a fixed number of monitoring sites within the region of study.

Actual exposures to an environmental hazard will depend on the temporal trajectories of the population's members that will take individual members of that population through a sequence of micro-environments, such as a car, house or street (Berhane, Gauderman, Stram, and Thomas, 2004). Information about the current state of the environment may be obtained from routine monitoring or through measurements taken for a specialized purpose. An individual's actual exposure is a complex interaction of behavior and the environment. Exposure to the environmental hazard affects the individual's risk of certain health outcomes, which may also be affected by other factors such as age and smoking behavior.

1.2.1   Estimating risks

If a study is carefully designed, then it should be possible to obtain an assessment of the magnitude of a risk associated with changes in the level of the environmental hazard. Often this is represented by a relative risk or odds ratio, which is the natural result of performing log-linear and logistic regression models, respectively. They are often accompanied by measures of uncertainty, such as 95% confidence (or in the case of Bayesian analyzes, credible) intervals. However, there are still several sources of uncertainty which cannot be easily expressed in summary terms. These include the uncertainty associated with assumptions that were implicitly made in any statistical regression models, such as the shape of the dose – response relationship (often assumed to be linear). The inclusion, or otherwise, of potential confounders and unknown latencies over which health effects manifest themselves will also introduce uncertainty. In the case of short-term effects of air pollution, for example, a lag (the difference in time between exposure and health outcome) of one or two days is often chosen (Dominici and Zeger, 2000), but the choice of a single lag doesn't acknowledge the uncertainty associated with making this choice. Using multiple lags in the statistical model may be used, but this may be unsatisfactory due to the high correlation amongst lagged exposures, although this problem can be reduced by using distributed lag models (Zannetti, 1990).

1.2.2 Dependencies over space and time

Environmental epidemiologists commonly seek associations between an environmental hazard Z and a health outcome Y. A spatial association is suggested if measured values of Z are found to be large (or small) at locations where counts of Y are also large (or small). Similarly, temporal associations arise when large (or small) values of Y are seen at times when Z are large (or small). A classical regression analysis might then be used to assess the magnitude of any associations and to assess whether they are significant. However, such an analysis would be flawed if the pairs of measurements (of exposures), Z and the health outcomes, Y, are spatially correlated, which will result in outcomes at locations close together being more similar than those further apart. In this case, or in the case of temporal correlation, the standard assumptions of stochastic independence between experimental units would not be valid.

An example of spatial correlation can be seen in Figure 1.2, which shows the spatial distribution of the risk of hospital admission for chronic obstructive pulmonary disease (COPD) in the UK. There seem to be patterns in the data with areas of high and low risks being grouped together, suggesting that there may be spatial dependence that would need to be incorporated in any model used to examine associations with potential risk factors.

1.2.3 Contrasts

Any regression-based analysis of risk requires contrasts between low and high levels of exposures in order to assess the differences in health outcomes between those levels. A major breakthrough in environmental epidemiology came from recognizing that time series studies could, in some cases, supply the required contrasts between levels of exposures while eliminating the effects of confounders to a large extent.

This is the standard approach in short-term air pollution studies (Katsouyanni et al., 1995; Peng and Dominici, 2008) where the levels of a pollutant, Z, varies from day-to-day within a city while the values of confounding variables, X, for example the age–sex structure of the population or smoking habits, do not change over such a short time period. Thus, if Z is found to vary in association with short-term changes in the levels of pollution, then relationships can be established. However, the health counts are likely to be correlated over time due to underlying risk factors that vary over time. It is noted that this is of a different form than that for communicable diseases, where it may be the disease itself that drives any correlation in health

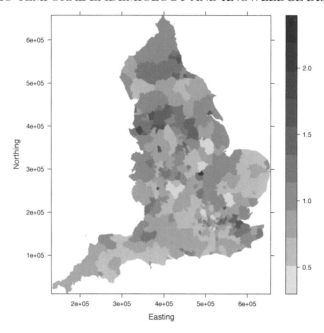

Figure 1.2: Map of the spatial distribution of risks of hospital admission for a respiratory condition, chronic obstructive pulmonary disease (COPD), in the UK for 2001. The shades of blue correspond to standardized admission rates, which are a measure of risk. Darker shades indicate higher rates of hospitalization, allowing for the underlying age–sex profile of the population within the area.

outcomes over time. This leads to the need for temporal process models to be incorporated within analyzes of risk. In addition, there will often be temporal patterns in the exposures. Levels of air pollution, for example, are correlated over short periods of time due to changes in the source of the pollution and weather patterns such as wind and temperature.

Missing exposure data, whether over space or time, can greatly affect the outcomes of a health analysis, both in terms of reducing sample size, but also in inducing bias in the estimates of risk. There is a real need for models that can impute missing data accurately and in a form that can be used in health studies. It is important that, in addition to predicting levels of exposure when they are not available, such models should also produce measures of associated uncertainty that can be fed into subsequent analyzes of the effect of those exposures on health. An example can be seen in Figures 1.3 and 1.4 and where a Bayesian spatio-temporal model was used to predict levels of fine particulate matter ($PM_{2.5}$) in 2016 for India, including areas where there was no monitoring. Figure 1.3 shows the medians of the posterior distributions of predictions on a 1 km × 1 km grid, and Figure 1.4 shows the coefficient of variation, a measure of uncertainty, associated with the predictions.

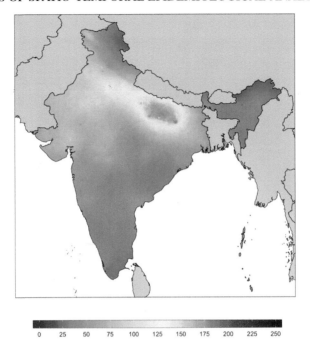

Figure 1.3: Predictions of fine particulate matter (PM$_{2.5}$) concentrations (μgm^{-3}) in 2016 in India. The predictions are from a Bayesian spatio-temporal model and are the medians of the posterior distributions of predictions on a 1 km × 1 km grid, based on measurements from approximately 650 monitoring sites throughout the country.

In addition to the issues associated with correlation over space and time, environmental epidemiological studies will also face a major hurdle in the form of *confounders*. If there is a confounder, X, that is the real cause of adverse health effects, there will be problems if it is associated with both Z and Y. In such cases, apparent relationships observed between Z and Y may turn out to be spurious. It may therefore be important to model spatio-temporal variation in confounding variables in addition to the variables of primary interest.

1.3   Examples of spatio-temporal epidemiological analyzes

Environmental exposures will vary over both space and time, and there will potentially be many sources of variation and uncertainty. Statistical methods must be able to acknowledge this variability and uncertainty and be able to estimate exposures at varying geographical and temporal scales in order to maximize the information available that can be linked to health outcomes in order to estimate the associated risks. In addition to estimates of risks, such methods must be able to produce measures of uncertainty associated with those risks. These measures of uncertainty should reflect

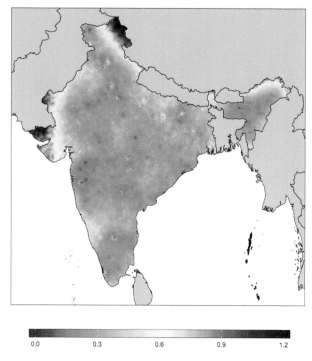

0.0   0.3   0.6   0.9   1.2

Figure 1.4: Coefficient of variation for the predictions of fine particulate matter (PM$_{2.5}$) concentrations (μgm^{-3}) in 2016 in India from a Bayesian spatio-temporal model.

the inherent uncertainties that will be present at each of the stages in the modeling process.

This has led to the application of spatial and temporal modeling in environmental epidemiology, in order to incorporate dependencies over space and time in analyzes of association. The value of spatio-temporal modeling can be seen in a number of major studies, and we give their examples here: (i) the Children's Health Study in Los Angeles; (ii) the MESA Air (Multi-Ethnic Study of Atherosclerosis Air Pollution) study and (iii) the Longitudinal Aging Study in India – Diagnostic Assessment of Dementia.

Example 1.2. *Children's health study – Los Angeles*

Children may suffer increased adverse effects to air pollution compared to adults, as their lungs are still developing. They are also likely to experience higher exposures as they breathe faster and spend more time outdoors engaged in strenuous activity. The effects of air pollution on children's health is therefore a very important health issue.

The Children's Health Study began in 1993 and is a large, long-term study of the effects of chronic air pollution exposures on the health of children living in Southern California. Approximately 4000 children in twelve communities were enrolled in the study although substantially more have been added since the initiation of the study. Data on the children's health, their exposures to air pollution and many other factors were recorded annually until they graduated from high school.

This study is remarkable, as the complexity of such longitudinal studies has generally made them prohibitively expensive. While the study was observational in nature, that is subjects could not be randomized to high or low exposure groups, children were selected to provide good contrast between areas of low and high exposure. Spatio-temporal modeling issues had to be addressed in the analysis since data were collected over time and from a number of communities which were distributed over space (Berhane et al., 2004).

A major finding from this study was that:

Current levels of air pollution have chronic, adverse effects on lung growth, leading to clinically significant deficit in 18-year-old children. Air pollution affects both new onset asthma and exacerbation. Living in proximity to busy roads is associated with risk for prevalent asthma. Residential traffic exposure is linked to deficit in lung function growth and increased school absences. Differences in genetic makeup affect these outcomes.

Example 1.3. *Air pollution and cardiac disease*

The MESA Air (Multi-Ethnic Study of Atherosclerosis and Air Pollution) study involves more than 6000 men and women from six communities in the United States. The study started in 1999 and continues to follow participants' health as this book is being written.

The central hypothesis for this study is that long-term exposure to fine particles is associated with a more rapid progression of coronary atherosclerosis. Atherosclerosis is sometimes called hardening of the arteries and when it affects the arteries of the heart, it is called coronary artery disease. The problems caused by the smallest particles is their capacity to move through the gas exchange membrane into the blood system. Particles may also generate anti-inflammatory mediators in the blood that attack the heart.

Data are recorded both over time and space, and so the analysis has been designed to acknowledge this. The study was designed to ensure the necessary contrasts needed for good statistical inference by taking random spatial samples of subjects from six very different regions. The study has yielded a great deal of new knowledge about the effects of air pollution on human health. In particular, exposures to chemicals and other environmental hazards appear to have a very serious impact on cardiovascular health.

Results from MESA Air show that people living in areas with higher levels of air pollution have thicker carotid artery walls than people living in areas with cleaner air. The arteries of people in more polluted areas also thickened faster over time, as compared to people living in places with cleaner air. These findings might help to explain how air pollution leads to problems like stroke and heart attacks. (http://depts.washington.edu/mesaair/)

Example 1.4. *Air pollution and cognitive function in the Longitudinal Aging Study in India (LASI)*

Indians experience some of the highest air pollution levels in the world. This study investigated whether ambient $PM_{2.5}$ levels are associated with poorer cognition in older Indians. In this study from the Longitudinal Aging Study in India – Diagnostic Assessment of Dementia (LASI-DAD) was used to explore possible associations between higher ambient $PM_{2.5}$ and poorer cognition (Adar et al., 2019). LASI-DAD is a study nested within a nationally representative sample of older (>45 years) Indians. During the first phase of LASI-DAD, a subsample of participants (>60 years) underwent a battery of cognitive tests, including verbal fluency, word recall, and the Hindi Mental State Examination (HMSE). Participants also self-reported sociodemographic data.

Ambient $PM_{2.5}$ for each participant's residence was estimated using a Bayesian spatio-temporal model, the Data Integration Model for Air Quality (DIMAQ), that was described in Section 1.1 of this Chapter. The estimated levels of $PM_{2.5}$ used in this study can be seen in Figure 1.3. This was used to produce estimates of $PM_{2.5}$. Regression models were then used to estimate associations between ambient $PM_{2.5}$ and cognitive scores, adjusting for age, gender, socioeconomic status, and region (North, Delhi, South). Among 1480 participants, the average age was 69±7 years and 55% were female. Greater $PM_{2.5}$ concentrations ($117 \pm 24 \ \mu gm^{-3}$) and lower cognitive scores (HMSE: 16±11) were found in northern India (excluding Delhi) as compared to southern India ($45\pm13 \ \mu gm^{-3}$ and 22±8, respectively). Ambient $PM_{2.5}$ was suggestively associated with worse cognition after adjustment for region and other sociodemographic confounders. Associations of -0.07 (95% CI:-0.2, 0.03) lower HMSE scores per 10 μgm^{-3} of $PM_{2.5}$.

Results from LASI-DAD show that among older adults living throughout India, associations were observed between higher ambient PM2.5 and poorer cognition, even after adjustment for individual sociodemographic characteristics and regional trends.

1.4   Good spatio-temporal modeling approaches

Often, spatio-temporal models are purpose-built for a particular application and then presented as a theoretical model. It is then reasonable to ask what can be done with that model in settings other than those in which it was developed. More generally, can it be extended for use in other applications? There are a number of key elements which are common to good approaches to spatio-temporal modeling. The approaches should do the following:

- Incorporate all sources of uncertainty. This has led to the widespread use of Bayesian hierarchical modeling in theory and practice.

- Have an associated practical theory of data-based inference.

- Allow extensions to handle multivariate data. This is vital as it may be a mix of hazards that cause negative health impacts. Even in the case where a single hazard is of interest, the multivariate approach allows strength to be borrowed from the other hazards which are correlated with the one of concern (W. Sun, 1998).

- Be computationally feasible to implement. This is of increasing concern as we see increasingly large domains of interest. One might now reasonably expect to see a spatial domain with thousands of sites and thousands of time points.

- Come equipped with a design theory that enables measurements to be made optimally for estimating the process parameters or for predicting unmeasured process values. Good data are fundamental to good spatio-temporal modeling, yet this aspect is commonly ignored and can lead to biased estimates of exposures and thus risk (Shaddick and Zidek, 2014; Zidek, Shaddick, and Taylor, 2014).

- Produce well calibrated error bands. For example, a 95% band should contain predicted values 95% of the time and thus have correct *coverage probabilities*. This is important not only in substantive terms, but also in model checking. There may be questions about the formulation of a model, related, for example, to the precise formulation of the assumed spatio-temporal process that is being used. However, that may be of secondary importance if good empirical performance of the model can be demonstrated. These criteria can really challenge the perceived efficacy of a model; 'All models are wrong but they can be useful' as George Box famously remarked (Box and Draper, 1987).

1.5   Knowledge discovery: acquiring information to reduce uncertainty

Knowledge about the world's natural processes has long been explored through a combination of two complementary information channels. The first, which could be called the 'knowledge channel', brings information derived through existing knowledge, information upon which theories can be built. Some of that knowledge comes from creative thought. For Newton, it was an apple he saw falling in an orchard he was visiting. That led to his laws of gravity and motion. For Einstein, it was the clock tower behind the bus on which he was riding. It dawned on him that time would appear to stand-still, were the bus to accelerate up to the speed of light. To him, that meant Newton's laws of motion would need to be amended to account for this relativistic effect. Of course, he also recognized that his theories would need to be empirically validated to be considered 'true'.

Things thought to be true, like Newton's Second Law of Motion, are commonly represented by 'models'. These, like the Second Law, are commonly mathematical in form, often with parameters that need to be fitted. Chapter 5, like those following, discusses how knowledge may be passed on through the knowledge channel and used to fit these models in ways that maximally reduce uncertainty about the natural phenomena they represent. The current chapter is about the data channel, through which flows information obtained from data. Its origins lie in the need for repeatability and replicability, fundamental principles enshrined in the Scientific Method. More precisely, it contributes to knowledge discovery and validation through model assessment and fitting. It is about initial data analysis and exploratory data analyzes using modern computational tools. Along with that, this chapter describes tools for communicating the information found in the data.

These two channels are not orthogonal, since knowledge can also be discovered in the data channel due to what might be called the 'a-ha' effect. In fact, the importance of knowledge discovery has made it an aspirational goal of modern statistical science, which has led to a gold-rush into domains where an 'a-ha' effect might be found. That quest comes with a need for caution and an understanding of the nature of now readily available datasets, since samples can also provide disinformation. At the same time, the knowledge channel may help guide the construction of the measurement model, for example where monitoring sites should be set up to collect the data. We will delve into those issues in Subsections 1.7 and 1.8. But the history of data science in one form or another goes back a long way. For completeness, Section 1.6 gives examples of early searches for the information data may provide.

1.6   Data collection: a brief history

Collecting data has a long history. In the physical sciences, it came long ago from experiments and the need for reproducibility. In contrast, survey sampling is comparably new. This section provides some of the background and current trends in the production of population surveys.

1.6.1   The census

The census was long seen as the way to accurately survey attributes of human populations. An early census is described in the Bible:

> 'Now in those days, a decree went out from Caesar Augustus, that a census be taken of all the inhabited earth. This was the first census taken while Quirinius was Governor of Syria.'   Luke 2:1-2.

Evidently, Quirinius saw this as the first step toward taxation, during the time of Christ. Others followed.

- The Domesday book came from a survey ordered by William I (William the Conqueror) in 1086. It was a census of all the shires, as they were called in what is now England and parts of Wales, after William invaded and conquered England in 1066 AD.

- Today, a great many nations carry out censuses to determine the state of their nation. In Canada, for example, a census of households is carried out every five years to collect information on the demographic, social and economic status of people across Canada. In the USA, it is a decadal census. In any case, the census is commonly supplemented by small area samples taken between censuses to update the census estimates. That is done in Canada and the USA.

The census would seem to be the ideal tool for characterizing a population's parameters of interest. But not so! Completing a census is expensive due to such things as the need to hire and train an army of surveyors to go out in the field, and ensure the quality of the records that these individuals obtain. In contrast, a well-designed random sample of one thousand or more items from that population will provide population estimates that are as good or better than the census estimates. The following example describes a famous experiment, which demonstrates that fact.

Example 1.5. *Surveys better than censuses*

Rao (1999) tells us about the seminal work of a famous Indian statistician named Prasanta Chandra Mahalanobis. It demonstrated the value of a sample survey over a complete census. To elaborate, at one time the important Indian jute crop was carefully monitored by a plot-by-plot enumeration. Mahalanobis took advantage of this fact and organized, as a test, a survey sample of the produce from that crop. At the same time, 'true' values could be obtained from administrative records kept by the Government of India.

Quoting the article by T.J. Rao:

'Mahalanobis' sample survey estimate of jute production was 7540 bales (1 bale = 400 lbs) obtained at a cost of 8 lakh rupees with a workforce of 600 while the plot-to-plot enumeration yielded a figure of 6304 bales at an expenditure of 82 lakh rupees and 33,000 employees which turned out to be an underestimate by 16.6%. This was evidenced by the alternative customs and trade figure of 7562 bales'.

That enshrined the survey as the instrument of choice and is now widely used.

As well, the census may be just a biased sample since inevitably, subgroups of the population will be missed. While small, these subgroups could be a very important part of the population from the perspective of an epidemiological study. Furthermore, the census is taken only periodically, thus missing temporal changes in the population during the inter-census period.

1.7 Discovering knowledge in data

A striking early application of data science that led to knowledge discovery, rather than mere information acquisition, is given in the next Example 1.6.

Example 1.6. *Florence Nightingale as a statistician*

Although Nightingale has long been recognized for her contributions to nursing, she is not so well known for those in data science (Magnello, 2012), She was sent to Crimea in 1854 to serve as a nursing administrator in a British Army hospital network during the war there. She witnessed the suffering of numerous sick soldiers, who were housed in very unsanitary conditions and 'suffered from frostbite, dysentery, extreme weakness and emaciation after which they encountered cholera and typhus epidemics', according to Magnello's account. Some died due to the injuries sustained in battle. But throughout her time in the Crimea, Nightingale carefully maintained records.

After returning to London in 1856, Nightingale with others completed an analysis of data compiled from her records, and learned that a great many wounded men had suffered in agony and died due to the diseases and infections they acquired while hospitalized. In particular, she learned that the latter caused far more casualties than the former. So she undertook to persuade the authorities of the need to reform in the way that the hospital facilities were managed. Realizing that tabular reports would not be very well understood, she decided to convey her findings through data visualizations. An example of her graphics is given in Figure 1.5. The diagram, which was presented in 1858, shows the causes of mortality.

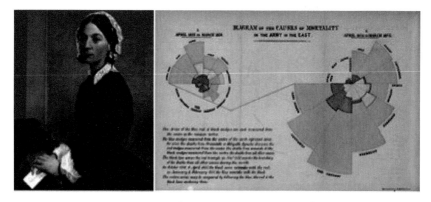

Figure 1.5: This graphic shows, on the left, Florence Nightingale: a young nurse about to leave England, with troops going off for service in the Crimean war. On the right is a polar bar chart that exemplifies Nightingale's use of data visualization. It shows what she learned and recorded about the causes of mortality among the British troops. In particular, the number of deaths due to preventable diseases (in blue) greatly exceeded those due to wounds (in red), and those due to other causes (in black). The blue wedges, for example, depict deaths due to preventable diseases, the red wedges measured from the center the deaths from wounds, and the black wedges measured from the center the deaths from all other causes.

Magnello's paper gives a fascinating and detailed account of Nightingale's struggle to get reforms in the way patients were treated. That struggle entailed a lot of further analyzes using her graphical tools to convince authors of the legitimacy of her claims. In the end she prevailed, the necessary commissions were set up, and reforms were made. Nightingale thus had a profound effect on the history of the World. And for that, she was recognized in 1912 by the Red Cross's establishment of The Florence Nightingale Medal. That medal is awarded to nurses for 'exceptional courage and devotion to the wounded, sick or disabled or to civilian victims of a conflict or disaster...'. She was also recognized in the statistical world by-election as the first female member of the Statistical Society (now the Royal Statistical Society) in 1858. That was just two years after returning from Crimea.

1.8   When things are not quite as they seem!

In modern times, data files may be a huge jumble of things. When crunched, they may lead to non-sensical discoveries that may be interpreted as an 'a-ha' discovery.

Example 1.7. *An urban myth?*

One of the largest UK grocery store chains saw a way of obtaining private data that could be connected to customer cash register receipts-the loyalty card. Customers were happy to oblige. The chain's data analysts were thus able to profile their customers, their purchases, and more importantly, what they did not purchase. Advertising could be then be better targeted and advertising costs reduced.

A story, which may be an urban myth, is described in the April 1998 edition of Forbes magazine. The store's data analysts had an 'a-ha' moment when they found that those who bought six-packs of beer, tended also to purchase diapers. The conclusion: 'a-ha', it is the fathers that buy the diapers and then reward themselves with the six-pack of beer. As the story goes, the store relocated their diapers next to the beer, and thus increased their market share of beer and diapers.

Although the story may well be a myth, it was plausible. And supported by data science! That led to the building of what were called 'data – warehouses' by companies large and small, according to Forbes, and the methodology sometimes worked. But then sometimes not the warehouses just became dust collectors. According to Forbes quoting 'informed sources', American Express spent 30 million in US dollars and got almost no benefit, at least by the time the Forbes article was written. The example teaches anew the age-old lesson that a careful investigation of the data including its sources is vital, before charging into an automatized number-crunching exercise.

1.9 The population

We now formalize the discussion above about the natural phenomenon of interest, assuming we have identified the population of items related to our inquiry. That population may be a finite set, for example a human subpopulation of individuals in a geographical subregion. Alternatively, it could be an infinite set, for example possible maximum temperatures at locations across a region at a given time. Sometimes, as an approximation, a finite population may be regarded as a sample from a super-population for technical convenience. For example, lung function might be measured at successive times, when the population itself will have changed. That population could then be viewed as a sample from an infinite superpopulation from which successive finite populations are drawn at successive times. Inference, in this case, could then turn to the stochastic model for that superpopulation. Measurable characteristics such as lung function may be viewed as having a continuous probability distribution.

A subset needs to be sampled and then their attributes measured. That subset may be randomly selected with a probability distribution P, which is known to the experimenter or known only to nature. Alternatively, the subset may be selected optimally in accordance with a model. These two are referred to respectively, as probability- or model-based sampling.

Some populations are created by convenience sampling. A class from a local school may visit a shopping center, informally survey voluntary respondents, and then place their data on the internet. Website surveys themselves relying on voluntary respondents are another example. A convenience sample could not be treated as a representative sample from a larger population.

1.10 The process model

Physical models of natural processes such as Newton's Second Law of Motion are deterministic. Another example is provided by a chemical transport model called MAQSIP, which consists of differential equations that lead to a numerical computer models, which predicts air pollution levels. But at best these models are only approximations of reality; the actual processes remain uncertain and may thus, in the Bayesian framework adopted in this book, be treated as random. The emerging field of uncertainty quantification embraces the idea of modeling that uncertainty, and Section 15.3 describes one way of doing just that.

Another stochastic source of uncertainty stems from the the aspirational goal of reproducibility in assessing physical models, which leads to the need to resample from the same population under completely unchanging conditions. But that goal is unattainable as it is never possible to control, completely, the conditions under which the experiment is performed. So that variation has come to be viewed as stochastic when a model for a natural process or an experiment is being fitted or assessed.

That view was manifest in the work of Gerolamo Cardano (circa 1500). He stated, without proof, what is nowadays called the 'law of large numbers'. Bernoulli (1713) gave a rigorous formal proof of that law, at least in the binary case. He thus helped lay the foundations of modern probability and statistical science, which embrace that stochastic variation. Hereafter, for simplicity in this chapter, we will use the term 'process' to include 'experiment' as well.

To embrace the considerations described in the previous paragraphs, let ω denote a possible outcome of the process and Ω the population of all possible outcomes to which the process could lead. Only a measurable attribute of ω, Z, is of interest and the experiment yields $Z = Z(\omega)$. But Z is not itself a measurement. It does possess a dimension such as 'length'. But it does not come with a 'scale' like 'metric' or 'imperial'. It most certainly does not possess units of measurement like mm or cm. However, Buckingham (1914) goes one step further in his famous paper and articulates the principle that any natural deterministic process model, even when expressed in terms of Z's, must be non-dimensionalizable, since nature itself does not recognize them. This principle does not require that a model, for example Newton's second law, be expressed in a non-dimensional form. Rather, it says it must be possible to represent it in a non-dimensional form. That principle would apply equally to stochastic process models. Moreover, the principle extends to the measurement model – the units of measurement should not determine the ultimate conclusions inferred from the data. That principle is implicitly recognized in the statistical invariance principle (Eaton and George, 2021), which concerns the data model. The latter will be taken up in more detail in Section 15.3, but for simplicity it will be ignored for now.

The random variables Z transform elements of Ω into its range space. These attributes and only known to lie on a physical scale, such as temperature, but these days they can come in much more complex forms such as linear operators, networks, images or snippets of text.

The distribution of Z is called the process model and denoted by P_Z. That distribution could be deterministic and put unit mass on a singleton. But here it will be a probability distribution on the range of Z and, for simplicity, be denoted by $p(z)$ or $p(z \mid \theta)$, according as the distribution is non-parametric or parametric. Also, p can either be a probability density function (PDF) or probability mass function (PMF), according to whether or not Z is a continuous or discrete random variable.

1.11 The process sampling model

A random sample of ω's is required $\{\omega_1, \ldots, \omega_n\}$, which in turn yields $Z_i = Z(\omega_i)$, $i = 1, \ldots, n$. For technical convenience, we assume these are arranged in the order in which they were obtained and represented by the column vector $\mathbf{Z} = (Z_1, \ldots Z_n)^T \in \mathscr{Z}$. The range of these vectors, will be denoted by the sample space $\mathscr{Z}$. Let $P_{\mathbf{Z}}$, or more simply, $p(\mathbf{z})$ or $p(\mathbf{z} \mid \xi)$ be the joint probability distribution of $\mathbf{Z}$, that is the process sampling distribution model. Let $(\mathscr{Z}, P_{\mathbf{Z}})$ be the process sampling space. Subsets of $\mathscr{Z}$ are called events.

The successive realizations of a process need not be independent. Respondents in a survey will not be selected with replacement, making the responses dependent. A more relevant example for this book is sampling from a spatial or temporal field. An example that illustrates the issues that can arise is given in the next subsection.

The set of all sampling distributions may be divided into three categories. The first involves sampling distributions that are known to the experimenter. The process of collecting such a sample is sometimes described as probability-based, while J. O. Berger and Wolpert (1988) speak of such processes as due to 'randomization' and their analysis as 'randomization analysis'. A sample survey exemplifies such a process, π_i being the known probability that a subject ω_i is drawn. The second category, which is sometimes called model-based sampling, consists of processes with unknown sampling distributions. Some designs are a mixture of model- and probability-based sampling distributions. Such a design is seen in controlled medical treatment trials. There subjects are assigned at random to a group, treatment or control with a known probability. Then a response with an unknown distribution is seen in each subject in each group. Finally, comes convenience-based sampling, which is usually quite inexpensive. In this case, the actual population would be the one that has to be inferred from a knowledge of how the convenience sample was created.

1.12   The data model

We now turn to a final major component of the database construction process, that is the measurement process. The complexity of this topic ensures that aspects of it often appear in ensuing chapters. Here we are just setting the stage for its first appearance ahead of the featured topic, which concerns how to deal with databases and the construction of the data channel described above.

For simplicity, we stick to the common measurement process where the output is a column vector of measurements $\mathbf{Y}$ that are expressions of the model (latent) process Z, or in short $\omega_i \rightarrow Z_i = Z(\omega_i) \rightarrow Y_i = Y(Z_i)$:

$$\mathbf{Y} \doteq (Y_1, \dots, Y_n)^T.$$

The measurement sampling distribution would be denoted by P_Y and be represented by $p(\mathbf{y} \mid \theta)$ or $p(\mathbf{y})$, according as there are or are not parameters involved. Each would be either a PDF or PMF, as appropriate. Note that θ may well contain both ξ and other parameters generated by the measurement process. Note as well that we have a joint distribution $p(\mathbf{y}, \mathbf{z} \mid \theta) = p(\mathbf{y} \mid \mathbf{z}, \theta) \times p(\mathbf{z} \mid \xi)$.

We start with a hypothetical example to avoid the complications of contextual detail that a more realistic example would introduce.

Example 1.8. *Infectious disease survey*

The example concerns a population of individuals, each coded by an identifier ω, who are susceptible to infection by a serious disease. Public health officers are concerned about the fraction ρ of the overall population Ω who are infected, that is those who are infected denoted by $\{+\}$. Then n members of that population are randomly selected by probability-based sampling to yield a sample $\mathbf{W} = (w_1, \dots, w_n)^T$, according to the order in which they are selected. All samples are possible and $\mathbf{W} \in \mathcal{W}$. However, since interest lies only in ρ, we may simplify the process model by replacing each ω_i by $Z_i \doteq Z_i(\omega_i) = +$ or $-$ according as a subject is infected or not $i = 1, \dots, n$. Note that Z is unknown to the investigator. The measurement process comes next, and it involves the measurement model, that is each of the randomly selected subjects is tested for the disease, yielding a measurement Y, a $+$ or $-$ according to the test result. But the measurement model must account for false positives and false negatives. We will leave that refinement as an exercise. In summary, we have the situation where $\Omega = \{\omega_1, \ldots, \omega_n\}$ with $\omega_i \in \{-, +\}$. The process outcomes are represented by the Z's. Finally, the sample measurements are represented by the Y's and the measurement vector itself would be $\mathbf{Y} = (\mathbf{Y_1}, \ldots, \mathbf{Y_n})$ with $Y_i = 1$ or $Y_i = 0$ according as $\omega_i = +$ or $\omega_i = -$. In this case, the sampling probability distribution space P, given by with $P(\omega) = p$ or $P(\omega) = 1 - p$ according as $\omega_i = +$ or $\omega_i = -$, the size of p being dependent on the severity of infection in the region. The distribution P_Y would depend on the accuracy of the result recorder.

Finally, we would have the distribution of the $\mathbf{Y}$-vector, P_Y, induced by P. Commonly, in the literature of statistical science, P_Y is called the sampling distribution and the process distribution is left as implicit. From our perspective, P_Y might more properly be called the measurement sampling distribution. And separating these two sources of randomness, due to the measurement and process, is important.

The next example raises some even more fundamental issues than did the previous example, ones that can arise in the spatio-temporal modeling and measurement of environmental processes.

Example 1.9. *Correlation and sample size?*

In 1997 Carroll et al. (1997) published an important paper that addressed the following question: 'What is the pattern of human exposure to ozone in Harris County (Houston) since 1980'? The paper concerns the relationship between the population density and atmospheric ozone concentrations. The paper argues for the need to interpolate the ozone field between the relatively small number of fixed monitors. So they develop and apply a spatio-temporal model of that field for the years 1980 to 1993, thus obtaining a very large dataset of measurements. They also rely on census data to get population densities, focussing on young children in particular and various measures of exposure. The paper concludes that exposure of young children to ozone decreased by approximately 2% from 1980 to 1993. But they also conclude that 'the current siting of monitors is not ideal if one is concerned with population exposure assessment'. Some other specific findings are reported, including that the model and estimation method are general and can be used in many problems with space-time observations.

Stein and Fang served as discussants for this paper and begin with their question 'Is this really a big dataset'? Although there were more than 1 million ozone measurements in the dataset, seemingly a lot, there were only 12 replicates for the so-called space–effect in any one year, not many. Not only that, they argue, the hourly measurements at any one site are pseudo-replicates due to their high autocorrelation, so accounting for the dependence is crucial. Finally, they provide some alternative analyzes while pointing to some deficiencies they see in the paper.

The paper featured in Example 1.9 points to a number of critical issues. To begin, note that the authors do not distinguish between ozone concentrations and their measured values. In fact, for air pollutants like ozone, there are in most cases, a variety of different ways of defining their concentrations (Hassler et al., 2014). For particulate air pollution that is smoke, $PM_{2.5}$ either mass μgm^{-3} or counts ppm can be used. The mass of the latter can be small when the counts are high, depending on what generates the smoke. In that case, the small particles can readily pass through the gas exchange member in the lung and into the bloodstream. The body reacts, tackling these invaders by generating anti-inflammatory mediators. High concentrations of the latter can in turn cause damage to the blood cardiovascular system (Wang et al., 2019). Thus, 'size' does truly matter.

Once a method for assessing the characteristic of interest is chosen, a variety of techniques are available for measuring the concentration. Beyond all that lies the inevitable measurement error problem, for example based on the quality of instruments being used. An important fundamental point is that stochastic dependencies in effect diminish the sample size. That loss must be accounted for in reaching conclusions based on the data these processes eventually yield.

One last point that the example raises, concerns a fundamental issue about the ozone fields and the data they eventually yield. Namely, why are these random, as both the authors and discussants assume? Since all the ozone fields that were involved in the analysis, have come and gone, why are they and the resulting measurements published in the data files random? A profound question. An answer is given by Wikle, Zammit-Mangion, and Cressie (2019):

'In the physical world phenomena evolve in space and time following deterministic perhaps chaotic, physical rules (except at the quantum level), so why do we need to consider randomness and uncertainty? The primary reason comes from the uncertainty resulting from the science and the mechanisms driving a spatio-temporal phenomenon'.

We agree. However, we go one step further by adopting the Bayesian paradigm in this book from among several paradigms that emerged for addressing it. The first such paradigm referred to at the beginning of this subsection is called probability-based sampling. The sampling probability distribution by which the sample is chosen is known. This approach was used in the United States Environmental Protection Agency's 2012 National Lakes Assessment, where the population consisted of a finite number of freshwater bodies. That approach was criticized since it could lead by chance to two adjacent lakes and thus waste resources. The second alternative is model-based sampling. The sample would be regarded as having been produced by an unknown process model, as in the case of a sample produced by nature. The latter would even cover the case of a repeated, controlled laboratory experiment, due to what might be considered random variation in the environmental conditions in the lab or in nature, when a process is sampled at several sites, for example. This paradigm also refers to the case where the sampling sites are selected optimally according to an inferred model for nature's true model. The latter two approaches, probability-based and model-based, have been compared (Wang et al., 2019) and they are discussed in detail in Chapter 13.

However, the authors' perspectives stem from the Bayesian foundations that lead to the rich theory for modeling the uncertainties about these processes with prior and posterior probability distributions. That would seem the only tenable choice of a paradigm for the stochastic models that were originally developed for application in geostatistics where orebodies were mapped from core samples taken at random locations. What could be less random than the rich bodies of gold ore buried beneath the surface of South Africa!

Within this book, we show examples of Bayesian analysis using different approaches to inference together with worked examples. In Chapter 6 we demonstrate the use of NIMBLE (de Valpine et al., 2017), a language which can be used for specifying Bayesian models, that allows the user to perform Markov chain Monte Carlo (MCMC) using hybrid Gibbs sampling, and R-INLA, which perform 'approximate' Bayesian inference based on integrated nested Laplace approximations (INLA) and thus do not require full MCMC sampling to be performed (Rue, Martino, and Chopin, 2009). INLA has been developed as a computationally attractive alternative to MCMC. In a spatial setting, such methods are naturally aligned for use with areal level data rather than the point level. However, by exploiting the fact that a Gaussian field (GF) with a Matern covariance function to be represented by a Gaussian Markov Random Field (GMRF) through Stochastic Partial Differential Equations models using point referenced data can be used within R-INLA (Lindgren, Rue, and Lindström, 2011).

1.13   Summary

This book provides a comprehensive treatment of methods for spatio-temporal modeling and their use in epidemiological studies. Throughout the book, we present examples of spatio-temporal modeling within a Bayesian framework and describe how data can be used to update knowledge, together with in-depth consideration of the role of uncertainty.

Throughout the book we will use the R statistical software. R is an object-oriented programming language and provides an integrated suite of software facilities for data manipulation, calculation and graphical display. It provides an environment within which almost all classical and modern statistical techniques are available. R can be used in a variety of ways, including directly from the command line or from within other programming environments. For many of the examples in this book we use RStudio (recently rebranded as posit), an integrated development environment (IDE) for R. It includes a console, syntax-highlighting editor that supports direct code execution, as well as tools for plotting, history, debugging and workspace management. Both R (cran.r-project.org) and RStudio (https://posit.co)

are open source and can be downloaded free of charge. They are both available for Windows, Mac OSX and Linux.

The base R environment provides a rich set of functions with many thousands of functions with many more provided as additional packages, including those which allow the manipulation and visualization of spatio-temporal data, performing epidemiological analysis and advanced spatio-temporal analyzes. These are available at The Comprehensive R Archive Network (CRAN) and can be downloaded from cran.r-project.org, a repository for R software. Additional packages need to be downloaded and installed.

From this book, the reader will have gained an understanding of the following topics:

- The basic concepts of epidemiology and the estimation of risks associated with environmental hazards;

- The theory of spatial, temporal and spatio-temporal processes needed for environmental health risk analysis;

- Fundamental questions related to the nature and role of uncertainty in environmental epidemiology, and methods that may help answer those questions;

- How data can be used to update knowledge and reducing uncertainty;

- A history of data collection and how databases may be constructed and how data is formally represented through the sample space and associated formal constructs such as the sample space and sampling distributions;

- Important areas of application within environmental epidemiology, together with strategies for building the models that are needed and coping with challenges that arise;

- Computational methods for the analysis of complex data measured over both space and time and how they can be implemented using R;

- Areas of current and future research directions in spatio-temporal modeling;

- Examples of R code are given throughout the book and the code, together with data for the examples, are available online on the book's GitHub site (https://spacetime-environ.github.io/stepi2);

- The book contains a variety of exercises, both theoretical and practical, to assist in the development of the skills needed to perform spatio-temporal analyzes.

Chapter 2

An introduction to modeling health risks and impacts

2.1 Overview

The estimation of health risks in epidemiology is most commonly performed using regression models with the aim of developing a realistic model of the system in question, to identify the variables of interest and to estimate the strength of their effect on a health outcome. Though an epidemiological regression model cannot itself prove causality (that can only really be provided by randomized experiments), it can indicate the change in the response variable that might be associated with changes in exposure which is a very useful tool in understanding and developing insight into possible causal relationships.

This chapter considers different methods for expressing the risks associated with exposures and their appropriateness given the type of study that is being performed. A number of aspects of model fitting are introduced, including the choice of distribution (e.g. Normal, Poisson or Binomial), the choice of the regression (e.g. linear, log-linear or logistic) and how the actual computation is carried out. There are many reasons for performing a regression analysis, and the intended use of the regression equation will influence the manner in which the model is constructed and interpreted. In the applications considered here, the interest is in explanation and prediction, but not prediction as is used in the stock market, where prediction of future events alone is often important.

2.2 Types of epidemiological study

Epidemiology is the study of why and how often diseases occur in different groups of people. A key feature of epidemiology is the measurement of disease outcomes in relation to a population at risk. Population studies aim to compare diseased and non-diseased individuals according to a common characteristic, such as age, sex or exposure to a risk factor. Cohort studies observe the progress of individuals over time and are useful for investigating and determining aetiological factors. A study may follow two groups with one group exposed to some risk factor while the other group is not exposed with the aim of seeing if, for example, exposure influences the occurrence of certain diseases. For rare conditions, very large samples will be

DOI: 10.1201/9781003352655-2

required to observe any cases. One insurmountable problem with cohort studies is that if the cohort has to be set up from scratch there may be a long delay before analysis can take place.

One solution to the problem of the small number of people with the condition of interest is the case-control study. In this type of study, we take a group of people with the disease, the cases, and a second group without the disease, the controls. We then find the exposure of each subject to the possible causative factor and see whether this differs between the two groups. The advantages of this method of investigation are that it is relatively quick, as the event of interest has already happened, and it is cheap, as the sample size can be small. However, there can also be difficulties with this method in terms of the selection of cases, the selection of controls and obtaining the data.

In collecting a set of controls, we want to look to gather a group of people who do not have the disease in question, but who are otherwise comparable to our cases. We must first decide upon the population from which they are to be drawn. There are many sources of controls; two obvious ones being the general population and patients with other diseases. The latter is usually preferred because of its accessibility. However, these two populations are not the same. While it is easier to use hospital patients as controls, there may be bias introduced because the factor of interest may be associated with other diseases.

Having defined the population from which to choose the sample, we must bear in mind that there are many factors, such as age and sex, which affect exposure to risk factors. The most straightforward way to choose the sample is to take a large random sample of the control population, ascertain all the sample's relevant characteristics, and then adjust for differences during the analysis, using for example logistic regression models. The alternative is to try to match a control to each case, so that for each case there is a control of the same age, sex, etc. If we do this, we can then compare our cases and controls, knowing that the effects of these intervening variables are automatically adjusted for. If we wish to exclude a case, we must exclude its control too or the groups will no longer be comparable. It is possible to have more than one control per case, but this can lead to the analysis becoming more complicated.

2.3   Measures of risk

Here, we consider measures of risk that are commonly estimated in epidemiological studies and that can be estimated using regression models. The choice of where risks are expressed, in terms of either relative risk or odds ratio, will largely be driven by the type of study that is being analyzed. Here we briefly describe three common designs: population, cohort and case-control studies. Each will produce a different type of outcome and, due to the intrinsic properties of their designs, different methods will be required for estimating risks.

Let D and $\bar{D}$ denote 'disease' and 'not disease', and E and $\bar{E}$ denote 'exposed' and 'unexposed', respectively. The risk of an event is the probability that an event will occur within a given period of time. The risk of an individual having a disease $(P(D))$ is estimated by the frequency with which that condition has occurred in a similar population in the past.

2.3.1 Relative risk

To compare risks for people with and without a particular risk factor, we look at the ratio. Suppose the risk for the exposed group is $\pi_1 = P(D|E)$ and the risk for the unexposed group is $\pi_0 = P(D|\bar{E})$.

The *relative risk* is

$$RR = \frac{\pi_1}{\pi_0}$$

Table 2.1: Number of diseased/non-diseased individuals by to a risk factor.

		Exposure to Risk Factor		
		Unexposed ($\bar{E}$)	Exposed (E)	
Disease	Absent ($\bar{D}$)	n_{00}	n_{01}	n_{0+}
	Present (D)	n_{10}	n_{11}	n_{1+}
		n_{+0}	n_{+1}	n_{++}

Given the number of diseased/non-diseased individuals who are in the exposed/non-exposed groups, as seen in Table 2.1, we can calculate the relative risk. The overall incidence, irrespective of exposure, will be n_{1+}/n_{++}.

From Table 2.1, we have

$$RR = \frac{n_{11}/n_{+1}}{n_{10}/n_{+0}} = \frac{n_{11}n_{+0}}{n_{+1}n_{10}}$$

In a population study, the total sample size n_{++} is fixed; in a cohort study, the margins n_{+0} and n_{+1} are fixed; and in a case-control study, the margins n_{0+} and n_{1+} are fixed.

Note that we cannot estimate the relative risk directly from a case-control study, as the n_{++} individuals are not selected at random from the population.

To construct confidence intervals we use

$$Var(\log RR) = \frac{1}{n_{11}} - \frac{1}{n_{+1}} + \frac{1}{n_{10}} - \frac{1}{n_{+0}}$$

Assuming that $\log RR$ is normally distributed, a 95% CI for log RR is

$$\log RR \pm 1.96\sqrt{\frac{1}{n_{11}} - \frac{1}{n_{+1}} + \frac{1}{n_{10}} - \frac{1}{n_{+0}}}$$

Example 2.1. *The risk of lung cancer associated with radon exposure in miners*

Table 2.2 gives the number of cases of lung cancer (diseased) in uranium miners in Beverlodge, Canada (Lubin et al., 1995) who were exposed to radon (exposed) and the number who were not exposed (unexposed).

Table 2.2: Number of cases of lung cancer in uranium miners who were exposed and unexposed to radon in a mine in Beverlodge, Canada. Here, the relative risk is 1.58 (95% CI: 0.90 – 2.76).

		Exposure to Risk Factor		
		No radon ($\bar{E}$)	Radon (E)	
Disease	No lung cancer ($\bar{D}$)	22204	30415	52619
	Lung cancer (D)	18	39	57
		22222	30454	52676

The relative risk of lung cancer is therefore $\frac{39/30415}{18/22204} = 1.58$, that is there is a 58% increase in the risk of lung cancer for miners (from this mine) when they are exposed to radon. The log of the relative risk is 0.46 and the 95% CI on the log scale is $-0.10 - 1.02$. Therefore, on the original scale of the data it is $0.90 - 2.76$, indicating that the observed increase in risk is non-significant.

2.3.2 Population attributable risk

If a relative risk is large but very few people are exposed to the risk factor, then the effect on the population will not be large, despite serious consequences for the individual. The effect of a risk factor on community health can be measured by *attributable risk*, which is related to the relative risk and the percentage of the population affected.

The attributable risk is the proportion of the population risk that can be associated with the risk factor:

$$\text{AR} = \frac{\text{population risk} - \text{unexposed risk}}{\text{population risk}} = \frac{P(D) - P(D|\bar{E})}{P(D)} = \frac{\theta(\text{RR} - 1)}{1 + \theta(\text{RR} - 1)}$$

where θ is the proportion of the population who are exposed to the risk factor, $P(E)$.

Example 2.2. *Population attributable risk of lung cancer associated with radon exposure*

Continuing the example of the miners exposed to radon, if the proportion of the population of miners who are exposed to radon is 5% then the attributable risk is 0.03 whereas if the proportion exposed rose to 10%, then the attributable risk would rise to 0.06. As more miners are exposed, the proportion of the risk for the entire population that can be attributed to radon exposure increases.

2.3.3 Odds ratios

An alternative to the risk is the *odds* of an event. If the probability of an event is p then the odds is,

$$\frac{p}{(1-p)}$$

This can be useful since it is not constrained to lie between 0 and 1. We often use the *log odds*:

$$\log\left(\frac{p}{(1-p)}\right)$$

Another way to compare people with and without a particular risk factor is to use the *odds ratio*. The odds ratio for disease given exposure is

$$\text{OR} = \frac{\text{odds of disease given exposed}}{\text{odds of disease given unexposed}} = \frac{P(D|E)\,(1-P(D|\bar{E}))}{P(D|\bar{E})\,(1-P(D|E))}$$

For a 2×2 table as in Table 2.1 the odds ratio is

$$\text{OR} = \frac{n_{00}n_{11}}{n_{10}n_{01}}$$

The odds ratio is a useful measure since it is independent of the prevalence of the condition.

Example 2.3. *Odds ratio of lung cancer associated with radon exposure in miners*

From the example of the miners exposed to radon seen in Table 2.2, the odds ratio will be $(39/30415)/(18/22204) = 1.58$. In this case, the odds ratios and the relative risk are very similar, as the risk of disease is small.

2.3.4 Relationship between odds ratios and relative risk

The odds ratio gives a reasonable estimate of the relative risk when the proportion of subjects with the disease is small.

The risk of disease for an exposed person is

$$\pi_1 = \frac{P(D \cap E)}{P(E)}$$

$$\approx \frac{P(E|D)P(D)}{P(E|\bar{D})}$$

Similarly,

$$\pi_0 \approx \frac{P(\bar{E}|D)P(D)}{P(\bar{E}|\bar{D})}$$

So

$$
\begin{aligned}
\text{RR} \quad &\approx \quad \frac{P(E|D)P(D)P(\bar{E}|\bar{D})P(\bar{D})}{P(E|\bar{D})P(\bar{D})P(\bar{E}|D)P(D)} \\
&= \quad \text{OR}
\end{aligned}
$$

2.3.5   Odds ratios in case-control studies

The odds ratio is particularly useful in a case-control study. Above, we have given the formula for the odds ratio for disease given exposure $\text{OR}_{D|E}$. From a case-control study, we can calculate the odds ratio for exposure given disease, $\text{OR}_{E|D}$ which can be shown to be equal to $\text{OR}_{D|E}$. So although we cannot calculate a relative risk for a case-control study, we can estimate its odds ratio, provided that the cases and controls are random samples from the same population.

In addition, for rare diseases, the odds ratio is close to the relative risk as seen previously. So in practice, the odds ratio from a case-control study can often be interpreted as if it were the relative risk.

2.4   Standardized mortality ratios (SMR)

When we are investigating differences in risk between populations, we can eliminate the effects of, for example, different age structures by looking at age-specific rates. However, this can be cumbersome, and it is often easier to make comparisons within a single summary figure. This is achieved by calculating standardized rates that allow for differing rates in specific groups, for example age and gender groups and the proportions of the population that are within those groups.

Let Y be the observed number of deaths in the population of interest and E be the expected number of deaths with respect to some reference population.

$$\text{SMR} = \frac{Y}{E}$$

The SMR is a ratio, not a rate or a percentage. An SMR of 1 means that the population of interest has the same number of deaths as we would expect from the reference population. If it is greater than 1, we have more deaths than expected; if it is less than 1 we have fewer deaths than expected.

2.4.1   Rates and expected numbers

A *rate* is defined as the number of events, for example, deaths or cases of disease, per unit of population, in a particular time span. To calculate a rate we require: a defined period of time, a defined population, with an accurate estimate of the size of the population during the defined period, the person-years at risk and the number of events occurring over the period.

$$\text{rate} = \frac{\text{No. events}}{\text{total person-time at risk}}$$

For a fixed time period Δt, an average size of the population at risk during that period $\bar{N}$ and the number of events A in the rate is

$$\text{rate} = \frac{A}{\bar{N} \times \Delta t}$$

The *crude mortality rate* is usually calculated as deaths per 1000 population per year. Let D be the number of deaths in a given time period of length Δt and $\bar{N}$ be the average size of the population at risk during that period (often approximated by the number in the population at the mid-point of the time period). Then the crude mortality rate is given by

$$r = \frac{d}{\bar{N} \times \Delta t} \times 1000$$

Rates may be required for particular sections of a community. Where the populations are *specified* these rates are referred to as *specific rates*. For example, age-specific or age- and sex-specific rates may be used for comparison of different populations. Other common specific rates are area, occupation or social class specific (and combinations of these).

For direct standardization, we use a standard population structure for reference. We then calculate the overall mortality rate that this reference population would have observed if it had the age – specific mortality rates of the population of interest.

Suppose the reference population has population counts $N'_k; k = 1, \ldots, K$ in each age-group k. We calculate the age-specific mortality rates r_k for the population of interest. The directly standardized rate is then given by

$$\text{directly standardized rate} = \frac{\sum_{k=1}^{K} N'_k r_k}{\sum_{k=1}^{K} N'_k}$$

For indirect standardization, we take the age – specific rates from the reference population and convert them into the mortality rate we would observe if those reference rates were true for the age-structure of the population of interest. This gives us the expected rate for the population of interest, if age-specific mortality rates were the same as for the reference population.

We calculate the age-specific mortality rates r'_k for the reference population. Suppose the population of interest has population counts $N_k; k = 1, \ldots, K$ in each age-group k.

The expected rate of deaths in the population of interest is

$$\text{expected rate} = \frac{\sum_{k=1}^{K} N_k r'_k}{\sum_{k=1}^{K} N_k}$$

Given the expected rate of deaths in the population of interest, the expected number of deaths is

$$E = \sum_{k=1}^{K} N_k r'_k$$

Example 2.4. *Risk of liver cancer and proximity to incinerators*

In a study of the association between the risk of liver cancer and living in proximity to a municipal incinerator in the UK (Elliott et al., 1996), the number of people with liver cancer living less than 3Â km from an incinerator was 152. The expected number of deaths for liver cancer based on national rates applied to the age–sex structure of the population living within 3 km of an incinerator was 118.10 and therefore the SMR was 1.29. This indicates there is a 29% increase in risk of liver cancer in those living in proximity to incinerators compared to what might be expected. Of course, there may be other factors that mean that the observed increase in risk is not wholly due to incinerators. In the next section, we see how the effects of other potential risk factors (covariates) can be used to adjust such risks by modeling SMRs using generalized linear models.

2.5   Generalized linear models

Data from epidemiological studies commonly consist of counts of disease in a defined geographical area and/or time-period, or of binary indicators of whether a subject is a case or control. The response variable is therefore going to be non-normal, being non-negative integers in the first case and constrained to be either 0 or 1 in the second. Linear regression is therefore unlikely to be appropriate. Any model used for estimating the association between such outcomes and possible explanatory variables (and subsequently estimates of associated risk) must therefore acknowledge the type of data coming from the study and accommodate suitable distributional assumptions. Examples include the Poisson distribution when predicting deaths and the Binomial when predicting the probabilities of being a case or control.

2.5.1   Likelihood

The likelihood, $L_n(\theta|y) = f(y|\theta)$ is a measure of the *support* provided for a particular set of the parameters, θ, of a probability model by the data, $y = (y_1,...,y_n)$. It is a relative measure and only determined by the values of the observed data, therefore any constants independent of θ can be omitted. It is often more convenient to consider the log likelihood, $l_n(\theta|y) = \log(L_n(\theta|y))$. If the response vector, y, consists of n independent and identically distributed observations, then the likelihood of θ is $L_n(\theta|y) = \prod_{i=1}^{n} L(\theta|y_i)$ and $l_n(\theta|y) = \sum_{i=1}^{n} l_n(\theta|y_i)$.

The first derivative of the log likelihood is known as the *score function*, U_n, which for a sample of size n is given by

$$U_n(\theta|y) = l'_n(\theta|y) = \frac{dl_n(\theta|by)}{d\theta} \qquad (2.1)$$

The maximum likelihood estimate (MLE) is found by solving the equation $U_n(\theta|by) = 0$.

For reasons of clarity, unless stated, the following descriptions consider a univariate unknown parameter, θ. In regular problems, analogous results for more than one parameter follow naturally using standard multivariate techniques such as those described in DeGroot and Schervish (2010) and in Chatfield and Collins (1980).

2.5.2 Quasi-likelihood

Quasi-likelihood only requires that the first two moments of the data generating distribution are specified, that is the mean and variance. The integral $Q(\mu|y) = \int_y^\mu \frac{y-t}{V(t)} dt$ acts like a *quasi*-likelihood even if it does not constitute a proper likelihood function, and estimates of the parameters of the model can be obtained by maximizing under certain conditions. Further details of the use of quasi-likelihood can be found in Section 2.7.2 (in relation to over-dispersion in Poisson models, where the variance is greater than the mean). Further technical details can be found in McCullagh and Nelder (1989).

2.5.3 Likelihood ratio tests

The likelihood ratio test is a useful way of comparing the fit of two competing nested models (where the set of parameters in one model is a subset of those in another). The models can be constructed to correspond to the null and alternative hypothesis of a test. If Ω is the parameter space of the larger model and Ω_0 is that of the smaller model, then the models are nested if $\Omega_0 \in \Omega$. The null hypothesis corresponds to $H_0 : \theta \in \Omega_0$ and the alternative $H_0 : \theta \in \Omega|\Omega_0$ (the set difference). The likelihood ratio test for comparing the two models, and thus testing the hypotheses, is twice the log of the difference between the maximized likelihoods under the two models.

$$2\left(\frac{\max_{\Omega|\Omega_0} l_n(\theta)}{\max_\Omega l_n(\theta)}\right)$$

In the case of regression models, if a particular model is compared to the 'full' or saturated model then the *scaled deviance* can be calculated

$$\begin{aligned}
\text{Deviance, } D &= -2\log(L_k/L_m) \\
&= -2(l_k - l_m) \qquad (2.2)
\end{aligned}$$

where l_k is the log of the likelihood of the model M_k and l_m is that for the saturated model, M_m, which contains all n parameters. In what follows, the scaled deviance will be referred to simply as the *deviance, D*.

Large values of the deviance ($L_k \ll L_m$) suggest that the current model does not fit well. If the model in question has r_k variables then the scaled deviance is asymptotically χ^2 distributed with $n - r_k$ degrees of freedom, if the model is appropriate. If the model fits poorly, then the deviance will be large.

Rather than make comparisons with the full model, M_m, it is generally more useful to make comparisons with another model with only one (or a few) extra parameters, that is comparing models M_k and M_q, with $r_k + 1$ and $r_q + 1$ parameters, respectively. This is because, for all but the Normal linear case, the χ^2 test for change in deviances is a much better asymptotic approximation than the one using comparisons with the full model (McCullagh and Nelder, 1989). If $r_k < r_q$ then M_k is said to be nested within M_q and if $D_k = -2(l_k - l_m)$ and $D_q = -2(l_q - l_m)$ then

$$D_k - D_q = -2(l_k - l_q) \sim \chi^2_{r_q - r_k} \tag{2.3}$$

These results assume that the number of parameters is fixed as $n \to \infty$. Further discussion of the selection of variables for use in regression models can be found in Chapter 7.

2.5.4 *Link functions and error distributions*

Generalized linear models (GLMs) are defined by the distribution of the errors and a link function which relates the linear predictor to the response. They can be used when data is an independent sample from an exponential family probability distribution; which includes the normal, binomial and Poisson distributions.

- The likelihood for a GLM has a general form for distributions in the exponential family of distributions; $f_y(y|\theta, \phi) = \exp\{(y\theta - b(\theta))/a(\phi)\} + c(y, \phi)\}$, where the expectation and variance of Y take the form $E(Y) = b'(\theta)$ and, $VAR(Y) = v_i = b''(\theta)a(\phi)$, respectively. The function $a(\phi)$ is often of the form $a(\phi) = \phi/w$, where ϕ is the dispersion parameter and w the prior weights.

- The effects of the explanatory variables are contained in the linear predictor, $\eta_i = \sum_{i=1}^{p} x_{ij}\beta_j$, which simplifies certain aspects of inference, both in terms of computation and properties of the resultant estimates.

- The link function links the mean function $\mu = E(Y)$ to the linear predictor, $g(\mu_i) = \eta_i$

In general, the link and error structure have to be explicitly defined. The parameters, β can be estimated by solving the estimating equations,

$$U_n(\beta) = \sum_{i=1}^{p} \frac{d\mu_i}{d\beta} v_i^{-1}(y_i - \mu_i(\beta)) = 0 \tag{2.4}$$

Linear models are a special case of GLMs with the following set up:

- $Y_i \sim N(\mu_i, \sigma^2)$, i.i.d. Normal observations
- $g(\mu_i) = \eta_i$, is the identity link function
- $\eta_i = \sum_{i=1}^{p} x_{ij}\beta_j$, a linear predictor

Example 2.5. *Poisson log-linear models*

In the majority of studies examining the effects of air pollution on health, the outcome, for example number of daily deaths, is assumed to follow a Poisson distribution. Poisson data, for example, take the form of counts and thus the outcome is in the range $[0, \infty)$. The natural link function is therefore $\log(\mu_i) = \gamma_i$, which restricts the outcome to the required range and assumes an underlying multiplicative relationship. In this case, $f_y(y|\theta) = (\mu, \phi)) = \exp\{y \log \mu - \mu - \log y!\}$, therefore $\log \mu = \theta, b(\theta) = \exp(\theta), c(y, \phi) = -\log y!$ and $a(\phi) = 1$.

2.5.5 Comparing models

Testing between competing nested models is achieved using the difference in deviance, as described in Section 2.5.3. The deviance will be of the form $\sum_{i=1}^{n} 2\{y_i(\tilde{\theta}_i - \hat{\theta}_i) - b(\theta_i) + b(\hat{\theta}_i)\}/\phi = D(y|\hat{\theta})$, where $\hat{\theta}$ is the MLE under the model in question and $\tilde{\theta}$ is the MLE under the saturated model. The deviance for Poisson data is, therefore $D = 2\sum_{i=1}^{n}\{y\log(\tilde{\theta}/\hat{\theta}) - (y - \hat{\theta})\}$.

The MLEs in all but the Normal case cannot be found by simply maximizing the log likelihoods numerically. Instead, they can be found using Iteratively Re-weighted Least Squares (IRLS) (McCullagh and Nelder, 1989).

2.6 Generalized additive models

Generalized additive models (GAMs) can be thought of as non-parametric extensions of GLMs. In Section 2.5 the form of the GLM was given as $g(\mu_i) = g(E(y)) = X\beta$. In a GAM, instead of assuming dependence on the sum of linear predictors, the outcome is assumed to be dependent on a sum of smooth functions of the predictors

$$g(E(Y)) = \sum_j S_j(X_i) \tag{2.5}$$

where S_j are smoothing functions. GAMs therefore provide a flexible framework for controlling for non-linear dependence on potential covariates (Hastie and Tibshirani, 1990; Wood, 2006).

GAMs are commonly used in epidemiological studies, especially in time series studies of the short-term effects of air pollution on health, where it is now almost the standard approach for studies of this type. For example, in analyzing the relationship between PM_{10} and SO_2 and hospital admission in New Haven and Tacoma,

U.S., Schwartz (1995) used a GAM to replicate the 19-day moving average used in Kinney and Ozkaynak (1991), modeling the outcome as a Poisson outcome rather than being restricted to the normal distribution as a consequence of using moving averages of the actual outcome variable. GAMs have also been used in this setting to allow for long-term patterns, such as seasonality, in time-series studies, enabling the associations between short-term changes in air pollution and health to be examined.

2.6.1 Smoothers

The class of potential smoothers is very large, and only a selection of the most commonly used ones are described here. For a more complete review, see Hastie and Tibshirani (1990). Possibly the most intuitive smoother is the moving average or running mean, in which the value of x_i is replaced by the average of that value together with those within a defined period around t

$$S(X_i) = \sum_{k=-p}^{p} w_p X_{i+k} : k = p+1, ..., n-p \qquad (2.6)$$

where w_k are the weights and $p > 0$. Here, $2p+1$ is the order of the moving average, that is the number of points which are included in calculating the average.

Unless the number of points included in the calculation of the average is large, in which case information will be lost, the resulting line is unlikely to be very smooth due to the sudden drop in weights as points are not included in the calculation. However, if the weights were specified to follow a probability distribution, as in *density estimation* (Silverman, 1986), then a smooth set of weights can be defined. An alternative approach is to calculate a least squares regression line within each set of neighboring points of the form

$$S(x_i) = \hat{\alpha}_{x_i} + \hat{\beta}_{x_i} x_i \qquad (2.7)$$

The fitted value at x_i is then used as the smoothed value. The regression can be fitted using weights, w_i, which can be constructed to be decreasing with distance from x_i, giving a *loess* smoother (Hastie and Tibshirani, 1990).

Another approach is to fit a polynomial to the data, for example

$$S(x_i) = \sum_{k=0}^{p} \beta_k x_i^k \qquad (2.8)$$

where the coefficients, β_k, are estimated from the data. As with the moving average approach, a choice of the extent of the smoothing (the order of the polynomial) has to be made. Simple polynomials are often useful as part of a model for the trend with additional terms describing the seasonality, but polynomials of higher order, whilst theoretically allowing very good fits to part of the data are likely to be too restrictive, especially if the model is to be used on another dataset or for forecasting out of the range of the current set.

2.6.2   Splines

Regression *splines* fit piecewise polynomials separated by *knots*, and are usually reforced to join smoothly at the knots. When the first and second derivatives are continuous, the piecewise polynomial is known as a *cubic spline*. A drawback of this approach is the need to choose the number and position of the knots, although attempts have been made to automate the procedure (Denison, Mallick, and Smith, 1998).

Splines provide a flexible technique for modeling non-linear relationships. They transform possible non-linear relationships into a linear form. They are formed by separating the data, $\mathbf{x}$, into $k+1$ sub-intervals. These intervals are defined by k knots, $k_1, ..., k_K$. The class of precise choice of splines and their basis functions is very large and further details can be found in Wahba (1990); Ruppert, Wand, and Carroll (2003); Wood (2006).

A spline, $f(x)$, is of the form

$$f(x) = \sum_{j=1}^{q} b_j(x)\beta_j \tag{2.9}$$

where $b_j(x)$ is the jth basis function and β_j are the basis parameters to be estimated. There are many ways to express the basis function which will represent the spline (Wood, 2006). A popular choice of spline are the cubic splines which have the following properties: (i) within each interval $f(x)$ is a cubic polynomial and (ii) it is twice differentiable and continuous at the knots. Cubic splines comprise cubic polynomials within each interval. Green and Silverman (1994) show a simple way to specify a cubic spline by giving four polynomial coefficients of each interval, that is

$$f(x) = d_i(x-x_i)^3 + c_i(x-x_i)^2 + b_i(x-x_i) + a_i, \quad x_i \le x \le x_{i+1}$$

where x_i are the knots and a_i, b_i, c_i and d_i are parameters representing the spline. A cubic spline on an interval $[a,b]$ is called a *natural cubic spline* (NCS) if its second and third derivatives are zero at a and b.

2.6.3   Penalized splines

The shape and smoothness of the spline depend upon the basis parameters and a term that represents smoothness, the latter of which can be represented in a number of ways. The most common of these is to use the number of knots, that is to space the knots equally throughout the data, and specify the smoothness by k the number of knots. However, too many knots may lead to over smoothness, whilst inadequate number of knots leads to rough model fit. Alternatively, a Ã§ approach can be adopted, which uses an overly large number of basis functions and penalizes excess curvature in the estimate using a penalty term.

Penalized splines control smoothness by adding a 'wiggliness' penalty to the least squares objective, that is fitting the model by minimizing

$$\|Y - X\beta\|^2 + \lambda \int_a^b \left[f''(x)\right]^2 dx$$

where the second part of this formula penalizes models that are too 'wiggly'. The trade-off between model fit and model smoothness is controlled by the smoothing parameter , λ. Since f is linear with parameters β_i, the penalty term can be written as a quadratic form in β:

$$\int_a^b \left[f''(x)\right]^2 dx = \beta^T S \beta$$

where S is a matrix of known coefficients.

Therefore, the penalized regression spline fitting problem is equivalent to minimize:

$$\|Y - X\beta\|^2 + \lambda \beta^T S \beta$$

In this case, the estimation of degree of smoothness becomes the issue of detecting the smoothing parameter λ. If λ is too high then the data will be over smoothed, and if it is too low then the data will be under smoothed. In both cases, this will mean that the spline estimate $\hat{f}$ will not be close to the true function f. Choosing λ may be done using data-driven criterion, such as cross validation (CV) and cross validation (GCV), details of which can be found in Wahba (1990); Gu (2002); Ruppert et al. (2003); Wood (2006).

Example 2.6. *The use of GAMs in time series epidemiology*

When assessing the short-term effects of an environmental exposure, for example air pollution, on health there will be a need to model underlying long-term trends in the data before shorter-term effects can be assessed. This can be performed within the framework of general additive models (see Section 2) with suitably chosen levels of smoothing over time. This is now the standard approach for epidemiological studies investigating the short-term effects of air pollution on health and we now describe some examples of this approach.

Examples of the use of GAMs to model underlying trends and long-term patterns in time-series studies can be found in Schwartz (1994a), where they were used to analyze the relationship between particulate matter and daily mortality in Birmingham (Alabama, U.S.), between particulate air pollution, ozone and SO_2 and daily hospital admissions for respiratory illness (Philadelphia, U.S.) and between ozone and particulate matter for children in six cities in the eastern U.S. In each of these analyzes, Poisson models were fitted using loess smoothers for time, temperature and a linear function of pollution, for example $\log(E(Y)) = \alpha + S_1(time) + S_2(temperature) + S_3(dewpoint) + \beta PM_{10} +$ day of the week dummy variables. A similar model was used in Schwartz (1997), but in this case the effect of weather was modeled using

regression splines. One of the major advantages of using non-linear functions could then be exploited, that of being able to include the possibility of
thresholds, without forcing the epidemiologist to specify a functional form. In
particular, there appeared to be a non-linear relationship between temperature
and mortality. However, unlike GLMs, there are no fixed degrees of freedom
and so although deviances can be calculated, and ways of approximating the
degrees have been proposed, there are no formal tests of differences between
models (Hastie and Tibshirani, 1990). Despite the possibility of using a non-
linear function for the variables of interest, namely air pollution, the final
results were always presented for a linear term, in order to produce a single
summary measure (relative risk per unit increase) and for comparability with
other studies.

2.7 Poisson models for count data

Poisson regression may be appropriate when the dependent, Y, variable is count data,
for example counts of mortality in a particular area and period of time, as opposed
to whether an individual has or does not have a disease (which would arise in a
case-control study). Often the interest is in comparing the rates of disease in different
areas. Here, we consider the estimation of relative risk in the case where observed
numbers of disease are available for a number of areas together with the *expected*
number of disease counts in those areas. It should be noted that these are not the
expected number of cases in the sense of statistical expectation, but instead are what
would be expected based on applying national rates of disease to the population
structure of those areas. The concept of expected numbers in this case is explained
in the following section.

2.7.1 Estimating SMRs

We can model the count Y in an area, i, with expected number E as Poisson, which
for fixed λ is

$$\Pr(Y = y|\lambda) = \frac{e^{-E\lambda}(E\lambda)^y}{y!}$$

for $y = 0, 1, \dots$. Here λ is the relative risk.
    For fixed y we have the likelihood function

$$l(\lambda) = \frac{e^{-E\lambda}(E\lambda)^y}{y!} \propto e^{-E\lambda}\lambda^y$$

for $\lambda > 0$.

Example 2.7. *The MLE of a Poisson rate*

The MLE of the relative risk is the SMR $= Y/E$

$$\begin{aligned}
log(l(\lambda|Y)) &\propto -(E\lambda) + Y\log(E) \\
\frac{\delta \log(l(\lambda|Y))}{\delta \lambda} &\propto -(E\lambda) + \frac{Y}{\lambda E} \\
0 &= -(E\hat{\lambda}) + \frac{Y}{\hat{\lambda} E} \\
\hat{\lambda} &= Y/E \qquad\qquad (2.10)
\end{aligned}$$

Estimating the MLE (and thus the SMR) can also be found by expressing the terms of a GLM, when it is assumed that $Y \sim P(E\lambda)$. If the rate is $\mu = E\lambda$, the linear predictor of a Poisson GLM would take the form

$$\log \mu = \log(E) + \beta_0 \qquad\qquad (2.11)$$

where $\log E$ is an offset, is a known multiplier in the log-linear mean function, $\mu = \exp(E) \times \beta_0$, and therefore will not have an associated coefficient in the results of the model.

Estimating the SMR using a Poisson GLM

We consider the observed and expected number of cases of respiratory mortality in small areas in the UK from a study examining the long-term effects of air pollution (Elliott, Shaddick, Wakefield, de Hoogh, and Briggs, 2007). Taking a single area (a ward) that had a population of 1601, the observed counts of deaths in people over 65 years old was 29 compared to the expected number which was 19.88. The SMR is therefore 29/19.88 = 1.46.

The R code for finding the MLE of the (log) SMR ($= \beta_0$) and its standard error would be

```
y <- 29; E <- 19.88
summary(glm(y ~ offset(log(E)),family=poisson))

Coefficients:
            Estimate Std. Error z value Pr(>|z|)
(Intercept)   0.3776     0.1857   2.033    0.042 *
```

Noting that the linear predictor, and thus the coefficient of interest, β_0, is on the log scale, the estimate of the SMR $= \exp(\beta_0) = \exp(0.3776) = 1.458$. The standard error of the estimate of β_0 can be used to construct a 95% confidence interval: $\hat{\beta}_0 \pm 1.96 \times se(\hat{\beta}_0) = (0.014, 0.741)$. Again this is on the log–scale and so the exponent is taken of both the lower and upper limits; $(\exp(0.014), \exp(0.741))$. The SMR in this case is therefore 1.458 (95% CI; $1.013 - 2.099$) meaning that the number of observed cases of disease in the area is significantly greater than that expected based on the age–sex profile of the population.

We now consider the estimation of the SMR over more than a single area; in this case, we use the observed counts and expected numbers for $N = 393$ areas. The parameter, β_0, now corresponds to the log of the overall SMR using data from all the areas, that is $\frac{\sum_{i=1}^{393} O_i}{\sum_{i=1}^{393} E_i}$. From the data, this is $8282/7250.2 = 1.142$ with the log of this being 0.133.

The R code to find the MLE in this case is

```
summary(glm(Y ~ offset(log(E)),family="poisson",
data=data))

Coefficients:
              Estimate Std. Error  z value Pr(>|z|)
(Intercept)   0.13305    0.01099    12.11    <2e-16 ***
---
Signif. codes:  0 '***' 0.001 '**' 0.01
'*' 0.05 '.' 0.1 ' ' 1
```

We can see that the estimate of the SMR will be $\exp(0.13305) = 1.142$, the overall SMR for all the areas. The 95% CI will be $\exp(0.112) - \exp(0.155) = 1.118 - 1.167$, indicating an overall increased risk of respiratory mortality in these areas compared to what might be expected if they experienced the same mortality rates (by age and sex) as the national population.

2.7.2   Over-dispersion

There is a strong possibility of over-dispersion in the Poisson models (i.e. where the variance is greater than the mean), arising from the presence of unmeasured confounders. These may be operating at the individual level, for example smoking, or at the area level, for example residual socio-economic confounding. Over-dispersion may also arise because of data anomalies such as errors in the numerators and/or denominators or due to migration.

The choice of a log link and variance that is proportional to the mean is the canonical one for the Poisson distribution and under regular Poisson assumptions, the variance is assumed to be equal to the mean, $VAR(Y_i) = E(Y_i)$, that is the dispersion parameter $\phi = 1$. When this is relaxed to proportionality, $VAR(Y_i) = \phi E(Y_i)$, the *dispersion*, or scale, parameter is assumed to be constant over all the data. The estimating equations for this will generally be different from those obtained by weighted least squares, but solutions can be found using quasi-likelihood techniques.

The likelihood-based approach theoretically allows the different models, and therefore the effect of different exposure scenarios, to be compared, but it makes no allowance for the extra-Poisson variability that may be present. This will lead to confidence intervals for the estimates of risk being too narrow and changes in deviances, used to compare models, being too small. An attempt to correct these effects, and to assess the degree of over-dispersion, can be made using a quasi-likelihood model (see Section 2.5.2), in which the usual Poisson assumption, that the variance is equal to the mean, is relaxed, allowing it to be a function of the mean and an unknown constant, that is $Var(Y_i) = cE(Y_i)$.

This *over-dispersion* may arise in a number of different ways, causing the variance to be greater than the mean. One example is when there is inter-subject variability where the Poisson mean parameter is not constant, but is a random variable. If a Gamma distribution, $Ga(a,b)$, were used for the distribution of the random effects, the marginal distribution of Y_{ti} is analytically tractable and takes the form of a negative binomial. Wakefield, Best, and Waller (2000) discuss the effect of different formulations of this Gamma distribution. Two cases are of particular interest, relating to the methods for allowing over-dispersion used here. In the first, the random effects follow a distribution of the form $\beta_{0i} \sim Ga(E_i a_i b, E_i b)$ (where E_i is the expected number of cases in area i), in which case the marginal variance of $Y_i|a_i,b$ is $E(Y_i|a_i,b)(1 + 1/b)$. This linear function of the mean is close to the quasi-likelihood approach described above, with $c = (1 + 1/b)$. If $\beta_{0i} \sim Ga(b, b/a_i)$ then $V(Y_i|a_i,b) = E(Y_i|a_i,b)(1 + E(Y_i|a_i,b))/b$. Here, the variance is a quadratic function of the mean. This quadratic form is also the case when a log-normal model is used for the random effects, as described in Chapter 7, Section 7.3. In that case, we might have the model $\log(Y_i) = \beta_0 + \beta_{0i} + \beta X_i$ with $\beta_{0i} \sim N(0, \sigma_{\beta_0}^2)$. In this case, the marginal distribution of Y_i is intractable but the mean and variance can be found and are

$$V(Y_i|\mu_i, \sigma_{\beta_0}^2) \quad = \quad E(Y_i|\mu_i, \sigma_{\beta_0}^2)\{1 + E(Y_i|\mu_i, \sigma_{\beta_0}^2))(\exp(\sigma_{\beta_0}^2)) \qquad (2.12)$$

where $E(Y_i|\mu_i, \sigma_w^2)E_i \exp(\mu_i + \sigma_{\beta_0}^2/2)$ and $\mu_i = \beta_0 + \beta X_i$

As with the example above, the variance is a quadratic function of the mean and so the results from the log-normal random effects model would not be expected to be the same as those from the quasi-likelihood model, where the variance is a linear function of the mean, although both will result in an increase in the variability of the estimates, and thus wider confidence/credible intervals.

Example 2.8. *Estimating the SMR using quasi-likelihood*

The R code for using quasi-likelihood to find the MLE of the $\log(\text{SMR}) = \beta_0$ and its standard error using the data from the previous example would be

```
summary(glm(Y ~ offset(log(E)),family="quasipoisson",
data=data))

Coefficients:
             Estimate  Std. Error  t value  Pr(>|t|)
(Intercept)   0.13305     0.02078    6.402  4.39e-10  ***

Dispersion parameter for quasipoisson family taken
to be 3.577536
```

Note that the estimate itself is the same as with the Poisson case, but the standard error has increased from 0.01099 to 0.02078, reflecting the over-dispersion which is present, with the dispersion parameter having been estimated to be over 3. The 95% confidence interval will therefore be wider; $\exp(0.092) - \exp(0.133) = 1.096 - 1.190$, with the increase in width reflecting the extra uncertainty that is present.

2.8   Estimating relative risks in relation to exposures

Consider an area i. If Y_i denotes the number of deaths in area i, it is assumed that $Y_i \sim P(E_i\mu_i)$, where E_i represents the pre-calculated age–sex standardized expected number of cases. The rate in each area, μ_i is modeled as a function of the exposures, X_{1i}, together with other area-level covariates, X_{2i},

$$\log \mu_i = \beta_0 + \beta_1 X_{1i} + \beta_d X_{2i} \tag{2.13}$$

where β_l represents the effect of exposure and β_d is the effect of the area-level covariate.

Example 2.9. *Modeling differences in SMRs in relation to differences in exposures*

We now consider the possible effects of air pollution in relation to the SMRs observed in the different areas; the exposure, X_{i1} for each area being the annual average of measurements from monitoring sites located within the health area. In addition, we consider the possible effects of a covariate; in this case, the covariate is a measure of deprivation known as the Carstairs score.

Smoking is known to be a major risk factor for respiratory illness, and it is known that smoking habits vary with social class (Kleinschmidt, Hills, and Elliott, 1995) and may therefore correlate with pollution levels, and act as a potential confounder. Although routine data on smoking levels at small area level are not available in Great Britain, strong correlations have, however, been demonstrated on several occasions between smoking rates and the Carstairs index of deprivation, which has also been shown to be a strong predictor of disease risk (Carstairs and Morris, 1989). The index is derived from a weighted aggregation of data on four census variables: unemployment, overcrowding, car ownership and social class.

The R code for fitting a model to estimate the relative risk associated with air pollution in this case is as follows:

```
summary(glm(Y ~ offset(log(E))+X1,family="poisson",
data=data_df))
# where data_df is a dataframe containing the health
    counts (Y), the expected numbers (E), the
    exposures (X1) and a measure of deprivation (X2)

Coefficients:
             Estimate  Std. Error  z value  Pr(>|z|)
(Intercept)  -0.04746     0.02603   -1.823    0.0683 .
X1            0.07972     0.01023    7.797  6.35e-15 ***
```

In this case, the effect of air pollution is highly significant and the associated relative risk will be $\exp(\beta_1) = \exp(0.07972) = 1.082$, indicating an increase in risk of 8.2% associated with every increase of one unit in air pollution (in this case, the units are $10\ \mu\mathrm{gm}^{-3}$).

Using a quasi-likelihood approach again results in the same estimate but with a larger standard error.

```
summary(glm(Y ~ offset(log(E))+X1,family="quasipoisson
    ",
data=data_df))

Coefficients:
             Estimate  Std. Error  t value  Pr(>|t|)
(Intercept)  -0.04746     0.04835   -0.982     0.327
X1            0.07972     0.01899    4.198  3.34e-05 ***

(Dispersion parameter for quasipoisson family taken
to be 3.449832)
```

The 95% CIs are $1.0615 - 1.1049$ for the Poisson case and $1.0434 - 1.1241$ when using quasi-likelihood; both indicating that the increase in risk is significant, with the wider intervals in the quasi-likelihood case again reflecting the extra uncertainty associated with the over-dispersion.

Adding the deprivation score, X_2, to the model might be expected to reduce the risk associated with air pollution as areas which are highly polluted are likely to also be deprived and deprived areas, with some exceptions, have higher rates of disease. It is therefore a confounder in the relationship between air pollution and health.

The R code for a model with both air pollution and deprivation is as follows:

```
summary(glm(Y ~ offset(log(E))+X1+X2,family="poisson",
data=data_df))

Coefficients:
            Estimate Std. Error z value Pr(>|z|)
(Intercept) -0.073589   0.027086  -2.717  0.00659 **
X1           0.025850   0.011023   2.345  0.01902 *
X2           0.051302   0.002582  19.871  < 2e-16 ***
```

It can be seen that adding deprivation to the model has resulted in a reduction in the size of the effect associated with air pollution, for which the RR has changed from 1.083 to 1.026 (95% CI; 1.004 – 1.049). The effect of deprivation is also significant, with an increase in risk of 5.3% (RR = exp(0.051302) = 1.053) associated with a unit increase in Carstairs score.

When using quasi-likelihood, the estimates of relative risk are the same, but again they have wider confidence intervals.

```
summary(glm(Y ~ offset(log(E))+X1+X2,family="
   quasipoisson",
data=data_df))

Coefficients:
            Estimate Std. Error t value Pr(>|t|)
(Intercept) -0.073589   0.040756  -1.806   0.0718 .
X1           0.025850   0.016585   1.559   0.1199
X2           0.051302   0.003885  13.206  <2e-16 ***

(Dispersion parameter for quasipoisson family taken
to be 2.264041)
```

This gives a RR for air pollution of 1.026 (95% CI; 0.993 – 1.060) and for deprivation a RR of 1.053 (95% CI; 1.045 – 1.061) which in this case leads to the effect of air pollution being non-significant. This suggests that it is deprivation that is playing a large part in the differences in SMRs observed in the different areas. Note the amount of the widening of the intervals is reduced as there is less over-dispersion; some of the extra-Poisson variability has thus been 'explained' by deprivation.

The effect of adding deprivation to the model can be assessed by calculating the change in deviance between two models: (i) with air pollution and (ii) with both air pollution and deprivation. A significant difference in deviance will indicate that deprivation is a significant risk factor.

The R code to perform a test between the deviances of the two models is as follows:

```
anova(glm(Y ~ offset(log(E))+X1,family="quasipoisson",
data=data_df),
glm(Y ~ offset(log(E))+X1+X2,family="quasipoisson",
data=data_df),
test="Chisq")

Analysis of Deviance Table

Model 1: Y ~ offset(log(E)) + X1
Model 2: Y ~ offset(log(E)) + X1 + X2
  Resid. Df Resid. Dev Df Deviance   Pr(>Chi)
1       391    1218.11
2       390     846.66  1   371.45 < 2.2e-16 ***
---
Signif. codes:  0 '***' 0.001 '**' 0.01
'*' 0.05 '.' 0.1 ' ' 1
```

This shows that deprivation has a highly significant effect on the risk of respiratory mortality. Using this method, the effect of taking air pollution out of the model can also be assessed, which proves to have a non-significant change in deviance; this indicates that when deprivation is included in the model the estimated risk associated with air pollution is non-significant.

```
anova(glm(Y ~ offset(log(E))+X1+X2,family="
   quasipoisson",
data=data_df),
glm(Y ~ offset(log(E))+X2,family="quasipoisson",
data=data), test="Chisq")

Analysis of Deviance Table

Model 1: Y ~ offset(log(E)) + X1 + X2
Model 2: Y ~ offset(log(E)) + X2
  Resid. Df Resid. Dev Df Deviance Pr(>Chi)
1       390     846.66
2       391     852.06 -1  -5.4054   0.1223
```

2.9   Modeling the cumulative effects of exposure

In order to assess the effect of environmental hazards on health, models are required that relate risk to the exposure, both in terms of the degree of exposure and the time over which exposure occurred. In cohort studies of individuals, such models need to account for the duration of exposure, time since first exposure, time since exposure ceased and the age at which first exposure occurred (Breslow and Day, 1980; Waternaux, Laird, and Ware, 1989). For the development of carcinogenesis, complex multi-stage models have been developed that use well-defined dose-response relationships (Dewanji, Goddard, Krewski, and Moolgavkar, 1999). However, when using aggregated daily mortality counts for a specific day or health period and a specified area, detailed exposure histories and other information are generally not available.

Considering, for ease of illustration, a generic area, if Y_t is the health outcome at time t, for example the number of respiratory deaths or on a single day or other period of time, and the true exposure history is $X(u), 0 \leq u \leq t$, then the outcome is modeled as a function of the exposure history.

$$E(Y_t) = f(X(u); \quad 0 \leq u \leq t) \tag{2.14}$$

As true personal exposure to air pollutants is unmeasurable over a lifetime, as it depends on ambient levels and integrated time activity, the term 'exposure' here relates to cumulative ambient outdoor concentrations of air pollutants, measured at the aggregate area level. The summaries of the exposure history are therefore constructed based on available data, X_t.

If it is assumed that $X(u)$ is piecewise continuous, then the cumulative exposure up to and including time t is

$$\int_0^t X(u)du \tag{2.15}$$

Rather than just considering the effect of the total exposure over a period of time, the contributions from intervals within the period may be of interest, in which case (2.15) can be expressed in the form of weighted integrals (Breslow, Lubin, Marek, and Langholz, 1983; Bandeen-Roche, Hall, Stewart, and Zeger, 1999).

$$C_t = \int_0^{u=t} W(t-u)X(u)du \tag{2.16}$$

where the weights, $W(t-u)$, determine the aspect of the exposure being summarized. For example, if the weights are of the form $W(u) = \min(1, u/b)$, then the exposures are phased in linearly over a period of length b until they reach their maximum. This can allow for delayed, as well as cumulative effects, depending on the form of the weights. In individual studies, the form of the cumulative exposure can be explicitly modeled. For example, in the case of exposure to asbestos fibers, the rate of elimination of the fibers from the lungs, λ, may be incorporated, and the model will take the form $W(u) = \{1 - \exp(-\lambda u)\}/\lambda$ (G. Berry, Gilson, Holmes, Lewinshon, and Roach, 1979).

Since exposure to air pollution starts in infancy, the lower limit of the integral will not be zero; instead, the sum is likely to be over a specified period of time. If the weights are of the form,

$$W(u) = \begin{cases} 1/(b-a) & \text{for} \quad a \leq u < b \\ 0 & \text{otherwise} \end{cases} \tag{2.17}$$

then the summary will represent the average for the period $(t-b,t-a]$, $0 \le a < b \le t$. For example, when studying the short-term effects of air pollution, if $a=0$ and $b=2$, then $W(t-u)$ would represent a three-day mean. An alternative is to model exposure-time-response relationships based on patterns seen in the data, for example using splines (Hauptmann, Berhane, Langholz, and Lubin, 2001).

When dealing with mortality counts, and exposure measurements, made at discrete times, the integral in Equation 2.16 can be approximated by a summation over a suitable discretization.

$$C_t = \sum_{k=0}^{t} W_{t-k}X_k \qquad (2.18)$$

If the probability of disease given cumulative exposure is assumed to be proportional to $\exp(\gamma C_t)$, that is a log-linear model in cumulative exposure, then a Poisson model can be used to estimate the weights, W_{t-k} in Equation 2.18. Assuming that $Y_t \sim P(E_t \mu_t)$, where E_t represents the expected number of cases, then

$$\log \mu_t = \alpha + \gamma \sum_{k=0}^{t} W_{t-k}X_k = \alpha + \sum_{k=0}^{t} \beta_{t-k}X_{t-k} \qquad (2.19)$$

Here the parameter, β_{t-k} represents the effect of exposure k time periods ago. Comparison with Equation 2.16 and 2.18 shows that $\beta_{t-k} = \gamma W_{t-k}$.

Example 2.10. *Modeling the risks associated with lagged effects of air pollution*

Following on from the previous example, we might fit the annual averages from the previous three years, $X_{it}, X_{i(t-1)}, X_{i(t-2)}$. The R code to do this is as follows:

```
glm(formula = Y ~ offset(log(E)) + X1 + X1t1 + X1t2,
family = "quasipoisson", data = data_df )


Coefficients:
              Estimate Std. Error t value Pr(>|t|)
(Intercept) -0.09740    0.04959   -1.964 0.050233 .
X1           0.02118    0.03223    0.657 0.511514
X1t1        -0.01415    0.03143   -0.450 0.652917
X1t2         0.04271    0.01251    3.414 0.000708 ***

(Dispersion parameter for quasipoisson family taken
to be 3.276761)
```

However, the measurements for areas in the individual years are likely to be highly correlated over this short period of time, leading to issues of collinearity. In this case, it has resulted in just one of the covariates being significant and in patterns in the effects over time that may not make much sense, that is a decrease in risk associated with the previous year (although this is non-significant). For this reason, where there are high levels of collinearity more sophisticated approaches may be required, such as those described in Chapter 7.

Developments have been made in specifying the shape of the distributions of the weights, W_{t-k}, within aggregate level studies examining the short-term effects of air pollution on health. Schwartz (2000) describes the use of a distributed lag model, where the weights fit a polynomial function (Harvey, 1993). This requires assumptions to be made, in terms of the polynomial used, on the maximum lags that are likely to have an effect, but has the advantage of increasing the stability of the individual estimates where there is high collinearity between the explanatory variables (Zanobetti, Wand, Schwartz, and Ryan, 2000).

2.10   Logistic models for case-control studies

In case-control studies, the response variable is whether an individual is a case or control and is therefore a binary variable. The most common link function in this case is the logistic link, $\log(y/(1-y))$, which will constrain the results of the linear predictor to produce values between zero and one representing the probability that an individual is a case (i.e. has the disease). This means that the estimates of the parameters in a logistic regression model will be on the log-odds scale.

If Y_i is an indicator of whether the ith individual is a case (one) or a control (zero) then $Y_i \sim Bi(1, \pi_i)$. A logistic regression model with just an intercept will take the form

$$\log(\pi/(1-\pi)) = \beta_0 \tag{2.20}$$

In this case, the intercept, β_0 represents the overall proportion of cases on the log-odds scale,

$$\begin{aligned} \log(\pi/(1-\pi)) &= \beta_0 \\ \pi &= \exp(\beta_0)/(1+\exp(\beta_0)) \end{aligned} \tag{2.21}$$

Example 2.11. *Estimating the odds ratio in a case-control study using a logistic model*

In a study of asthma of whether children living near main roads require higher levels of asthma treatment than those who live further away, cases and controls were grouped according to whether or not they lived within 150 m of a main road (Livingstone, Shaddick, Grundy, and Elliott, 1996). Of the 1066 cases, 172 lived within 150 m of a main road with the corresponding number of controls being 464 (out of 6233).

The MLE of the probability that an individual is a case can be found using R as follows:

```
summary(glm(formula = Y ~ 1, family = "binomial", data
    = data_df2))
# where data_df2 is a dataframe with the health
    outcome (1 or 0) in Y and the exposure in X

Coefficients:
            Estimate Std. Error z value Pr(>|z|)
(Intercept) -1.76594    0.03314   -53.28  <2e-16 ***
```

The estimate -1.76594 is on the log-odds scale. Using 2.21 this can be converted back to the probability scale as, $\frac{\exp(-1.76594)}{(1+\exp(-1.76594))} = 0.146$ which is the same as the proportion of cases (1066/6233).

Including the effect of exposure, X_i in the model gives

$$\log(\pi_i/(1-\pi_i)) = \beta_0 + \beta_1 X_i \qquad (2.22)$$

where β_1 is the estimated increase in log odds per unit increase in X_1. It is the difference between two log odds, with and without an increase of one unit in X_1 and is, $\log(p_0/(1-p_0)) - \log(p_1/(1-p_1)) = \log\{p1/(1-p1)\}$ which is the log of the odds ratio. Therefore, taking the exponent of the estimate of β_1 gives us the odds ratio associated with a unit increase in X_1.

Example 2.12. *Estimating the odds ratio of asthma associated with proximity to roads*

We now estimate the effects of living near to a main road on asthma. The R code to do this is as follows;

```
summary(glm(Y~X, family="binomial", data=data))

Coefficients:
            Estimate Std. Error z value Pr(>|z|)
(Intercept) -1.86455   0.03594   -51.875  <2e-16 ***
X            0.87216   0.09623    9.063   <2e-16 ***
```

Here, the odds ratio associated with living close to a main road is $\exp(0.87216) = 2.391$ (95% CI; 1.981 − 2.889. This indicates that there is a significant increase in risk of asthma in the children under study associated with their living close to a main road. Of course there may be confounders, such as parental smoking, which may affect this. If available, these confounders could be added to the model in the same way as seen in the Poisson example.

2.11 Summary

This chapter contains the basic principles of epidemiological analysis and how estimates of the risks associated with exposures can be obtained. This chapter also provides an introduction to R and provides worked examples of how to estimate epidemiological risks and health impacts. From this chapter, the reader will have gained an understanding of the following topics:

- Methods for expressing risk and their use with different types of epidemiological study;
- Calculating risks based on calculations of the expected number of health counts in an area, allowing for the age–sex structure of the underlying population;
- The use of generalized linear models (GLMS) to model counts of disease and case-control indicators;
- The basics of R, including how to import data and how to use packages;
- How to use R to fit regression models in R and estimate epidemiological risks;
- Modeling the effect of exposures on health and allowing for the possible effects of covariates.

2.12 Exercises

Exercise 2.1. Show that the odds ratio for exposure given disease, $OR_{E|D}$, can be equal to the odds ratio for disease given exposure $OR_{D|E}$.

Exercise 2.2. Express the probability density for the normal distribution with mean μ and variance σ^2 in the exponential family form

$$f(y) = \exp\left\{\frac{y\theta - b(\theta)}{a(\phi)} + c(y,\phi)\right\}, y \in S$$

State the general formula for the mean and variance of an exponential family distribution and check that they hold for a normal random variable.

Exercise 2.3. In the case of logistic regression, express $fy(y|\theta)$ in the form of the exponential family and find expressions for $b(\theta), c(y, \phi)$ and $a(\phi)$.

Exercise 2.4. Show that for a Binomial (n, p) variable, the MLE of p is $\sum_{i=1}^{n} Y_i/n$.

Exercise 2.5. The observed Y_i counts of mortality in N areas all assumed to be Poisson distributed with the mean in each area being $E_i\lambda$ where E_i is the (age–sex adjusted) expected number of deaths and λ_i is the relative risk in that area. Show that MLE of the risk for all areas combined is equal to the overall SMR $= \frac{\sum_{i=1}^{N} O_i}{\sum_{i=1}^{N} E_i}$.

Exercise 2.6. It is thought that there is a relationship between air pollution and respiratory deaths. The table below contains data from two cities, A and B. The first city (A) had much lower pollution measurements than the second (B). A sample of residents from each city was followed and their ages at death were recorded. The number of deaths in 10 year age groups and the number of person-years at risk (PYR) are given for each city.

Number of deaths and person-years (PYR) for two factories manufacturing rubber under different operating conditions.

Age range	City A		City B	
	Deaths	PYR	Deaths	PYR
20–29	3	6000	1	3000
30–39	3	5000	4	4000
40–49	5	4000	5	3500
50–59	7	4045	8	3701
60–69	27	3571	43	3702
70–79	30	1777	40	1818
80–89	8	381	10	350

It is thought that the death rate in the city B might be higher than that in city A and that this might be due to the differences in air pollution. A regression model was used to assess the effect of city on death rate.

(a) Explain why simple linear regression might not be appropriate in this case, and suggest an alternative model, giving reasons for your choice.

(b) Use the data in the table to calculate the $\log_e$ of the death rates (LDR) by age group for each city. Plot them against age group, labelling the points according to city. What does the plot suggest?

The results of a Poisson regression model including just the intercept term are as follows.

Model 1

```
Coefficients (standard error)
 Intercept           -5.443109        0.100000
 Degrees of Freedom: 14 Total; 13 Residual
 Residual Deviance: 120.0000
```

(c) Calculate the overall death rate in the two cities from data in the table, and show that you could have produced the same result using the output from the model.

A city term was then added to Model 1, giving the following results.

Model 2

```
Coefficient (standard error)
 Intercept           -5.00000     0.100000
 City  B              0.400002     0.150000

 Degrees of Freedom: 14 Total; 12 Residual
   Residual Deviance: 110.000
```

(d) Calculate a relative risk with a 95% confidence interval comparing city B with city A. What do you conclude about the relative risk of living in city B compared to city A?

(e) Explain how you would assess the effect of adding the city term on the fit of the model. Show that there is a significant effect in this case.

Chapter 3

The importance of uncertainty: assessment and quantification

3.1 Overview

Uncertainty is a topic that permeates all scientific inquiry and its importance is magnified when the results are applied in decision-making, which in this setting will involve legislation, regulations and designing public policy.

Despite the general importance of the concept of 'uncertainty', its meaning lacks a universally agreed on definition. In fact, it shares its general lack of definition with 'information', as described by the late Debabrata Basu (Basu, 1975):

'But what is information? No other concept in statistics is more elusive in its meaning and less amenable to a generally agreed definition'.

It has been described in various ways, including 'incomplete knowledge in relation to a specified objective' which arises 'due to a lack of knowledge regarding an unknown quantity' (Bernardo and Smith, 2009). However, the lack of a clear-cut definition has not stopped people from taxonomizing it! Thus, we have for example the distinction between *aleatory* (stochastic) and *epistemic* (subjective) uncertainty (Helton, 1997). It seems generally agreed that some aspects of uncertainty are quantifiable while others are inherently qualitative, that is, not subject to quantification. The latter would, for example, include framing the problem to be investigated by defining the system boundaries and explicating the role of values (van der Sluijs et al., 2005). Both qualitative and quantitative aspects of uncertainty need to be taken into account within environmental risk analyzes.

There will often be intangible sources of uncertainty which will arise through the subjective judgements that are sometimes required to estimate the nature and magnitude of empirical quantities where other methods are not appropriate. Uncertainty may arise as a result of imprecise language in describing the quantity of interest and disagreement about interpretation of available evidence. There may also be uncertainty about the actual methods being used to assess policy changes, whether the data available to implement them is suitable for the purpose and the extent to which the results can be generalized.

Where models are used to mathematically represent real-life processes, there are a number of potential sources of uncertainty. These may include concerns about the

DOI: 10.1201/9781003352655-3

input data, uncertainties in the model description, how well the chosen models represent spatial and other variation and of course the stochastic nature of the physical processes being described. Uncertainty in one part of a model will also propagate to other parts of the model, and if multiple models are implemented then uncertainty will propagate through these as well. Often, such systems become so complex that the identification and characterization of uncertainty will need to be prioritized, looking at the most sensitive and most important parameters for the uncertainty assessment.

This chapter considers various aspects of uncertainty, from initial characterization to methods for quantification where appropriate. Methods for considering and handling uncertainty range from the philosophical and qualitative in nature (Walker et al., 2003; Briggs, Sabel, and Lee, 2009) to more quantitative approaches based on probabilistic or statistical methods (Cullen and Frey, 1999).

3.2 The wider world of uncertainty

Post-normal science (see Chapter 1) called for a search for new approaches to dealing with uncertainty, one that recognized the diversity of stakeholders and evaluators needed to deal with these challenges. New tools were needed to facilitate the conduct of post-normal scientific investigations in an organized way. One such tool is the Numerical–Units–Spread–Assessment–Spread (NUSAP) matrix (Funtowicz and Ravetz, 1990). It was designed to facilitate the analysis and diagnosis of the uncertainties in the knowledge base underlying a complex environmental issue, and in particular those expressed in the assumptions made by modelers. The NUSAP matrix consists of five columns, the first three of which comprise the quantitative elements involved in generating the knowledge base. For example, these might be the estimated relative risks of unit changes in air pollution calculated by an environmental epidemiologist, the units of measurement involved and the degree of uncertainty, for example standard errors (Funtowicz and Ravetz, 1990). In short, the first three columns capture the information that is available from standard statistical approaches.

However, this does not capture the underlying uncertainty that may arise from many other sources. In an epidemiological investigation, there is typically a hypothesis to be tested that will ideally be based on some preconceived theory or understanding of the aetiological processes involved. However, there will be uncertainty inherent in this understanding (Briggs et al., 2009). In risk and impact assessment, there will be uncertainty arising from the specification of the risks or policy, the question(s) to be analyzed, and the conditions, for example scenarios and study areas, under which the analyzes will be performed. Uncertainty may arise according to the extent, both spatially and temporally, of the analysis, what aspects to include and which to ignore, and, fundamentally, the underlying 'model' of the system under study (Briggs et al., 2009). There will also be uncertainty in the definition of the key relationships of interest and the processes that they represent. The scope for uncertainty is therefore very large, and its implications will run throughout the analysis, results and interpretation.

The final two columns of the NUSAP matrix act as an aid to recording this more general uncertainty. This may record the result of a 'pedigree analysis'. This pedigree analysis, summarized in the final column, would be based on an organized discussion amongst experts, possibly from a wide variety of subject areas and interests, charged with determining the uncertainty in the relevant knowledge base related to the overall objectives of the analysis.

Example 3.1. *Concerns about high levels of dioxin*

Controversy arose about the potential human health effects of a waste incinerator located near Antwerp when an unusually high number of children were found to have congenital defects (van der Sluijs et al., 2005). Members of the local population suggested that the cause was dioxin emissions from the incinerator. However, the operators, supported by local officials, disagreed and argued that the claims were not supported by scientific evidence. Years of debate ensued due to the uncertainties involved.

A workshop was held in which structured discussions about the uncertainties took place based on the findings from three scientific studies. The first was a spatio-temporal epidemiological analysis to determine if there were increased health risks among children whose parents lived, or had lived, in the region at risk. The second was an exposure assessment of how much dioxin might have been absorbed by people living in that region during the period of the study. The third was a biomonitoring study comparing the region in question with other similar regions which were used as 'controls'. A pedigree matrix (van der Sluijs et al., 2005) was used to evaluate each of the three components of this investigation, each having a specifically designed matrix.

One of the outcomes of the workshop was a recognition that the way the problem had been framed played a strong role in the ensuing debate (van der Sluijs et al., 2005). This pointed to the need for an extension to the pedigree matrix to include factors such as 'problem framing', 'research design' and 'extended review'. The NUSAP process of structured dialogue was shown to lead to insights that can go deeper than relying solely on statistical calculations of uncertainty.

3.3   Quantitative uncertainty

As noted in the introduction, quantitative uncertainty can be dichotomized as that which is unknown, *epistemic* and that which is unknowable, *aleatory uncertainty*. The first refers to a lack of knowledge about the processes which generate estimates of the parameters of interest, while the second refers to intrinsic uncertainty associated with the estimates. Though the distinction between the two may sometimes be blurred, the overall aim is the same; to reduce the uncertainty associated with the underlying processes and information required in order to perform estimation and prediction. In addition, a natural requirement of any estimate or prediction is a characterization and quantification of the uncertainty associated with them, without which the estimate/prediction has little use in reality.

Example 3.2. *Aleatory and epistemic uncertainty*

As a simple example, let A denote the event that shaking a die results in a six showing. Whether A will occur is uncertain, it may or may not. If it were known that the die is perfectly balanced, then the uncertainty in this case could be characterized by saying there is one chance in six of its being correct. This uncertainty can never be reduced even if a long string of repeated tosses is observed.

However, if it were not known if the die is balanced and that the likelihood of a six in this case is θ, one might say the chances of correctly predicting that A occurs is θ. But if θ is unknown, we have an example of epistemic uncertainty. This uncertainty can be eliminated by observing repeated tosses so that eventually uncertainty about θ would be eliminated.

3.3.1   Data uncertainty

Uncertainty will arise when attempting to obtain information about empirical quantities which have some true value that could, in principle at least, be measured. Uncertainty arises when these quantities are inaccurately measured. For example, data may be missing or incomplete, either spatially or temporally. These missing values may be ignored completely, inducing uncertainty as data are not available. Alternatively, values of the missing data may be imputed, for example by using an average of existing values. This will introduce uncertainty due to (unknown) differences between the true unknown value and the imputed value. In some cases no data may be available, in which case we may make use of surrogate or proxy variables. In the case of air pollution, for example, the full ambient pollution field cannot be completely measured but instead monitors are located at selected points in time and space. Interpolating to other locations, in either time, space or both, will introduce uncertainty due to assumptions that will be required in order to fit statistical models. Interpolating will be further hampered by missing values at the monitoring sites and the non-random placement of monitors. Monitoring stations may be situated in response to suspected 'hot-spots' of pollution, whereas methods of interpolation will assume that the sites are located randomly or will require some information on how the non-randomness operates. Even apparently appropriate data can be subject to inherent randomness. This may be subject to measurement error arising as a result of variability arising from measurement instruments and methods. If continuous variables are discretized this often requires some subjective assessment of the boundary, for example between hot and cold temperatures.

3.3.2   Model uncertainty

The basis of a statistical analysis is the formation of a statistical model that is intended to represent the associations between the variables of interest. However, a model will always be a simplified approximation of underlying causal structure. Different choices of the model could include different parameters or structural form, as well as statistical choices such as frequentist versus Bayesian methods and choice of Bayesian priors. There will be many possible choices of model and many methods are available for selecting between candidate models as described in Chapter 7. In addition to statistically based approaches, the choice will to some extent be pragmatic and will be based on the availability of data and what is computationally feasible. Uncertainty about the model can arise through uncertain data as discussed in Section 3.3.1 and factors such as measurement error or missing values can influence the choice of model. Mathematical models, even those involving physical laws, as described in Chapter 15, will have uncertainty associated with them through the use of approximations and dependence on parameters that must be estimated using experimental data. The latter will be subject to all the sources of data uncertainty described in Section 3.3.1 and these will be propagated through the process and manifest themselves in the output.

3.4   Methods for assessing uncertainty

There are many methods for assessing the effects of quantitative uncertainty, and we describe a selection of them here. An underlying concept behind many of them is the idea of changing the inputs to a system and observing the effects on the outputs, and often this is done in order to identify the components that are likely to have the greatest effect on the overall uncertainty. Other methods are based on mathematical approximations to the uncertainty characterization.

3.4.1   Sensitivity analysis

Sensitivity analysis aims to assess how changes in model inputs, either one at a time or in combination, can affect outputs from a model. The model is run a number of times with different input values in order to observe the resulting change in the output. It allows parameters that have large (or small) effects to be identified. Possible procedures for such sensitivity analysis include the following:

- Parameters varied one at a time – local sensitivity analysis, which sees how changes in one parameter affect the result.
- Parameters varied in combinations – global sensitivity analysis, where several parameters are varied together.
- Extreme values – all parameters are set at their maximum/minimum values.

The identification of variables that may have a substantial effect on model output is an important step in any analysis of uncertainty, as it is these variables which are liable to contribute most to the final uncertainty. This is especially important when the models are complex and computationally expensive to run, and it may be infeasible to fully incorporate full uncertainty modeling for every variable. Sensitivity analysis can therefore be used to inform decisions as to which input variables might be suitable candidates for the application of more complex or computationally demanding methods, such as the Taylor expansion or Monte Carlo simulation.

3.4.2 Taylor series expansion

This is a mathematical technique that approximates the underlying distribution which characterizes uncertainty in a process (MacLeod, Fraser, and Mackay, 2002; Oden and Benkovitz, 1990; Morgan and Small, 1992). Once such an approximation is found, it can provide a computationally inexpensive way of characterizing the uncertainty in model output and so is useful when dealing with large and complex models for which simulation-based methods may prove to be infeasible. Firstly, a set of important input variables have to be identified using sensitivity analysis by performing model runs with a set of pre-defined values of all the candidate variables and computing a coefficient indicating their relative sensitivity (RS). The final distribution of uncertainty, based on a log-normal distribution, is constructed by combining the uncertainties from each of the variables weighted by their RS. It is important to note that in identifying dominant sources of uncertainty for a model output, it is the combination of the sensitivity and uncertainty of the parameters that is important, and they cannot be considered in isolation, except in the unlikely case that they can all be considered independent.

3.4.3 Monte Carlo sampling

This replaces single values of input variables for a model with repeated samples from probability distributions (Metropolis and Ulam, 1949; Sobol, 1994; Rubinstein and Kroese, 2011). This results in uncertainty being propagated through the model, resulting in a distribution for the output. This distribution gives a value for the most likely value (the mean or median) together with a measure of its uncertainty, often represented by quantiles of the distribution. This is a very useful technique where models are highly non-linear, with many input variables, although it can be computationally expensive, especially in cases where models are large and incorporate large amounts of data.

The classic form of Monte Carlo simulation implies the use of the simple random sample technique; however, it is possible to apply other sampling methods to improve the coverage and efficiency of the Monte Carlo methods. Latin Hypercube Sampling (LHS) is an example of such a method (McKay, Beckman, and Conover, 2000; Stein, 1987). Instead of randomly generating realizations of the prior distributions, this approach divides the distribution up into areas of equal probability, for example using percentile bands of interest and selecting from the median of these bands only, known as 'Median LHS', or alternatively selecting randomly from within the specified probability range. The order of the sampling is usually random. LHS can be applied to reduce the number of realizations, particularly when accumulated distributions are to be assessed. For a general overview, see example Cullen and Frey (1999). LHS has been used in a variety of applications where correlation between parameters exists, for example Iman and Conover (1982); Pebesma and Heuvelink (1999). This is a particularly important point when assessing the uncertainty between two different scenarios, where there can be a large degree of correlation.

3.4.4   Bayesian modeling

Bayesian analysis is the subject of Chapters 5 and 6 but we briefly discuss it here in the context of a framework for quantifying uncertainty. The Bayesian philosophy considers that uncertainty can be described by means of probability distributions, and is thus highly parametric. The basic concept of Bayesian philosophy is that of the conditional distribution (Bernardo and Smith, 2009). Data, if available, are actively used and are assigned a probability distribution that will be conditional on a set of parameters. For example, data may be assumed to be Gaussian, conditional on the values of the mean and the variance. Moreover, each parameter has a probability distribution, known as a prior, that can incorporate differing degrees of subjectivity. If expert opinion or information from the literature are available, the prior distribution will reflect this, giving higher probability to suggested values. The prior distribution and the data are combined according to Bayes' theorem, leading to the posterior distribution of the parameters of interest. The uncertainty associated with the parameters is included in the model via the prior distributions and is propagated through to the posterior distribution. The output is not a single number but an entire probability distribution from which both measures of central tendency and uncertainty can be obtained. Often however the posterior distribution is not a known probability distribution or it is difficult to treat it analytically and so simulation or approximations are often used. This is the subject of Chapter 6.

3.5   Quantifying uncertainty

Although uncertainty is a fundamental concept, it is somewhat absent from the mainstream of statistical science and the best ways to define and quantify it remain unclear (Chen, van Eeden, and Zidek, 2010; Chen, 2013). The importance of random variability has led statisticians to model it, seek its causes and its relative importance. Following from this, statistical scientists have traditionally seen the identification of sources of uncertainty, its quantification and reduction through measurement and modeling as hallmarks of their discipline.

As described in Section 3.4.4 and more fully in Chapter 5, Bayesian theory represents uncertainty through probability (Oh and Li, 2004). That seems satisfactory for the uncertainty associated with the occurrence of a chance event such as $A = Heads$ on the toss of a coin. In this case, $p = P(A) = 0.9$ would imply a high degree of certainty in that case whereas $p = 0.5$ would reflect a state of complete uncertainty. However, in more complex situations where uncertain quantities T are involved, probabilities would need to be expressed as distributions to adequately describe the uncertainties (Frey and Rhodes, 1996). In other words, $p = P(T \leq t)$ would work for a single t but it would not characterize the degree of overall uncertainty about T. For that, a metric calculated from that distribution is required. The topic is an important one, as any contemplated action or decision must take into account uncertainty associated with the result. For example, deciding which smelters to close because of the high levels of arsenic they were generating could be based on spatial predictions of soil deposits produced through the methods seen in Chapter 10. Such decisions would then depend critically on the degree of confidence that could be placed on predictions made in the vicinities of the various smelters.

Various metrics have been proposed, notably the variance of and entropy of T's distribution, and these will be the topic for this section. Notably, both of these are additive when independent random variables are combined appropriately, but little is known about their behavior when additional information about T itself becomes available. One would heuristically expect uncertainty about it to go down, but does it? Starting with the simplest case above, where probability is the index of uncertainty, we see that such heuristics can often be too simplistic.

Example 3.3. *Uncertainty as probability*

Let $P(Y \in C)$ represent our uncertainty about the event, $A = \{Y \in C\}$. Now we learn that, in fact $Y \in A$, $A \cap C \neq \phi$ will our uncertainty about the event decrease as our heuristics suggest?

The answer can be 'no' when the new information conflicts with our prior beliefs. In fact $P(Y \in C | Y \in A)$ may be closer to $1/2$ than $P(Y \in C)$ as shown by J. V. Zidek and van Eeden (2003). In their example, if $Y \sim U[0, 1]$, C=[0,c], and A=[a,1] with $0 < a < c < 1$, then $P(Y \in C | Y \in A) = (c-a)/(1-a) = 1/2$ when $a = 2c-1$. If $c = 7/8$ and $a = 3/4$ we would move from a state of near certainty about the event to one of complete uncertainty (conditional probability $1/2$) about whether it has occurred. So new information need not reduce our uncertainty with this simple measure of uncertainty.

3.5.1 Variance

Suppose T denotes an uncertain quantity, for example an estimate of the long-run annual average temperature, μ_T, or a prediction of an unmeasured pollutant at a spatial location. How might the degree of our uncertainty about T be indexed? A common approach is to use the variance $Var(T)$ and it, or rather the standard deviation, σ_T, is used for example by The U.S. National Institute of Standards and Technology, to express measurement uncertainty. The institute's web page (http://physics.nist.gov/cuu/Uncertainty/basic.html) states that 'Each component of uncertainty, however evaluated, is represented by an estimated standard deviation, termed *standard uncertainty*?'. Perhaps a preferable alternative would be the coefficient of variation $CV_T = \sigma_T/\mu_T$ which does not depend on the scale on which T is measured, making this a more intrinsic property. Expressed as a percentage (which will also be unitless), CV_t, it is even used as a metric for assessing the quality of the data from which the estimate was produced, assuming the latter is obtained in a principled way (Bergdahl et al., 2007). Unless that metric is under a specified percentage, statistical agencies may not publish the estimates, meaning that for example national estimates may be published while those for small areas may not since the samples are too small. In the authors' experience, 20% is a challenging target to reach in practice with samples of a realistic size.

When T is in fact an estimate, σ_T is referred to as the standard error se_T. The se_T has been so well accepted as an appropriate measure of an estimate's uncertainty that it (or an estimate of it) is routinely quoted in most all scientific literature together with the estimate.

Example 3.4. *Uncertainty as variance*

Here, interest is in making inference about $T \sim N(\mu_T, \sigma_T^2)$. The variance $\sigma_T^2 = 1$ indexes the uncertainty about T. Some feedback reveals to the investigator that $|T| < C$ for a known constant C. Thus, the uncertainty index has to be recalculated as $Var(T \mid\mid T \mid < C)$. Heuristics suggest that the new information should reduce uncertainty about T. But does it? The answer is that it does, and in fact $Var(T \mid\mid T \mid < C) < 1$ for any μ_T and $0 < C$. Moreover, the new index is a monotone increasing function of C. In other words, the result is quite striking!

The result seems plausible when $\mu_T = 0$ for then the condition $|T| < C$ tells us at least if C is small that $T \approx \mu_T$. However, it does not seem plausible when $\mu_T \neq 0$ since the new information puts T in a place very different from where the distribution is centered.

The results in Example 3.4 are true in great generality (Chen, 2013), at least when new information comes in a relatively simple form. However, nothing seems to be known beyond these simple cases. Simple counterexamples show that they do not always hold, as in Exercise 3.4. Apart from the fact that as an estimate or predictor, T would need to be unbiased for the variance to play the role of an uncertainty index, it is not even clear whether it will generally pass the simple test of downward revision under increasing information.

These considerations, and other doubts about the suitability of the variance as an index of uncertainty, lead us to consider another index of uncertainty in the following Section (3.5.2).

3.5.2 Entropy

Entropy's role as an index of aleatory uncertainty has a long history, but it has relevance in many modern applications, including that encountered in Chapter 14 where it is used in monitoring network design to select sites where uncertainty (entropy) is highest.

To describe this index, we begin by letting E be a random event and $\overline{E}$ its complement. Furthermore, $T = E$ if E occurs and $T = \overline{E}$ if not. Next $p = Pr(E)$ denotes the probability that the event E occurs, so that $1 - p$ is the probability that $\overline{E}$ occurs. Concentrating on E for the moment, we are uncertain about whether it does or does not occur. Letting $\phi(.)$ represent as reduction-in-uncertainty function to be determined below, we get a reduction of $\phi(p)$ in that uncertainty if E does occur. In the same way, we get a reduction of $\phi(1-p)$ if $\overline{E}$ occurs. The idea is that if $p = 0.9$ we would get a smaller reduction $\phi(p)$ in our uncertainty if E does occur than we would get $\phi(1-p)$ if $\overline{E}$ occurs, the latter being quite a surprise. Thus, the expected reduction in uncertainty for observing $\mathbf{T}$ is

$$H(T) = p\phi(p) + (1-p)\phi(1-p)$$

To specify ϕ we need to impose some requirements and these are: $\phi \in [0,1]$; $H(T_1, T_2) = H(T_1) + H(T_2)$ when T_1 and T_2 are independent. Then it turns out that $\phi(p) = -log(p)$ in this simple case.

We now turn to the more general case of discrete random variables, T where $T \in \{t_i, \ldots, t_n\}$. In that case, with $p_i = P(T = t_i)$, we obtain

$$H(T) = \sum_{i=1}^{n} -p_i \log p_i \qquad (3.1)$$

as the average reduction of uncertainty for observing T.

In the case of a continuous random variable T, things are a bit more complicated. A naive approach would be to first partition the continuous domain of T into n equiprobable discrete subsections, S_i, with $n^{-1} = p_i = P(T \in S_i) = \int_{S_i} f_T(u)du$ where f_T denotes the pdf of T. With this approximation, we get the result in Equation 3.1 namely

$$H(T) \approx = -\sum_{i=1}^{n} n^{-1} \log n^{-1} = \log n$$

as an approximation. Letting the width of those subsections go to zero, and $n \to \infty$ we get ∞ in the limit. Obviously, this approach does not work.

The next approach is by analogy:

$$H(T) \equiv -E[\log f(T)] = -\int \log f(t) f(t)dx.$$

However, this proves unsatisfactory in more subtle ways. Firstly, the probability density function PDF is not invariant under transformations from say Celsius to Fahrenheit if T were temperature. Uncertainty should ideally be an intrinsic property of an uncertain quantity, and in fact should be invariant under any 1:1 transformation of the scale of measurement. Recognizing this problem, Jaynes (1963) introduces the idea of a reference measure with PDF $h(x)$:

$$H(T) \equiv -E\left[\log \frac{f(T)}{h(T)}\right] \qquad (3.2)$$

In fact Jaynes gives an ingenious argument, which shows that if h is defined correctly Equation 3.2 can be obtained from Equation 3.1 by an approximation argument similar in spirit to the failed naive argument above. However, commonly in practice h is taken to be $1(T\text{units})$ so that it cannot be explicitly seen. However, it does mean that the units of measurement cancel in f_T/h, making this a unitless quantity as it must be if its logarithm is to be taken (see Section 10.3).

3.5.3   Information and uncertainty

It is not clear precisely how information and uncertainty are related. At one time uncertainty seems to have been thought of exclusively as aleatory uncertainty and then entropy was seen as a way of quantifying the uncertainty in the probability distribution of a random variable (Harris, 1982). When the variable was observed, all uncertainty was gone, so the entropy could then be thought of as the amount of information that had been gained by observing the variable (Shannon, 2001; Renyi, 1961).

That was all well and good until it was recognized that not all quantitative uncertainty could be considered to be due to chance (aleatory) and that some of it had to be ascribed to a lack of knowledge (epistemic) (Helton, 1997). In this case, the latter is knowable, meaning that with enough data that uncertainty would disappear.

The approach in Section 3.5.2 fails when epistemic uncertainty is introduced, meaning that aleatory uncertainty (corresponding to the amount of information) forms just one component of a decomposition. The other corresponds to epistemic uncertainty when the uncertainty about the model is expressed as a probability distribution.

Example 3.5. *Aleatory and epistemic uncertainty*

Recall that epistemic uncertainty is that component of uncertainty related to the truth of a proposition, and that it is reduced or eliminated given enough data. Let the indicator function $Z = I\{ace\}$ represent the truth of the proposition 'the next toss of this die will be an ace' when the probability of an ace p is uncertain. Repeated tosses of the die would resolve this uncertainty. However, even if eventually $p = 1/6$ came to be known for certain, the value of Z would not be known. This uncertainty due to chance variation is aleatory uncertainty. To get a better understanding of what is going on, let's consider the example within a Bayesian setting and assign a beta prior distribution on p with prior density proportional to $p^{\alpha-1}(1-p)^{\beta-1}$. After n repeated tosses we would have a posterior density proportional to $p^{\alpha+r-1}(1-p)^{\beta+n-r-1}$ where r is the number of times a six turned up in these independent tosses.

Although it is not clear that the variance is the correct way to quantify uncertainty (Chen et al., 2010), we consider it here because it is commonly used. The posterior variance of Z is approximately

$$Var[Z \mid r] = Var\{E[Z \mid p,r]\} + E\{Var[Z \mid p,r]\} \tag{3.3}$$

$$\approx \frac{\hat{p}(1-\hat{p})}{n}\} + \hat{p}(1-\hat{p}) \tag{3.4}$$

where $\hat{p} = r/n$ (Chen et al., 2010). The first term represents the epistemic uncertainty, which declines to zero as $n \to \infty$ while the second represents the aleatory uncertainty.

We may ask 'what happens if a 7 turns up on the second toss of the die'? Unfortunately, we are stuck since all our calculations were done conditional on a six-sided die. In this case, our uncertainty would increase. Bayesian theory can allow for the 'known unknowns' to be accommodated by acknowledging model uncertainty. Here, if we had allowed a die with an unknown number of faces into our model, we could have dealt with the '7'. An insurmountable problem arises from the 'unknown unknowns' as there is no formal theory that allows us to represent the increase in uncertainty that arises due to a surprise outcome. Nevertheless, it is important to recognize that information can both increase or decrease our uncertainty.

So what lessons does Example 3.5 teach us about spatio-temporal modeling? First, it tells us that additional data may increase rather than decrease our uncertainty when the initial class of models is insufficiently rich. The analyst should try to ensure a class of models that is big enough to admit even seemingly unrealistic scenarios to the maximum feasible extent, leading to a restatement of the late Dennis Lindley's version of Cromwell's rule: 'don't put a probability of zero on anything'. Secondly, we learn that spatio-temporal models must be able to retain the aleatory component of uncertainty in a dynamic system. A meteorologist with sufficient data would be able to estimate the correlation between temporally stationary responses seen at two sites, say $Y_{s_1 t}$ and $Y_{s_2 t}$, due to chance variation in things like variable wind direction. There is no model here. A naive Bayesian approach might model the process like this (Chen et al., 2010): $Y_{st} = \beta_{st} + \varepsilon_{st}$ or in vector form $\mathbf{Y}_s = \beta_s + \epsilon_s$ with $\beta_s \sim N_p(\mu_0 \mathbf{1}_{T+1}, \sigma_\beta^2 \mathbf{I}_{T+1})$ and $\mu_0 \sim N(\mu^*, \sigma_\mu^2)$. It is easily shown that conditional on the data

$$Corr(Y_{s_1(T+1)}, Y_{s_2(T+1)}) = [\sigma_\mu^{-2} + pT\sigma^{-2}]^{-1} \to 0, \text{ as } T \to \infty \qquad (3.5)$$

in contradiction to the meteorologist's calculation. This is because the Bayesian failed to distinguish between the two forms of uncertainty and built the model accordingly. Even in less extreme cases, uncertainties will shift between components of a Bayesian posterior distribution when the marginal distribution of the process responses are fixed and reflect aleatory uncertainty.

3.5.4 Decomposing uncertainty with entropy

In this section we return to the problem of decomposing uncertainty into the part that is aleatory and the part that is epistemic, with entropy playing the role of the uncertainty index. The latter means in this section that uncertainty about the model parameters is represented by a probability distribution, as in Chapter 5. To begin, assume $T \sim f(. \mid \theta)$. Given data D

$$H(T, \theta) = H(T \mid \theta) + H(\theta) \qquad (3.6)$$

where

$$
\begin{aligned}
H(T \mid \theta) &= E[-\log(f(T \mid \tilde{\theta}, D)/h_1(T)) \mid D] \\
H(\theta) &= E[-\log(f(\tilde{\theta} \mid D)/h_2(\theta)) \mid D] \\
h(T, \theta) &= h_1(T) h_2(\theta)
\end{aligned}
$$

with $\tilde{\theta}$ meaning that the expectation is being computed over a random θ (Caselton, Kan, and Zidek, 1992; Le and Zidek, 1994). An important example of this decomposition, for an application detailed in Chapter 14 is given in Appendix B.

3.6 Summary

This chapter contains a discussion of uncertainty, both in terms of statistical modeling and quantification, but also in the wider setting of sources of uncertainty outside those normally encountered in statistics. The reader will have gained an understanding of the following topics:

- Uncertainty can be dichotomized as either qualitative or quantitative, with the former allowing consideration of a wide variety of sources of uncertainty that would be difficult, if not impossible, to quantify mathematically.

- Quantitative uncertainty can be thought of as comprising both aleatory and epistemic components, the former representing stochastic uncertainty and the latter subjective uncertainty.

- Methods for assessing uncertainty including eliciting prior information from experts and sensitivity analysis.

- Indexing quantitative uncertainty using the variance and entropy of the distribution of a random quantity.

- Uncertainty in post-normal science derives from a wide variety of issues and can lead to high levels of that uncertainty with serious consequences. Understanding uncertainty is therefore a vital feature of modern environmental epidemiology.

3.7 Exercises

Exercise 3.1. Referring to Example 3.2, give a reasonable expression of your uncertainty about the prediction of a six when θ is unknown. How is this case different from the case when θ was known to be $1/6$?

Exercise 3.2. Referring to Example 3.4,

(i) determine in explicit form both $E(T \mid\mid T \mid < C)$ and $Var(T \mid\mid T \mid < C)$

(ii) numerically evaluate and plot both functions of C in (i).

Exercise 3.3. Repeat Exercise 3.2, but this time for the uniform distribution where $T \sim U[-1, 1]$

Exercise 3.4. The results in Exercise 3.2 do not always hold. Give two counterexamples.

EXERCISES   65

Exercise 3.5. You are to predict the outcome T of the toss of a die, but you do not know if the die is fair.

(i) Model both the aleatory and the epistemic uncertainty in this situation, and show how the total uncertainty can be decomposed using your model.

(ii) You are to bet on the event $T = 1$ occurring and asked to state the best odds you can offer me, below which you will refuse to bet. What are those odds?

(iii) The die is tossed and a 7 turns up. What are the best odds you would be willing to give me now?

Exercise 3.6. Using the notation of Appendix A, $Z \sim N_p(\mu, \Sigma)$,

(i) find the entropy of the distribution of Z.

(ii) interpret your result from (i) when $p = 2$.

Exercise 3.7. RESEARCH QUESTION: How does the entropy of the distribution of T $H(T)$ change if it learned that $|T| < C$ for a known C?

Chapter 4

Extracting information from data

4.1 Overview

There is a rich history of collecting environmental data and recently there has been an explosion in quantity and complexity of data related to the physical and natural world around us, from monitoring, satellite remote sensing, climate modeling, social media and contributions from citizen science. In addition to a consideration of the type of data that is available, we show how R can be used to process data to ensure it is in a suitable form for analysis, visualization and modeling.

Data is increasingly available from Internet sources, including as the GitHub repository which is associated with this book. The award-winning book of Wikle, Zammit-Mangion and Cressie (Wikle et al., 2019) also provides a convenient source of tools and other things through its website for general spatio-temporal modeling. That book notes that the NOAA's National Climate Data Center data can be obtained from the IRI/LDEO Climate Data Library at Columbia University (https://iridl.ldeo.columbia.edu/)

Data products may include:

1. metadata
2. raw data;
3. models developed specifically for preprocessing the data;
4. spatial-temporal data files;
5. data from controlled experiments;
6. remote sensing data including images along with descriptive notes interviews and codebooks; laboratory analysis outputs (text files, .csv);

Generally, unlike books, articles, and other such works, data and code cannot be copyrighted, so they can be cited in the traditional way, for example, through a BibTeX listing. Yet many readers will be downloading these things for analyzes that appear in their documents. And in that case, they will wish to cite their sources for those users, as well as a way of giving credit to those who created those sources. So how can this be done? The DOI (Digital Object Identifier) system has been created for that purpose. In fact, whole GitHub repositories can be so designated. When this book's revision was being written, DOI's may be obtained for these repositories from Zenodo, an organization offered by CERN.

DOI: 10.1201/9781003352655-4

4.2   Using R to process and analyze data

4.2.1   Importing a dataset

Using RStudio we can import datasets using the 'Import Dataset' option in the 'Environment' window (as can be seen in Figure 4.1). You can choose whether you want to import a .csv file, an Excel file or files from SPSS, SAS or stata. You can import many more file types by installing an appropriate package and writing code to read in the files (see the next section).

Try the following with the file `WHO_GM_Database.csv`. Note that this is a cut down and tidied up version of the third of the files listed above. It is used here as an example of how to import data into R as the original files are quite large and can take a while to load (as well as being a little messy in places)

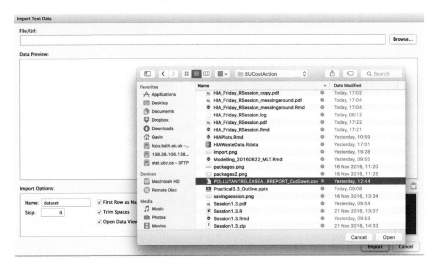

Figure 4.1: Importing a file into RStudio using the dropdown menus in the Environment pane.

You will then see a preview of your data together with an example of the code that R will use to read in the data (as can be seen in Figure 4.2). You can choose what the dataset will be called when it has been imported and set other options. These options can be very useful if a dataset isn't quite as clearly formatted, as is the case with the original files. For example, you can decide to skip a certain number of rows at the beginning of the file which is often useful or to use different text delimiters (things that indicate the gap between columns in the data).When you are ready, press 'Import'.

Importing a data file using code

To read a CSV file into R we use the `read.csv()` function.

```
# Read in a .csv file
mydata <- read.csv(file='<filepath_and_filename>.csv')
```

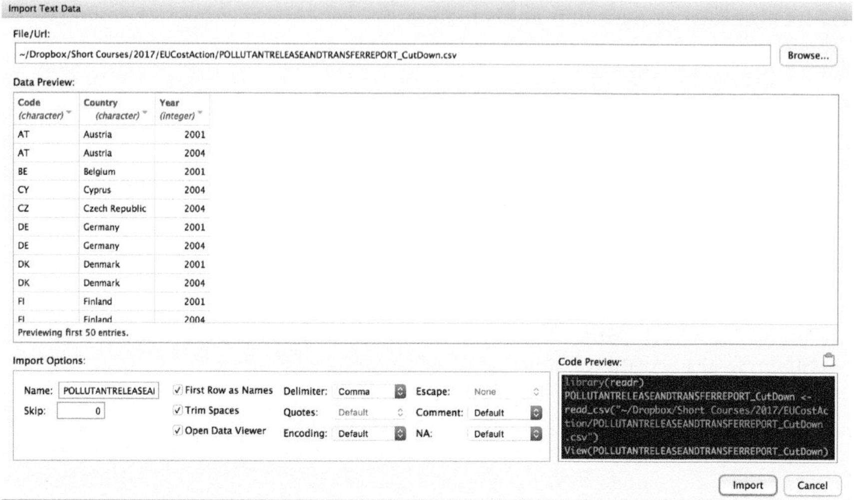

Figure 4.2: Previewing the data and choosing options in RStudio.

Note that we should put in the full path to the file when using `read.csv`. Or we can set a **working directory**. The function `getwd()` will tell you the file path of the current working directory of the R process.

```
getwd()
[1] "/Users/gavin/Desktop/Book/Chap4"
```

The function `setwd()` is used to set the working directory to your chosen location.

```
setwd("Chosen_Directory_Path")
```

Or you can use the files Pane in 'RStudio' and choose the working directory from the 'Session' menu (Session->Set Working Directory->Files Pane Location). Once we have set the working directory, we don't have to repeatedly type the path to the folder.

Getting to know the structure of dataframes

Once a dataframe has been loaded into R we can examine it and perform analysis. Initially, we can understand our dataset by finding the number of observations and variables in data frames by using the `nrow()` and `ncol()` functions, respectively.

We will load and analyze data from the World Health Organization's Global Air Pollution database. The data is open source and can be downloaded from the WHO's website in `.csv` format. It contains over 11,000 measurements of fine particulate matter air pollution ($PM_{2.5}$ and PM_{10}) for the years 2010-2019 and details of the locations of monitoring sites. We can import this into R and convert it to a dataframe either by using the `read.csv` function.

```
# reading in a .csv file into R
# set the working directory
setwd("~/Desktop/Book/Chap4/")
# import the dataset from a .csv file
WHO_GM_Database <- read.csv("WHO_GM_Database.csv")
# Viewing the structure of the variables within the WHO Air
    Pollution dataset
str(WHO_GM_Database)
'data.frame':   65428 obs. of  10 variables:
$ ISO3 : chr "AFG" "AFG" "AFG" "ALB" ...
$ CountryName: chr "Afghanistan" "Afghanistan" "Afghanistan
    " "Albania" ...
$ Year : chr "2009" "2009" "2019" "2015" ...
$ Longitude : num 67.1 69.2 69.2 19.4 19.4 ...
$ Latitude : num 36.7 34.5 34.5 41.3 41.3 ...
$ PM25 : num 68 86 119.8 NA 14.3 ...
$ PM10 : num 334 260 NA 17.6 24.6 ...
$ SDG1Region : chr "Central Asia and Southern Asia" "
    Central Asia and Southern Asia" "Ce $ SDG2Region : chr
    "Southern Asia" "Southern Asia" "Southern Asia" "Europe
    " ...
$ SDG3Region : chr "Southern Asia" "Southern Asia" "
    Southern Asia" "Southern Europe" ...
```

A quick way of viewing the dataset to see the data are using the `names()`, `str()` and `head()` functions. The `names()` function will display the variable names within a dataframe. The `str()` function will display the structure of the dataset, and the `head()` function will display the first 6 rows in the dataframe.

```
# Display the variable names
names(WHO_GM_Database)
 [1] "ISO3"          "CountryName" "Year"          "Longitude"
     "Latitude"
 [6] "PM25"          "PM10"          "SDG1Region"  "SDG2Region"
     "SDG3Region"

# View the first 6 rows of the WHO Air Pollution dataset
head(WHO_GM_Database)
  ISO3 CountryName Year Longitude Latitude       PM25
     PM10
1  AFG Afghanistan 2009  67.11667 36.70000  68.00000
     334.0000
2  AFG Afghanistan 2009  69.19128 34.53076  86.00000
     260.0000
3  AFG Afghanistan 2019  69.19051 34.53581 119.77360
     NA
```

```
4   ALB      Albania 2015   19.44920 41.31990        NA
    17.6483
5   ALB      Albania 2016   19.44920 41.31990  14.32325
    24.5591
6   ALB      Albania 2014   19.48620 40.40309        NA
    15.2537
                    SDG1Region      SDG2Region
                         SDG3Region
1 Central Asia and Southern Asia Southern Asia    Southern
    Asia
2 Central Asia and Southern Asia Southern Asia    Southern
    Asia
3 Central Asia and Southern Asia Southern Asia    Southern
    Asia
4    Northern America and Europe        Europe Southern
    Europe
5    Northern America and Europe        Europe Southern
    Europe
6    Northern America and Europe        Europe Southern
    Europe

# tail(WHO_GM_Database) will show the last 6 rows of the
    dataset
```

Extracting and creating variables

Data within dataframes can be extracted using '[]'. As dataframes are two-dimensional objects, we need to specify two things, the row and/or the column, separated with a comma, for example [,]. Lets extract (i) the variable Year from WHO_GM_Database and assign it to a new variable called YearOfMeasurement, (ii) the first row from of WHO_GM_Database and assign to a variable called FirstRow (iii) 3rd row for variable CountryName from WHO_GM_Database.

```
# Extracting the variable Year from WHO_GM_Database and
    assign to a new variable called Year
YearOfMeasurement <- WHO_GM_Database[,'Year']
```

```
# show the first 5 entries in YearOfMeasurement
YearOfMeasurement [1:5]
[1] "2009" "2009" "2019" "2015" "2016"

# Extracting the row (or observation) from WHO_GM_Database
    and assign to a new variable called FirstRow
FirstRow <- WHO_GM_Database [1,]

# Show the first 10 entries in FirstRow
FirstRow [1:10]
   ISO3 CountryName Year Longitude Latitude PM25 PM10
1  AFG Afghanistan 2009   67.11667     36.7   68  334
                         SDG1Region      SDG2Region
                         SDG3Region
1 Central Asia and Southern Asia Southern Asia Southern
    Asia
# Extracting the 3rd row for Year from WHO_GM_Database
WHO_GM_Database [3,'Year']
[1] "2019"
```

Alternatively, you can extract variables from the dataframes by using the $ operator. We first specify the dataset, then give the name of the variable that we want. Let's extract the variable Year from WHO_GM_Database.

```
# Extracting the variable a from WHO_GM_Database , and show
    the first 3 entries
WHO_GM_Database$Year [1:3]
[1] "2009" "2009" "2019"
```

Creating a new variable within a dataframe is straightforward. Let's create a variable TimeSince2010 within WHO_GM_Database which is the difference between Year and 2010. For this we ex- tract the variable Year from WHO_GM_Database and subtract 2010. In the dataframe, Year is a character variable (which you can see using str(WHO_GM_Database)) and we will need to convert this to a numeric variable before performing the calculation.

```
# convert Year to a numeric variable

WHO_GM_Database$Year <- as.numeric(WHO_GM_Database$Year)

# Extracting Year a from WHO_GM_Database ,subtract 2000 and
    make a new variable in the WHO_GM_Database dataframe.
    For clarity, we will only show the first 3 entries

WHO_GM_Database$TimeSince2010 <- WHO_GM_Database$Year -
    2000
WHO_GM_Database$TimeSince2010 [1:3]
[1]  9  9 19
```

4.3   Data wrangling and the Tidyverse

It is estimated that data scientists spend around 50–80% of their time cleaning and manipulating data. This process, known as data wrangling, is a key component of modern statistical science, particularly in the age of big data. The Tidyverse incorporates a suite of packages, such as `tidyr` and `dplyr` that are designed to make common data wrangling tasks not only easier to achieve, but also easier to decipher. Readability of the code is a core ideal in the philosophy underpinning the packages.

The architect behind the Tidyverse, Hadley Wickham, distinguishes between two types of data set: tidy and messy. This is not to be pejorative towards different ways in which people store and visualize data; rather it is to make a distinction between a specific way of arranging data that is useful to most R analyzes, and anything else. In fact, Hadley has a neat analogy to a famous Tolstoy quote: 'Tidy datasets are all alike, but every messy dataset is messy in its own way' (Hadley Wickham). Specifically, a tidy data set is one in which: rows contain different observations; columns contain different variables; and cells contain values.

According to Hadley (2014), a *tidy* dataset will have three characteristics: (1) each row is an observation; (2) each column is a single variable; (3) each value occurs in a single cell. This kind of data frame makes analysis easy, but data are commonly stored in an untidy way as it can be more compact. Thus you might have variables U, V and W in a form like seen in the adjoining short table.

Long Table		
U	V	W
U_1	V_1	W_{11}
U_2	V_1	W_{21}
U_3	V_1	W_{31}
U_4	V_1	W_{41}
U_1	V_2	W_{12}
U_2	V_2	W_{22}
U_3	V_2	W_{32}
U_4	V_2	W_{42}
U_1	V_3	W_{13}
U_2	V_3	W_{23}
U_3	V_3	W_{33}
U_4	V_3	W_{43}

Short Table			
	V_1	V_2	V_3
U_1	W_{11}	W_{12}	W_{13}
U_2	W_{21}	W_{22}	W_{21}
U_3	W_{31}	W_{31}	W_{31}
U_4	W_{41}	W_{41}	W_{41}

The short table was lengthened by *pivoting* on V, but we could also have pivoted on U.

However, the analysis of data stored in a short table can generally be made easier to analyze by converting it into a long table like that seen above. For example, W becomes easier to regress on U and V. In fact, since these tables represent data frames, not matrices, more complicated analyzes of association like logistic regression become relatively easy. Tidyverse provides the pivot_longer function for lengthening the table.

The short table cannot only be lengthened, but it can be widened in an analogous way using the *pivot_wider* tool where new columns are added to represent new variables while dropping some rows from the long table. Other tools are available for tidying the data and for these we refer the reader to Timbers, Campbell, and Lee (2022). Tidyverse greatly assists with the management and preliminary analysis of data files. It is not just a single package. Instead, it is an *R meta package* that installs and loads a collection of R packages, each of which can be be installed and run individually.

The idea of *tidy* data gives rise to the nomenclature of the Tidyverse. We will explore a number of ways in which datasets can be manipulated to and from the tidy format.

4.3.1 Simple manipulations using Tidyverse

Again, we will use the WHO_GM_Database dataframe and will start by looking at some basic operations, such as subsetting, sorting and adding new columns.

Filter rows in Tidyverse

One operation we often want to do is to extract a subset of rows according to some criterion. For example, we may want to extract all rows of the iris dataset that correspond to the versicolor species. In Tidyverse, we can use a function called filter(). For clarity, we will show the first 3 rows of the output

```
filter(WHO_GM_Database, Year == 2019)[1:3,]
   ISO3           CountryName Year Longitude Latitude
       PM25 PM10
1  AFG           Afghanistan 2019  69.19051 34.53581
   119.77360    NA
2  ALB                Albania 2019  19.48620 40.40309
   10.31525    NA
3  ARE United Arab Emirates 2019  54.37730 24.45390
   NA   100
                              SDG1Region      SDG2Region
                                SDG3Region TimeSince2010
1    Central Asia and Southern Asia Southern Asia    Southern
      Asia              19
2       Northern America and Europe          Europe Southern
      Europe              19
3 Western Asia and Northern Africa   Western Asia     Western
      Asia              19
```

Sorting rows

Using Tidyverse, the arrange() function will sort the WHO_GM_Database data by CountryName (alphabetically) and then by Year (numerically). Again, for clarify we will show only the first few rows of the data (9 rows)

```
arrange(WHO_GM_Database, CountryName, Year)[1:9,]
    ISO3 CountryName Year Longitude Latitude      PM25
       PM10
1   AFG Afghanistan 2009   67.11667 36.70000   68.00000
    334.00000
2   AFG Afghanistan 2009   69.19128 34.53076   86.00000
    260.00000
3   AFG Afghanistan 2019   69.19051 34.53581  119.77360
            NA
4   ALB      Albania 2011   19.82177 41.33027   27.53000
    52.36900
5   ALB      Albania 2011   19.85167 41.34560   37.49400
    112.44400
6   ALB      Albania 2012   19.82177 41.33027   20.20700
    33.99500
7   ALB      Albania 2012   19.85167 41.34560   24.52900
    37.85900
8   ALB      Albania 2013   19.82177 41.33027   16.06237
    31.61542
9   ALB      Albania 2014   19.48620 40.40309         NA
    15.25370
                        SDG1Region      SDG2Region
                          SDG3Region TimeSince2010
1  Central Asia and Southern Asia Southern Asia    Southern
   Asia               9
2  Central Asia and Southern Asia Southern Asia    Southern
   Asia               9
3  Central Asia and Southern Asia Southern Asia    Southern
   Asia              19
4      Northern America and Europe         Europe Southern
   Europe             11
5      Northern America and Europe         Europe Southern
   Europe             11
6      Northern America and Europe         Europe Southern
   Europe             12
7      Northern America and Europe         Europe Southern
   Europe             12
8      Northern America and Europe         Europe Southern
   Europe             13
9      Northern America and Europe         Europe Southern
   Europe             14
```

Select columns

Now let's say that we wish to select just the CountryName, Year and PM25 columns from the data set and assign it to a new dataset, WHO_GM_Database_reduced. In Tidyverse we can use the select() function:

```
WHO_GM_Database_selectcolumns <- select(WHO_GM_Database,
    CountryName, Year, PM25)
head(WHO_GM_Database_selectcolumns)
  CountryName Year       PM25
1 Afghanistan 2009   68.00000
2 Afghanistan 2009   86.00000
3 Afghanistan 2019  119.77360
4     Albania 2015         NA
5     Albania 2016   14.32325
6     Albania 2014         NA
```

There is even a set of functions to help extract columns based on pattern matching, for example

```
WHO_GM_Database_selectcolumns2 <- select(WHO_GM_Database,
    starts_with("Country"))
head(WHO_GM_Database_selectcolumns2)
  CountryName
1 Afghanistan
2 Afghanistan
3 Afghanistan
4     Albania
5     Albania
6     Albania
```

Note that we can also remove columns using a – operator, for example

```
WHO_GM_Database_selectcolumns3 <- select(WHO_GM_Database, -
    starts_with("SDG"))
head(WHO_GM_Database_selectcolumns3)
  ISO3 CountryName Year Longitude Latitude       PM25
     PM10 TimeSince2010
1  AFG Afghanistan 2009  67.11667 36.70000   68.00000
     334.0000             9
2  AFG Afghanistan 2009  69.19128 34.53076   86.00000
     260.0000             9
3  AFG Afghanistan 2019  69.19051 34.53581  119.77360
     NA               19
4  ALB     Albania 2015  19.44920 41.31990         NA
     17.6483            15
5  ALB     Albania 2016  19.44920 41.31990   14.32325
     24.5591            16
6  ALB     Albania 2014  19.48620 40.40309         NA
     15.2537            14
```

```
WHO_GM_Database_selectcolumns4 <- select(WHO_GM_Database, -
   SDG1Region, -SDG2Region, SDG3Region)
head(WHO_GM_Database_selectcolumns4)
  ISO3 CountryName Year Longitude Latitude        PM25
     PM10        SDG3Region
1  AFG Afghanistan 2009   67.11667 36.70000   68.00000
   334.0000    Southern Asia
2  AFG Afghanistan 2009   69.19128 34.53076   86.00000
   260.0000    Southern Asia
3  AFG Afghanistan 2019   69.19051 34.53581  119.77360
   NA    Southern Asia
4  ALB      Albania 2015   19.44920 41.31990          NA
   17.6483 Southern Europe
5  ALB      Albania 2016   19.44920 41.31990   14.32325
   24.5591 Southern Europe
6  ALB      Albania 2014   19.48620 40.40309          NA
   15.2537 Southern Europe
  TimeSince2010
1              9
2              9
3             19
4             15
5             16
6             14
```

Adding columns

Finally, let's add a new column representing the different between Year and 2000 as before, but using the Tidyverse. To avoid over-riding the first version we will call it TimeSince2010_tidy and for clarity will only show the first three rows.

```
WHO_GM_Database$Year <- as.numeric(WHO_GM_Database$Year)
mutate(WHO_GM_Database, TimeSince2010_tidy = Year - 2000)
   [1:2,]
  ISO3 CountryName Year Longitude Latitude       PM25 PM10
1  AFG Afghanistan 2009   67.11667 36.70000   68.0000  334
2  AFG Afghanistan 2009   69.19128 34.53076   86.0000  260

                    SDG1Region       SDG2Region
                    SDG3Region TimeSince2010
1 Central Asia and Southern Asia Southern Asia Southern
   Asia              9
2 Central Asia and Southern Asia Southern Asia Southern
   Asia              9

  TimeSince2010_tidy
1                  9
2                  9
```

Why is the Tidyverse so useful?

1. These functions are all written in a consistent way. That is, they all take a data.frame (or a `tibble` object) as their initial argument, and they all return a revised data.frame or `tibble object`.

2. Their names are informative. In fact, they are verbs, corresponding to us doing something specific to our data. This makes the code much more readable.

3. They do not require lots of extraneous operators: such as $ operators to extract columns, or quotations around column names.

4. Functions adhering to these criteria can be developed and expanded to perform all sorts of other operations, such as summarizing data over groups.

Pipes

Piping comes from Unix scripting, and simply means a chain of commands, such that the results from each command feed into the next one. It can be helpful in making code more succinct, and uses the pipe operator %>% to chain functions together.

For example, the following will filter the dataframe to extract rows when the year is 2019 and then how the first 6 rows using the head function.

```
WHO_GM_Database %>% filter(Year == 2019) %>% head()
    ISO3          CountryName Year Longitude Latitude
        PM25    PM10
1   AFG           Afghanistan 2019  69.19051 34.53581
    119.77360     NA
2   ALB                Albania 2019  19.48620 40.40309
    10.31525      NA
3   ARE United Arab Emirates 2019  54.37730 24.45390
    NA 100.00
4   ARE United Arab Emirates 2019  54.37730 24.45390
    NA 102.29
5   ARE United Arab Emirates 2019  54.37730 24.45390
    NA 104.69
6   ARE United Arab Emirates 2019  54.37730 24.45390
    NA 112.58
                        SDG1Region       SDG2Region
                            SDG3Region TimeSince2010
1    Central Asia and Southern Asia Southern Asia     Southern
     Asia                19
2        Northern America and Europe         Europe Southern
     Europe                19
3 Western Asia and Northern Africa  Western Asia      Western
     Asia
```

When we did this without piping we would write something like filter(WHO_GM_Database, Year == 2019) and assign it to a new variable and then use the head() function (or we could have added [1:6] to the end). The pipe operator %>% passes the outcome from the left-hand side of the operator, that is the result of the `filter`, as the first argument to the right-hand side function. This makes the code more succinct, and easier to read (because we are not repeating pieces of code).

Chaining pipes

Pipes can be chained together multiple times. For example:

```
WHO_GM_Database$Year <- as.numeric(WHO_GM_Database$Year)

WHO_GM_Database %>%
filter(Year == 2019) %>% select(CountryName, Year, PM25, -
    starts_with("SDG")) %>% mutate(TimeSince2010_tidy =
    Year - 2000) %>% arrange(CountryName, Year) %>%
head()
  CountryName Year       PM25 TimeSince2010_tidy
1 Afghanistan 2019 119.77360                 19
2      Albania 2019  10.31525                 19
3      Algeria 2019  21.53338                 19
4    Australia 2019        NA                 19
5    Australia 2019        NA                 19
6    Australia 2019        NA                 19
```

Notice that the pipe operator must be at the end of the line if we wish to split the code over multiple lines.

In essence, we can read what we have done in much the same way as if we were reading prose. Firstly we take the `WHO_GM_Database` data, filter to extract just those rows corresponding to `CountryName`, `Year`, `PM25`, mutate the data frame to contain a new column that is the difference between the Year and 200 and finally arrange in order of `CountryName` and `Year`.

Note: we can also pass the result of the right-hand side using the assignment operator `<-` to make a new variable of the result, for example `NewData <- WHO_GM_Database %>%filter(Year == 2019) %>% select(CountryName, Year, PM25, -starts_with("SDG")) %>% mutate(TimeSince2010_tidy = Year - 2000) %>% arrange(CountryName, Year)`. Note that if you do not make another variable, it would overwrite the original data to produce a new data set with only the selected entries.

4.4   Grouping and summarizing

A common thing we might want to do is to produce summaries of some variable for different subsets of the data. For example, we might want the mean values of PM25 for each `CountryName`. The `dplyr` package (which is part of the Tidyverse) provides a function `group_by()` that allows us to group data, and `summarize()` that allows us to summarize data.

In this case, we can think of what we want to do as grouping the data by `CountryName` and then averaging the PM25 values within each group. Note that there are missing values in PM25, as in some locations only PM10 is measured, and vice-versa. We use mean(PM25, na.rm=TRUE) to exclude missing values when calculating the mean.

```
WHO_GM_Database %>%
  group_by(CountryName) %>%
summarize(mn = mean(PM25, na.rm=TRUE))
# A tibble: 127 Ã- 2
   CountryName      mn
   <chr>         <dbl>
 1 Afghanistan   91.3
 2 Albania       22.3
 3 Algeria       21.5
 4 Andorra       11.0
 5 Argentina     10.2
 6 Australia      8.11
 7 Austria       14.2
 8 Bahamas        4.16
 9 Bahrain       55.4
10 Bangladesh    76.8
# ... with 117 more rows
```

4.5 Summarize

The summarize() function applies a function to a dataframe or subsets of a dataframe. For example, we can produce a table of estimates for the mean and variance of both PM25 lengths and PM10, within each CountryName.

```
WHO_GM_Database %>%
  group_by(CountryName) %>%
summarize(MeanPM25 = mean(PM25, na.rm=TRUE), MeanPM10 =
    mean(PM10, na.rm=TRUE), VarPM25 = var(PM25, na.rm=TRUE)
    , VarPM10 = var(PM10, na.rm=TRUE))
# A tibble: 127 Ã- 5
   CountryName MeanPM25 MeanPM10  VarPM25 VarPM10
   <chr>          <dbl>    <dbl>    <dbl>   <dbl>
 1 Afghanistan    91.3      297    691.     2738
 2 Albania        22.3     36.4    77.9      655.
 3 Algeria        21.5      NaN      NA       NA
 4 Andorra        11.0     19.2    0.276     1.09
 5 Argentina      10.2     27.4    0.0103    1.45
 6 Australia       8.11    17.7    54.2      58.4
```

```
 7  Austria         14.2      20.4    11.2        25.8
 8  Bahamas          4.16      4.65    1.04         1.19
 9  Bahrain         55.4      176.    103.       4844.
10  Bangladesh      76.8      142.    690.       1784.
#  ... with 117 more rows
```

Example 4.1. *Example: Health impacts associated with outdoor air pollution*

We now demonstrate how using dataframes and the `Tidyverse` can allow us to perform a health impact analysis of air pollution very efficiently. We will be calculating the annual number of deaths attributable to $PM_{2.5}$.

Preliminaries

We wish to estimate the annual number of deaths attributable to $PM_{2.5}$ air pollution. In order to do this, we need

- a relative risk (RR),
- the population at risk for the areas of interest,
- the overall mortality rate (OMR) and
- a baseline value for air pollution (for which there is no associated increase in risk).

In this example, we use a RR of 1.06 per 10 μgm^{-3}, the population at risk is 1 million and an overall mortality rate of 80 per 10000. We first enter this information into R by assigning these values to a series of variables.

```
# Relative Risk
RR <- 1.06

# Size of population
Population <- 1000000

# Unit for the Relative Risk
RR_unit <- 10

# Overall mortality count, used for calculating the
   overall mortality rate
OMR_count <- 80

# Denominator (population at risk), used for
   calculating the overall mortality rate.
OMR_pop <- 10000
```

```
# Mortality rate
OMR = OMR_count/OMR_pop
OMR
[1] 0.008

# Baseline value of PM2.5 for which there is no
    increased risk
baseline <- 5

# Population attributable fraction
#PAF = (Proportion of population exposed*(RR-1))/(
    Proportion of population exposed*(RR-1)+1).
#In this case the proportion of the population exposed
    is one.

PAF = (RR-1)/RR
PAF
[1] 0.05660377
```

In this example, we will calculate the attributable deaths for increments of 10 μgm^{-3}, however the following code is general and will work for any increments.

```
# PM2.5 categories
PM2.5.cats <- c(5,15,25,35,45,55,65,75,85,95,105)

# Create a dataframe containing the PM2.5 categoriess
Impacts <- data.frame(PM2.5.cats)
```

Calculating Risks

We now calculate the increases in risk for each category of $PM_{2.5}$. For each category, we find the increase in risk compared to the baseline.

For the second category, with $PM_{2.5} = 15$, the risk will be 1.06 (the original RR) as this is 10 μgm^{-3} (one unit) greater than the baseline.

For the next category, $PM_{2.5}$ is 10 μgm^{-3} higher than the previous category (one unit in terms of the RR) and so the risk in that category again be increased by a factor of 1.06 (on that of the previous category). In this case, the relative risk (with respect to baseline) is therefore 1.06 * 1.06 = 1.1236.

For the next category, $PM_{2.5} = 25$ which is again 10 μgm^{-3} (one unit in terms of the RR) higher, and so the relative risk is 1.06 multiplied by the previous value, that is 1.06 * 1.1236 = 1.191016.

We can calculate the relative risks for each category (relative to baseline) in R. For each category, we find the number of units from baseline and repeatedly multiply the RR by this number. This is equivalent to raising the RR to the power of (Category-Baseline)/Units, for example

$$RR^{\left(\frac{\text{Category-Baseline}}{\text{Units}}\right)}$$

We add another column to the Impacts dataframe containing these values.

```
# Calculating Relative Risks
Impacts <- mutate(Impacts, RR = RR^((Impacts$PM2.5.
    cats - baseline)/RR_unit))
```

Once we have the RR for each pollution level, we can calculate the rate for each category. This is found by applying the risks to the overall rate. Again, we add these numbers to the Impacts dataframe as an additional column using `mutate`. To use this function, we need to add columns which contains replications of the OMR and `Population`.

```
# Create an additional column containing replication
    of the OMR
Impacts$OMR <- rep(OMR, nrow(Impacts))
Impacts$Population <- rep(Population, nrow(Impacts))

# Calculating the rates in each category
Impacts <- mutate(Impacts, Rate = RR * OMR)

# Add the PAFs for each category
Impacts <- mutate(Impacts, PAF = RR * (RR-1)/RR)

# Add the number of (expected) deaths  per year for
    each category
Impacts <- mutate(Impacts, DeathsPerYear = Rate *
    Population)
```

For each category, we need to calculate the extra deaths (with reference to the overall rate). The number of deaths for the reference category is the first number in the `DeathsPerYear` column.

```
# The reference number of deaths
Impacts$DeathsPerYear[1]
[1] 8000
```

```
# make into a vector by using the rep (replicate)
    function and add to the dataframe
Impacts$ReferenceDeaths <- rep(Impacts$DeathsPerYear
    [1], nrow(Impacts))

# We can then calculate the excess numbers of deaths
    for each category
Impacts <- mutate(Impacts, ExtraDeaths = DeathsPerYear
    - ReferenceDeaths)
```

For each category, we then want to calculate the number of deaths gained. These are the difference between the values in each category. We can find these using the diff() function. This will produce a set of differences for which the length is one less than the number of rows in our Impacts dataframe. We need to add a zero to this to ensure that they line up when we add them as another column.

```
# Calculate the number of deaths gained
diff(Impacts$ExtraDeaths)
 [1]  480.0000 508.8000 539.3280 571.6877 605.9889
      642.3483 680.8892 721.7425
 [9]  765.0471 810.9499

# We can now add these gains to the main Impacts
    dataframe
Impacts$Gain <- c(0,diff(Impacts$ExtraDeaths))

# Show the results
Impacts
    PM2.5.cats          RR    OMR Population          Rate
              PAF DeathsPerYear
1            5 1.000000 0.008       1e+06 0.008000000
  0.0000000      8000.000
2           15 1.060000 0.008       1e+06 0.008480000
  0.0600000      8480.000
3           25 1.123600 0.008       1e+06 0.008988800
  0.1236000      8988.800
4           35 1.191016 0.008       1e+06 0.009528128
  0.1910160      9528.128
5           45 1.262477 0.008       1e+06 0.010099816
  0.2624770     10099.816
6           55 1.338226 0.008       1e+06 0.010705805
  0.3382256     10705.805
7           65 1.418519 0.008       1e+06 0.011348153
  0.4185191     11348.153
8           75 1.503630 0.008       1e+06 0.012029042
  0.5036303     12029.042
```

```
9                85  1.593848  0.008           1e+06  0.012750785
       0.5938481           12750.785
10               95  1.689479  0.008           1e+06  0.013515832
       0.6894790           13515.832
11              105  1.790848  0.008           1e+06  0.014326782
       0.7908477           14326.782
      ReferenceDeaths  ExtraDeaths         Gain
1                8000        0.000     0.0000
2                8000      480.000   480.0000
3                8000      988.800   508.8000
4                8000     1528.128   539.3280
5                8000     2099.816   571.6877
6                8000     2705.805   605.9889
7                8000     3348.153   642.3483
8                8000     4029.042   680.8892
9                8000     4750.785   721.7425
10               8000     5515.832   765.0471
11               8000     6326.782   810.9499
```

4.6   Visualizing data

The second edition of Tufte's classic on the visual display of quantitative information (Tufte, 1942) lists the criteria for excellence for graphical displays of statistical
information. Tufte (1942) suggests the following as good visualization criteria:

- show the data;
- induce the viewer to think about substance rather the technicalities and methodology associated with the data and display;
- avoid distorting the data;
- present numbers in a compact space;
- make large datasets coherent;
- encourage the viewer's eye to compare different pieces of data;
- reveal the data at several levels of data from broad to fine;
- serve a clear purpose;
- be integrated with other descriptions of he data.

He presents as a 'classic', the figure seen in the Example 4.2. It was drawn by Charles
Joseph Minard (1871-1870), a French Engineer, in 1861, according to Tufte, who
concludes that it may well be the 'best statistical graphic ever drawn'.

Example 4.2. *Napolean's army is defeated*
Like Example 1.6, this example concerns a famous historical event,
Napolean's march on Moscow, and like the previous example, it also shows

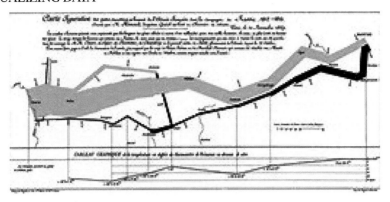

Figure 4.3: Napoleon wages war on Russia in 1812. Making their way east towards Moscow the yellow path shows the army's numbers, initially 500,000 in numbers dropping. The black path shows that the numbers that returned declined to near zero.

the power of data visualization. But it goes one step further by showing the temporal dynamics of the march on a spatial map – a remarkably imaginative illustration. In particular, the example shown in Figure 4.3 shows the size of the outbound army in yellow, initially 500,000 in number. As the march wears on that number declines due to starvation, desertion, disease and other factors. On arrival, Napolean finds a deserted city burned to the ground by its citizens. The return path in black shows the size of the army continuing to diminish in size on its return journey. The continuing losses were now due also, in part, to attacks by Russian troops as well as cold weather of winter – the temperatures got as low as -30 degree Celsius. In the end, the entire army was annihilated (Austen, 2012).

Example 4.3. *Mapping cancer incidence in Southern and Eastern Serbia*

In this example, we will see how to use R to create maps and then map the values of data within a dataframe. We will create a map of South and East Serbia. and creating expected number of cases and SIRs of cancer in City of Bor. To create maps, we use something called 'shapefiles'. Shapefiles contain location, shape and attributes of geographic features such as country borders. The files SE_Serbia.shp, and SE_Serbia.dbf contain the location, shape and attributes of South and East Serbia by district. These were obtained from http://www.gadm.org. On this website you can download administrative boundaries for almost every country in the world.

We will use the following files

- shapefiles and information for South and East Serbia split by administrative district (SE_Serbia.shp, SE_Serbia.dbf)

- population counts and density for South and East Serbia split by administrative district (SE_Serbia.csv)
- population counts and incidence rates of all cancers, by age group and sex in City of Bor (Bor_Rates.csv),
- observed counts of all cancers cancer, by age group and sex in City of Bor (Bor_Observed.csv)

These need to be in the working directory, which can be set using the setwd() function.

```
setwd("Chosen_Directory_Path")
```

Alternatively use Session > Set Working Directory > Choose Directory in the toolbar on the top of the top right panel in RStudio.

For this example, we need the following packages

- sp – Package to use spatial objects.
- spdep – Package to use spatial objects.
- rgdal – Package to load and manipulate spatial data.
- CARBayes – Package to fit spatial GLMMs which contains some useful functions for manipulating spatial data
- RColorBrewer – Package to give scaled colours for plots.
- raster – Package to work with rasters.
- rworldmap – Package to plot maps.

Use the install.packages() function or the packages window in the bottom right pane of RStudio to download and install the packages that we need. We use the library() function to load the required packages into the R library.

```
# Loading required packages
library(spdep)
library(shapefiles)
library(sp)
library(CARBayes)
library(rgdal)
library(RColorBrewer)
library(raster)
library(rworldmap)

# a function from a previous version of CarBAYES that
    we use here
source("combine.data.shapefile.R")
```

Before reading in any data for this example you will need to ensure that you are in the correct folder. You can use the setwd() function to do this.

```
setwd("Chosen_Directory_Path")
```

If you cannot get the `setwd()` to work, go to `Session > Set Working Directory > Choose Directory` in the toolbar on the top.

Creating maps of Southern and Eastern Serbia

creating-maps-of-southern-and-eastern-serbia

To create maps, we use something called 'shapefiles'. Shapefiles contain location, shape and attributes of geographic features such as country borders. The files `SE_Serbia.shp` and `SE_Serbia.dbf` contain the location, shape and attributes of South and East Serbia by district. These were obtained from `http://www.gadm.org`. The functions `read.shp()` and `read.dbf()` will read these shapefiles into R.

```
# Reading in borders
shp_Serbia <- read.shp(shp.name = "SE_Serbia.shp")
dbf_Serbia <- read.dbf(dbf.name = "SE_Serbia.dbf")
```

The file `SE_Serbia.csv` contains the population of South and East Serbia by district and we will use this to create maps. These are in csv format, so we use the `read.csv()` function.

```
# Read population data for Serbia
pop_Serbia <- read.csv('SE_Serbia.csv')
```

To check that the data has been read into R correctly, we can use the `head()` and function, which prints the first six rows of a dataset.

```
# Printing first six rows
head(pop_Serbia)
  CountryName ISO3  District  Area_KM2 Pop_2011 Pop_Per
     _KM2_2011
1     Serbia   SRB       Bor     3510   124992
          35.61026
2     Serbia   SRB Branicevo   3865   183625
          47.50970
3     Serbia   SRB Jablanica   2770   216304
          78.08809
4     Serbia   SRB     Nisava   2727   376319
  137.99743
5     Serbia   SRB    Pcinja   3520   159081
          45.19347
6     Serbia   SRB     Pirot   2761    92479
          33.49475
```

We can see that this dataset contains the following variables:

- `CountryName` – Name of Country,
- `ISO3` – ISO country code

- `District` – Name of district,
- `Area_KM2` – Area of district (in km²),
- `Pop_2011` – Population count in 2011,
- `Pop_Per_KM2_2011` – Population density in 2011 (in km²)

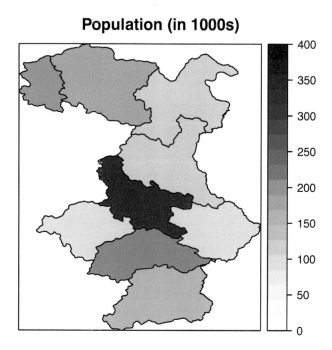

Figure 4.4: Populations in different administrative areas in Serbia

Let's create a map of population in 2011 for Southern and Eastern Serbia. To plot the population data in a map, we need to attach them to the shapefiles. The function `combine.data.shapefile()` allows us to combine shapefiles to plot later.

```
# Combining population data and the shapefile
Serbia <- combine.data.shapefile(data = pop_Serbia, #
    Dataset to attach
                          shp   = shp_Serbia, #
                                Shapefile
                          dbf   = dbf_Serbia) #
                                Database file
```

We use downloaded population data to create the map seen in Figure 4.4. To plot the map, we use the `spplot()` function. To obtain the colours for the plot, we use the package `RColorBrewer`, which gives a comprehensive set of colours to use in our plots. For more information on these colour schemes, see `http://colorbrewer2.org/`.

```
# Scaling population counts (to 1000s)
Serbia$Pop_2011 <- Serbia$Pop_2011/1000

# Creating map of population counts in Serbia
spplot(obj  = Serbia, # Spatial object to be plotted
       zcol = c("Pop_2011"), # Choice of the column
          the object you are plotting.
       main = "Population (in 1000s)", # Plot title
       at   = seq(0,400, length.out=20), # Break
          points for legend
       col = 'black', # Colour for borders
       col.regions = colorRampPalette(brewer.pal(9, '
          Blues'))(20)) # Create a set of colours
```

Example 4.4. *Cancer in Bor*

We will work through an example of creating expected counts and a standarized morbidity ratio (SMR) using data on all types of cancer (except skin) in the Muncipality of Bor, Serbia between 2001 and 2015.

Expected Numbers

In order to calculate SMRs, we need to estimate the number of cases we expect in Bor per year, based on their age–sex profiles. To calculate expected numbers, we use indirect standardization.

For indirect standardization, we take the age and sex-specific rates from the reference population (in this example, Serbia) and convert them into the mortality rate we would observe if those reference rates were true for the age and sex-structure of the population of interest (in this example, Bor). Therefore, we require

- population counts by age and sex for Bor
- the age and sex-specific incidence rates for cancer in Serbia.

The file `Bor_Populations.csv` contain the populations and incidence rates required by age and sex. These are in csv format, so we use the `read.csv()` function.

```
# Reading in observed numbers of hospital admissions
    in England by local authority
Bor_Rates <- read.csv(file="Bor_Rates.csv")
```

To check that the data has been read into R correctly, and to familiarise ourselves with the data, we can summarize it using the summary() function. This will allow us to check for anomalies in our data.

```
# Summarising first six rows of the Rates and
    populations of Bor
summary(Bor_Rates)
      City                    Sex
 Length:32               Length:32
 Class :character        Class :character
 Mode  :character        Mode  :character




   AgeGroup                   Pop
 Length:32               Min.    : 506.0
 Class :character        1st Qu.: 853.5
 Mode  :character        Median :1101.0
                         Mean    :1067.5
                         3rd Qu.:1232.0
                         Max.    :1482.0

 Incidence_Serbia         Incidence_SE_Serbia
 Min.   :0.0001243        Min.    :0.0001088
 1st Qu.:0.0002873        1st Qu.:0.0002470
 Median :0.0015951        Median :0.0015305
 Mean   :0.0044163        Mean    :0.0039337
 3rd Qu.:0.0080899        3rd Qu.:0.0072949
 Max.   :0.0173886        Max.    :0.0149553
```

We can see that Bor_Rates has the following variables:

- City – Name of City,
- Sex – Sex category,
- AgeGroup – Age categories, in 5-yearly groups,
- Pop – Population count,
- Incidence_Serbia – Incidence rates of cancer in Serbia per year
- Incidence_SE_Serbia – Incidence rates of cancer in South and East Serbia per year

Now that we have read in the population and the incidence rates required, we calculate the expected number as follows

$$E = \sum_k N_k \times r_k$$

where r_k are the age- and sex-specific rates of obtaining cancer in Serbia and N_k are the population counts by age and sex in Bor.

In R we can calculate each of the $N_k \times r_k$ by multiplying the columns containing the Serbian incidence rates and the population profile of Bor. We add another column to the `Bor_Rates` dataframe containing these values. Remember that to extract and assign columns in a dataframe we use the `$` operator.

```
# Calculating the expected number by Settlement, age
    and sex
# using the Serbian incidence rates and Bor population
    profiles
Bor_Rates$Expected <- Bor_Rates$Incidence_Serbia * Bor
    _Rates$Pop
```

Calculating SMRs

The observed number of cases of cancer by sex in the Municipality of Bor need to be read into R. These are in csv format, so we use the `read.csv()` function.

```
# Summing all expected cases by
aggregate(Expected ~ City + Sex, # Variable to
    aggregate ~ Variables to Stratify
            data = Bor_Rates, # Dataset name
            sum) # Function to summarize over
   City    Sex Expected
1  Bor Females 68.30022
2  Bor   Males 71.45852
```

To check that the data has been read into R correctly, we can use the `head()` function, which prints the first six rows of a dataset.

```
# Printing first six rows of the observed counts
head(Bor_Observed)
   City    Sex Observed
1  Bor   Males     1581
2  Bor Females     1540
```

We can see that `Bor_Observed` has the following variables:

- `City` – Name of City,
- `Sex` – Sex category,
- `Observed` – Observed number of cases of cancer between 2001 and 2015

```
# Summing all expected cases by Settlement and Sex
Bor_Expected <- aggregate(Expected ~ City + Sex, #
    Variable to sum over ~ Variables to Stratify by
                    data = Bor_Rates, # Dataset
                    name
                    sum) # Function to summarize
                    over
```

Remember, we calculated expected numbers for one specific year, whereas the observed counts are over 10 years (2001-2015). For the SMRs, we assume that the population remains the same across that time period and multiply the expected cases by 15.

```
# Multiplying the number of cases by 15 to obtain
    expected cases between 2001 and 2015
Bor_Expected$Expected <- 15 * Bor_Expected$Expected
```

To compare the observed and expected counts, we need to merge the two datasets `Bor_Expected` and `Bor_Observed` together. We do this using the `merge()` function.

```
# Merging files together
Bor <- merge(Bor_Expected, # First file to merge
             Bor_Observed, # Second file to merge
             by = c('City','Sex')) # Variables to
                 merge
```

Now that we have observed and expected numbers of cancer cases, we can calculate raw SMRs. Remember that

$$SMR = \frac{observed}{expected}$$

We add another column to the Bor dataframe containing these values.

```
# Calculating SMR by sex
Bor$SMR <- Bor$Observed / Bor$Expected
```

```
# Printing the results
Bor
   City    Sex Expected Observed      SMR
1  Bor Females 1024.503     1540 1.503167
2  Bor   Males 1071.878     1581 1.474982
```

4.7 Summary

There is a rich history of collecting environmental data and recently there has been an explosion in quantity and complexity of data related to the environment, from monitoring, satellite remote sensing, numerical modeling and many other sources. This chapter provides an introduction to the variety of different sources of data that are available and methods for obtaining, manipulating and processing data using the Tidyverse in R so that it is a form that can be readily used for analysis. The reader will have gained an understanding of the following topics:

- How the Tidyverse can be used for data wrangling;
- The importance of visualization in communication and understanding;

- How R can be used to summarize and visualize data;
- The use of shapefiles to produce maps in R;
- How to calculate expected numbers and SMRs in practice;
- How to perform health impact analysis.

4.8 Exercises

Exercise 4.1. Using the WHO ambient air quality database, extract the data for a region (SDG3Region) of your choice.

 (i) Produce summaries of the air pollution for each country within your chosen region

 (ii) Use an appropriate statistical test to assess whether there any significant differences in air pollution between the countries in 2016? What reasons do you think there might be for any differences? What additional data might you want to collect to test your hypotheses?

(iii) Produce graphical summaries of the level of air pollution in each country over time. Do you see any trends? Are the trends the same for each country?

Exercise 4.2. In Example 4.1 an analysis of the health impacts associated with increased levels of air pollution was presented.

 (i) Repeat this example using a lower and a higher relative risk and present the results from all three analyzes (including the one given in the example) on a graph. What do you conclude about the relationship between the relative risk and the number of deaths per year?

(iii) The question of whether there is a lower bound for the effect of air pollution, that is it still harmful at very low levels, is a current research question. Repeat your analyzes using different baseline risks (i.e. smaller and greater than the 5 given in the example). What do you conclude?

Exercise 4.3. For a country of your choice, repeat the exercise shown in 4.3 to produce a map of the country. You can download shapefiles for administrative areas for different countries at http://www.gadm.org.

 (i) Extract the monitoring site locations from the WHO Ambient Air Quality database and plot them on your map.

 (ii) What do you think about the spatial pattern of air pollution monitoring in the country that you have chosen? Is the entire country covered by the monitoring network? What effects, if any, do you think this might have on your summaries of air pollution for this country?

Chapter 5

Embracing uncertainty: the Bayesian approach

5.1 Overview

The paradigm described in Chapter 4 for modeling a process of interest leads to combining information coming through two channels, the first, which relies on prior knowledge, yields information that may be expressed as process models. These models will usually represent unobserved quantities. For example, temperature can be felt and modeled by a process model in the terminology of Berliner (1996), but not observed. The second channel brings in the information obtained by the measurement process, in Berliner's terminology. Ultimately, the Scientists must combine these two sources of information in a maximally informative way that then maximally reduces uncertainty about the process of interest. That will mean fitting the process model using the data described by the measurement model in ways that will depend on the statistical paradigm adopted by the modeler.

In Bayesian statistics, probability describes all types of uncertainty, both through unpredictability and through imperfect knowledge. Uncertainty is described by means of probability distributions that are assigned to uncertain quantities. When estimating the values of unknown parameters, which are often related to characteristics of the process under study, these values will be uncertain due to lack of knowledge rather than due to random variation. In the Bayesian setting, parameters are treated in the same way as all other uncertain quantities; they are treated as random variables and assigned probability distributions. As such, probability statements can be made about them, such as 'an interval that has 95% probability of containing the true value' or 'the probability that a null hypothesis is true is...'. This is in contrast to the frequentist approach under which statements about probability are based on the idea of repetition, for example '95% of all confidence intervals calculated under repeated sampling will cover the true parameter value' or 'the p-value for a hypothesis test is the probability that we would observe this, or something more extreme (under the assumption that the null hypothesis is true)'. Bayesian statistics may be thought of as *subjective* in the sense that prior knowledge and beliefs about what we expect to see can be incorporated into the inferential process. Frequentist statistics on the other hand is based solely on observed data and is therefore referred to as *objective*.

DOI: 10.1201/9781003352655-5

This chapter introduces the Bayesian approach, upon which the majority of the methodology introduced in this book is based, while making comparisons to the likelihood approach. The choice of prior distributions, central to the idea of Bayesian statistics, is considered together with the ways in which prior distributions then combine with information from data to obtain posterior distributions. A posterior distribution captures our beliefs about a particular quantity and will be the basis of interpretation and possible further inference. In the following chapter, we consider methods for implementing these ideas in practice.

5.2 Introduction to Bayesian inference

When considering the effects of a set of covariates on a response variable, interest often lies in drawing conclusions about the unknown parameters, θ. In the case of a regression model, unknown parameters might include the set of coefficients, β and the variance, σ^2. Interest might lie in predicting values, Z, one of the process variables, also called response variables, for particular values of the explanatory variables. When data, y, are observed, such inference will be expressed as $p(\theta|y)$ and $p(Z|y)$ for the cases of parameter estimation and prediction, respectively.

In the frequentist setting, the combination of the process and measurement models would lead to a model for the random sample of measurements $\mathbf{y} = (y_1,\ldots,y_n)^T$ made in accordance with the measurement model. However, that model would involve p unknown quantities $\theta = (\theta_1,\theta_2,\ldots,\theta_p)^T$ and these would need to be estimated to complete the model specification, called the sampling distribution $p(\mathbf{y}|\theta)$. The estimates might well be obtained through maximum likelihood estimation: first, one obtains the estimator $\widehat{\theta}$ that maximizes the likelihood function. The idea is that $\widehat{\theta}$ is the value most likely to have generated the observed data. As $\widehat{\theta}$ is a function of the data, before observing a sample, $\widehat{\theta}$ is a random variable. Under the frequentist approach, the uncertainty about $\widehat{\theta}$ is described through its sampling distribution. Commonly, the distribution of the MLE does not have a closed form and frequentists resort to large sample theory and use the fact that, asymptotically, the distribution of $\widehat{\theta}$ follows a normal distribution.

In the Bayesian setting, there are three key elements:

(i) $p(\theta)$ is the prior distribution for the parameters;

(ii) $p(\mathbf{y}|\theta)$ is the likelihood of the data given the parameters;

(iii) $p(\theta|\mathbf{y})$ is the posterior distribution of the parameters given the data.

Before we collect any data, we formulate our *a priori* beliefs about the values of θ. These may be based on previous studies that suggest, for example, a range of values we expect θ to take. These beliefs are expressed in terms of a probability density function, $p(\theta)$. After data, $\mathbf{y}$, have been observed, we again specify a model $p(\mathbf{y}|\theta)$ for how the data depend on θ. Now the question is how our beliefs about θ can take into account both the prior beliefs and the information from the data. These *posterior* beliefs are expressed in terms of the *posterior* distribution $p(\theta|\mathbf{y})$. This posterior distribution can be found using Bayes theorem:

$$p(\theta|\mathbf{y}) = \frac{p(\mathbf{y}|\theta)p(\theta)}{p(\mathbf{y})}. \tag{5.1}$$

When $p(\theta)$ and $p(\mathbf{y}|\theta)$ are proper densities, $p(\theta|\mathbf{y})$ will also be a probability density function.

The distribution of the data, $p(\mathbf{y}|\theta)$, is related to the frequentist likelihood, since $l(\theta|\mathbf{y}) \propto p(\mathbf{y}|\theta)$ and this is often used to obtain the density $p(\theta|\mathbf{y})$ up to proportionality:

$$
\begin{aligned}
p(\theta|\mathbf{y}) &\propto p(\mathbf{y}|\theta)p(\theta) \\
&\propto l(\theta|\mathbf{y})p(\theta) \text{ or equivalently,} \\
\text{posterior} &\propto \text{likelihood} \times \text{prior, that is,} \\
p(\theta|\mathbf{y}) &= c \times l(\theta|\mathbf{y})p(\theta).
\end{aligned}
$$

The constant c is known as the *normalizing constant*. We will see in Chapter 6 that it is not always needed in practice but where it is needed, such as when using Bayes factors (Chapter 7, Section 7.9.1), it can be found by using the fact that the posterior distribution must integrate to one, that is $\int p(\theta|\mathbf{y}) \, d\theta = 1$ and therefore $c = [\int l(\theta|\mathbf{y})p(\theta) \, d\theta]^{-1}$. A useful definition is that of a *kernel* of a distribution. Assume a probability function for a random variable W is given by $p(w|\theta) = a(\theta)k(\theta,w)$, for some functions $a(\cdot)$ and $k(\cdot)$, where $a(\theta)$ does not depend on W. Then $k(\theta,w)$ is said to be the *kernel* of the distribution, and $p(w|\theta) \propto k(\theta,w)$.

Although the prior distribution allows knowledge from previous studies or experiments to be incorporated, it can introduce an increased level of complexity into the calculations. There may be cases where there are actual data available with which to construct priors, but decisions often have to be based on knowledge of the literature and other sources. In such cases, there may be doubts as to the accuracy of the prior distributions, and it is important to assess the sensitivity of the posterior to the choice of priors.

5.3 Exchangeability

Given n observations, $\mathbf{y} = (y_1, y_2, \ldots, y_n)^T$ and a joint distribution $p(\mathbf{y}|\theta) = p(y_1, y_2, \ldots, y_n|\theta)$, in frequentist statistics *independence* is often assumed, that is $p(\mathbf{y}) = \prod_{i=1}^{n} p(y_i)$. However, this assumption does not really seem so reasonable in a Bayesian setting. Independence implies that, $p(y_{m+1}, \ldots, y_n|y_1, \ldots, y_m) = p(y_{m+1}, \ldots, y_n), 1 \leq m < n$ and hence there is no learning experience. In this case, the first m values tell us nothing about what might happen next, which is in contrast to the ideas underpinning Bayesian statistics, those of incorporating prior information. In this setting, a more reasonable assumption may be that of *exchangeability*, which means that for a finite set of random variables $(Y_1, \ldots, Y_n)^T$ every permutation $(Y_{\pi(1)}, \ldots, Y_{\pi(n)})^T$ has the same joint distribution as every other permutation.

Similarly, an infinite collection of random variables is exchangeable if every finite subcollection is exchangeable.

If Y_i; $i = 1, \ldots, n$ are independent and identically (IID) distributed, then they are exchangeable.

$$
\begin{aligned}
p(y_1, \ldots, y_n) &= p(y_1) \ldots p(y_n) \\
&= p(y_{\pi(1)}) \ldots p(y_{\pi(n)}) \\
&= p(y_{\pi(1)}, \ldots, y_{\pi(n)}).
\end{aligned}
$$

However, a sequence of exchangeable random variables does not rely on an IID sequence. being exchangeable does not necessarily imply IID. Exchangeable Y_i s have the same marginal distribution, but they need not be independent; exchangeability is a weaker assumption than IID.

This can cause a problem in specifying the joint distribution $p(\mathbf{y})$. We can use de Finetti's Representation Theorem to help this specification (Bernardo and Smith, 2009). If $Y_1, \ldots, Y_n$ is an exchangeable sequence of 0-1 random variables with joint mass, $p(y_1, \ldots, y_n)$ then there exists a distribution function $q(\cdot)$ such that we can write $p(y_1, \ldots, y_n) = \int_0^1 \prod_{i=1}^{n} \theta^{y_i} (1 - \theta)^{1 - y_i} q(\theta) \, d\theta$ where $\theta = \lim_{n \to \infty} \left(\frac{1}{n} \sum_{i=1}^{n} y_i \right)$ is the 'long-run average number of 1s'. The theorem provides justification for the Bayesian approach of conditioning on prior information. The idea is that Y_i are independent Bernoulli random variables and are conditional on the value of some random quantity θ where θ represents the limiting relative frequency of 1s and $q(\theta)$ represents beliefs about θ. If Y_i are exchangeable Bernoulli variables, then they can be treated as if they were conditionally independent Bernoulli trials, conditional on θ. If θ has prior distribution $q(\theta)$, then $p(y_1, \ldots, y_n | \theta) = \prod_{i=1}^{n} p(y_i | \theta) = \prod_{i=1}^{n} \theta^{y_i} (1 - \theta)^{1 - y_i}$.

Analogous results are available for situations other than Bernoulli and provide justification for conditional independence in these cases (Bernardo and Smith, 2009).

Example 5.1. *Normal distribution with unknown mean and known variance*

Suppose $Y_1, \ldots, Y_n$ are exchangeable observations that are normally distributed with unknown mean θ, and known variance σ^2, that is, $Y_i | \theta \sim$ i.i.d. $N(\theta, \sigma^2)$.

As θ is the mean of a normal distribution and $\theta \in \mathbb{R}$, it is reasonable to assign a normal prior distribution to θ, such that $\theta \sim N(\theta_0, \sigma_0^2)$ with known constants θ_0, σ_0^2. In this case,

$$
\begin{aligned}
p(\theta) &= (2\pi\sigma_0^2)^{-1/2} \exp\left\{ -\frac{1}{2\sigma_0^2} (\theta - \theta_0)^2 \right\} \\
&\propto \exp\left\{ -\frac{1}{2\sigma_0^2} (\theta^2 - 2\theta\theta_0) \right\}.
\end{aligned}
$$

The distribution of the data is $p(\mathbf{y}|\theta) = \prod_i^n p(y_i|\theta)$. Since Y_i are treated as conditionally independent, it follows that

$$p(\mathbf{y}|\theta) = \prod_{i=1}^n \left[(2\pi\sigma^2)^{-1/2} \exp\left\{ -\frac{1}{2\sigma^2}(y_i - \theta)^2 \right\} \right]$$

$$= (2\pi\sigma^2)^{-n/2} \exp\left\{ -\frac{1}{2\sigma^2} \sum_{i=1}^n (y_i - \theta)^2 \right\}$$

$$l(\theta|\mathbf{y}) \propto p(\mathbf{y}|\theta)$$

$$\propto \exp\left\{ -\frac{n}{2\sigma^2}(\theta^2 - 2\bar{y}\theta) \right\}.$$

The posterior distribution of θ is then given by:

$$p(\theta|\mathbf{y}) \propto p(\theta)l(\theta|\mathbf{y})$$

$$\propto \exp\left\{ -\frac{1}{2\sigma_0^2}(\theta^2 - 2\theta\theta_0) - \frac{n}{2\sigma^2}(\theta^2 - 2\bar{y}\theta) \right\}$$

$$\propto \exp\left\{ -\frac{n}{2w\sigma^2}\left(\theta^2 - 2\theta(w\bar{y} + (1-w)\theta_0) \right) \right\}.$$

It can be seen that the posterior distribution is also Normal, $\theta|\mathbf{y} \sim N(w\bar{y} + (1-w)\theta_0, \frac{w\sigma^2}{n})$ with mean $w\bar{y} + (1-w)\theta_0$ where the weights are $w = \frac{\sigma_0^2}{\sigma_0^2 + \sigma^2/n}$. This is a weighted average and the mean of the data $\bar{y}$. Note that $n = 0$ corresponds to having no data, in which case the posterior is the same as the prior distribution and when $n \to \infty$, $E[\theta|\mathbf{y}] \to \bar{y}$; that is all the information comes from the data. Note that the posterior distribution was obtained by just looking at the kernel of $p(\theta|\mathbf{y})$ and recognizing the kernel of a normal distribution; that is, it was not necessary to explicitly compute the constant c (which involves an integral over θ) to understand that the posterior distribution of θ follows a normal distribution. In this case, we say that the normal distribution is a conjugate family with respect to the class of normal sampling distributions when the variance is known. Conjugate families are discussed in more detail in Section 5.7.1.

Example 5.2. *Over-dispersion in a Poisson model*

Here we revisit over-dispersion as seen in Chapter 2, Section 2.7.2 in a Bayesian setting by using a Gamma prior for the rate of disease. Suppose we are interested in studying the incidence of a disease. As discussed in Chapter 2, a Poisson may be a plausible model for such count data,

$$Y_i|\theta \sim Po(E_i\lambda), i = 1,...,N, \tag{5.2}$$

where Y_i is the observed number of cases of disease, λ is the disease rate and E_i is the expected number of cases based on the age–sex structure of the underlying population.

Using a Gamma(a,b) prior distribution, $p(\lambda) \propto \theta^{a-1} \exp^{-b\lambda}$, the posterior distribution will be a Gamma$(\sum y_i + a, \sum n_i + b)$ distribution.

The marginal mean and variance of Y_i can be obtained using properties of the conditional expectation and the total law of variance, that is,

$$
\begin{aligned}
E[Y_i|a,b] &= E_\lambda[E[Y_i|\lambda]|a,b] \\
&= E_\lambda[E_i\lambda|a,b] \\
&= E_i E_\lambda[\lambda|a,b] \\
&= = \frac{aE_i}{b}.
\end{aligned}
\tag{5.3}
$$

$$
\begin{aligned}
var(Y_i|a,b) &= E_\lambda[var(Y_i|\lambda)|a,b] + var_\lambda(E[Y_i|\lambda]|a,b) \tag{5.4} \\
&= E_\lambda[E_i\lambda|a,b] + var_\lambda(E_i\lambda)|a,b) \\
&= E_i E_\lambda[\lambda|a,b] + E_i^2 var_\lambda(\lambda)|a,b) \\
&= \frac{aE_i}{b} + \frac{aE_i^2}{b^2} \\
&= \frac{aE_i}{b}\left(1 + \frac{E_i}{b}\right) \\
&= E[Y_i|a,b]\left(1 + \frac{E_i}{b}\right). \tag{5.5}
\end{aligned}
$$

So the over-dispersion is of the form $(1 + \frac{E_i}{b})$, which is always positive; and, for fixed E_i, the smaller the value of b in the prior distribution, the larger the over-dispersion parameter.

5.4   Using the posterior for inference

Strictly speaking, there is no need for point estimates within a Bayesian framework as a parameter is considered a random variable and a lot more information is available from examining the entire (posterior) distribution.

In practice, however, it is useful to summarize the posterior distribution through a single point estimate. From a Bayesian point of view, this is seen as a decision problem. The Bayes estimator $\hat{\theta}$ is obtained after defining a loss function, say $L(\theta, a)$, which takes values on $\mathbb{R}^+$. The loss function measures the loss in estimating the parameter θ through the value a, for every value of a. After observing a sample $\mathbf{y}$, the Bayes estimator is the value of a that minimizes the expected loss with respect to the posterior distribution, that is,

$$
\hat{\theta} = \min_{\forall a} E_{p(\theta|\mathbf{y})}[L(\theta,a)] = \min_{\forall a} \int_\theta L(\theta,a)p(\theta \mid \mathbf{y})d\theta. \tag{5.6}
$$

There are in the literature some common loss functions that are used. The most common is the squared loss which penalizes in a quadratic fashion values of a that are far from θ, that is, $L(\theta, a) = (\theta - a)^2$. It can be shown that in this case, the value of a that minimizes the expected loss is the posterior mean of θ. Note that this is true regardless of the prior specification and resultant posterior distribution for θ. Another commonly used loss function is the absolute one, $L(\theta, a) = |\theta - a|$, which penalizes values of a that are far from θ linearly. The Bayes estimator in this case is the posterior median of θ. A third loss function that is commonly used is the $0 - 1$ loss function, that is, $L(\theta, a) = 1$ if $\theta = a$, and 0 otherwise. In this case, it can be shown that the Bayes estimator is given by the posterior mode. Different loss functions give different Bayes estimators. Although the ones described above are the most used loss functions, there might be situations that overestimating the value of θ might induce greater loss than underestimating it by the same amount. See Section 7.4 of DeGroot and Schervish (2010) for further details.

Posterior beliefs are captured by a whole distribution, and typically we want to summarize this distribution. This can be achieved in a variety of ways, including the following:

- Using graphs and plots of the shape of the distribution.

- Calculating summaries such as the mean, median, variance and intervals that contain most of the values.

- Calculating posterior probability that θ is greater than some value.

Credible intervals are in some sense the Bayesian analogue of confidence intervals or rather the way in which confidence intervals are commonly interpreted. They comprise an interval that captures the most likely values of θ. A $(1 - \alpha)100\%$ credible interval (θ_l, θ_u) is an interval within which $(1 - \alpha)100\%$ of the posterior distribution lies, that is $P(\theta_L < \theta < \theta_U | \mathbf{y}) = 1 - \alpha$. Of course, this could define an infinite number of possible intervals and typically the $\alpha/2$ and $1 - \alpha/2$ percentiles of the posterior distribution are used such that $P(\theta < \theta_L | \mathbf{y}) = \alpha/2, P(\theta > \theta_U | \mathbf{y}) = \alpha/2$. Hence, there is a $(1 - \alpha)100\%$ probability that θ is between θ_L and θ_U. When the posterior distribution is unimodal and symmetric, this interval results in the one with the shortest range among all possible intervals with probability $1 - \alpha$. Although equal-tail intervals are the most used ones, they do not always provide the interval with the shortest range. The highest posterior density (HPD) interval is the one that provides θ_L and θ_U that minimizes $\theta_L - \theta_U$ among all possible intervals with probability $1 - \alpha$. If a sample from the posterior distribution of θ is available, the HPD can be computed through the R package HDInterval.

5.5 Predictions

Let Z be a process value that has not been measured. Since Z is unknown, within the Bayesian framework it is considered a random variable with an associated distribution. In performing prediction, there are two cases to consider, both before and after data have been observed. In the case of the former, the *marginal* or *prior predictive distribution* $p(y)$ is a distribution that does not depend on any previous observations.

After the data have been observed, a predicted value, Z, is obtained,

$$p(z|\mathbf{y}) = \int p(z|\theta)p(\theta|\mathbf{y})\, d\theta,$$

where $p(z|\theta)$ is the distribution of the data given the value of θ, the same distribution we assumed for the rest of the data $p(y_i|\theta)$ and $p(\theta|\mathbf{y})$ is the posterior distribution, reflecting the uncertainty about the true value of θ. The posterior predictive distribution is averaged over all possible values of θ accounting for the posterior uncertainty about θ.

Example 5.3. *A predictive distribution for normally distributed data with unknown mean and known variance*

Given normally distributed data $Y_1, \ldots, Y_n$ with unknown mean θ, and known variance σ^2 and prior distribution $\theta \sim N(\theta_0, \sigma_0^2)$ where θ_0, σ_0^2 are known constants, the posterior distribution is $\theta|\mathbf{y} \sim N(w\bar{y} + (1-w)\theta_0, \frac{w\sigma^2}{n})$. In this case, the distribution of predictions of a new observation, Z, will be normal,

$$Z|\mathbf{y} \sim N\left(w\bar{y} + (1-w)\theta_0, \sigma^2 + \frac{w\sigma^2}{n}\right).$$

5.6 Transformations of parameters

Sometimes we may be more interested in a function of the parameter rather than in the parameter itself. For example, with Binomial data the interest may be in the odds of success, $\theta/(1-\theta)$ rather than in the probability θ directly. In this situation, we need to transform the prior and/or posterior distribution from one parameterization to another.

5.6.1 Prior distributions

Given a function g and prior distribution for θ, in order to find the corresponding prior beliefs, $p_\phi(\phi)$ we use change of variables. For a discrete θ, we have $p_\phi(\phi) = p_\theta(g^{-1}(\phi))$ and for the continuous case, $[p_\phi(\phi) = |J|p_\theta(g^{-1}(\phi))$ where J is the Jacobean matrix with $(i,j)^{th}$ element $J_{ij} = \frac{\partial \theta_i}{\partial \phi_j}$ the partial derivative of $\theta = g^{-1}(\phi)$ with respect to ϕ_j.

5.6.2 Likelihood

The likelihood is *invariant* to transformation of the parameters; and so $g^{-1}(\phi)$ may be substituted for θ, that is $p(\mathbf{y}|\phi) = p(\mathbf{y}|\theta = g^{-1}(\phi))$. The likelihood will be $l_\phi(\phi|\mathbf{y}) \propto p(\mathbf{y}|\phi) = p(\mathbf{y}|\theta = g^{-1}(\phi)) \propto l_\theta(g^{-1}(\phi)|\mathbf{y})$ and the maximum of $l(\theta|\mathbf{y})$ occurs at the same point as the maximum of $l(\phi|\mathbf{y})$. The maximum likelihood estimator for ϕ is $\hat{\phi} = g(\hat{\theta})$.

5.6.3   Posterior distributions

If the posterior distribution of θ is denoted by $p_\theta(\theta|\mathbf{y})$ the corresponding prior beliefs of ϕ will be expressed as $p_\phi(\phi|\mathbf{y})$. For a continuous θ, we have:

$$
\begin{aligned}
p_\phi(\phi|\mathbf{y}) &\propto l_\phi(\phi|\mathbf{y})p_\phi(\phi) \\
&\propto l_\theta\left(g^{-1}(\phi)|\mathbf{y}\right)p_\theta\left(g^{-1}(\phi)\right)|J| \\
&= |J|p_\theta\left(g^{-1}(\phi)|\mathbf{y}\right).
\end{aligned}
$$

In general, posterior moments are not invariant under parameterization, unlike maximum likelihood estimators. The posterior mean for θ is $E_{\theta|\mathbf{y}}[\theta|\mathbf{y}]$ but, unless $g(\theta)$ is a linear transformation, $E_{\phi|\mathbf{y}}[\phi|\mathbf{y}] = E_{\theta|\mathbf{y}}[g(\theta)|\mathbf{y}] \neq g(E[\theta|\mathbf{y}])$. If the posterior distribution for θ is approximated through simulation methods, as will be discussed in Chapter 6, posterior summaries of any non-linear one-to-one transformation of θ are easily obtained. One just needs to apply the transformation $g(\theta)$ to the sampled values of $p_\theta(\theta|\mathbf{y})$.

Posterior quantiles are invariant to transformations. In particular, this means that the median and credible intervals based on quantiles are also invariant to transformations. If m is the median of the posterior distribution, $P(\theta \leq m|\mathbf{y}) = 0.5$ then $0.5 = P(\theta| \leq m|\mathbf{y}) = P(g(\theta) \leq g(m)|\mathbf{y}) = P(\phi \leq g(m)|\mathbf{y})$. Therefore, $g(m)$ is the median of the posterior distribution expressed in terms of ϕ. More generally, if $s(\theta,q)$ is the quantile of the posterior distribution such that $P(\theta \leq s(\theta,q)|\mathbf{y}) = q$ then $P(\phi \leq g(s(\theta,q))|\mathbf{y}) = q$.

The mode, $\tilde{\theta}$, occurs at the maximum of the posterior distribution and so maximizes the log posterior: $\log p_{\theta|\mathbf{y}}(\theta|\mathbf{y}) \propto \log p(\mathbf{y}|\theta) + \log p_\theta(\theta)$ which takes the form $\log p_{\theta|\mathbf{y}}(\theta|\mathbf{y}) \propto \log p(\mathbf{y}|\theta = g^{-1}(\phi)) + \log p_\theta(g^{-1}(\phi)) + \log|J|$. In this case, $\tilde{\phi} = g(\tilde{\theta})$ only if $J = \frac{\partial \theta}{\partial \phi}$ does not depend on ϕ. In general, posterior modes are not invariant to transformations.

5.7   Prior formulation

5.7.1   Conjugate priors

When the prior and the likelihood are from the same family of distributions, they are called *conjugate prior distributions*.

As seen in Chapter 2, the exponential family of distributions has the form, $p(y_i|\theta) = f(y_i)g(\theta)\exp\{\phi(\theta)^T\mathbf{u}(y_i)\}$. Given a sufficient statistic for θ, the likelihood can be written $l(\theta|\mathbf{y}) \propto g(\mathbf{t},\theta)$ and the posterior can be written as $p(\theta|\mathbf{y}) = p(\theta|\mathbf{t}) \propto g(\mathbf{t},\theta)p(\theta)$. If Y_i, $i = 1,\ldots,n$ are exchangeable, then the likelihood is $l(\theta|\mathbf{y}) = g(\theta)^n\exp\{\phi(\theta)^T\mathbf{t}(\mathbf{y})\}$ where $\mathbf{t}(\mathbf{y})$ is the sufficient statistic $\mathbf{t}(\mathbf{y}) = \sum_{i=1}^n u(y_i)$.

The conjugate prior will have the same form as the likelihood, $p(\theta) \propto g(\theta)^\eta\exp\{\phi(\theta)^T v\}$ for some η and v. This general form specifies the distributional family, whilst specific choices of η and v characterize the moments of the prior.

The posterior can be found as follows:

$$p(\theta|\mathbf{y}) \quad \propto \quad g(\theta)^n \exp\left\{\phi(\theta)^T \mathbf{t}(\mathbf{y})\right\} g(\theta)^\eta \exp\left\{\phi(\theta)^T \mathbf{v}\right\}$$
$$= \quad g(\theta)^{\eta'} \exp\left\{\phi(\theta)^T \mathbf{v}'\right\},$$

with $\eta' = \eta + n$ and $\mathbf{v}' = \mathbf{v} + \mathbf{t}(\mathbf{y})$. This has the same form as $p(\theta)$ so the prior is conjugate.

Note that the Poisson-Gamma of Example 5.2 is an example of a conjugate family, as the posterior distribution falls within the same family as the prior distribution.

5.7.2 Reference priors

Although one of the central premises of the Bayesian approach is the ability to capture subjective beliefs about parameters, through *informative priors* there may be times when *non-informative* or *reference* priors may be useful. The idea is to perform Bayesian inference based on a minimum of subjective prior information. When using non-informative priors, all the information comes from the data.

Example 5.4. *Reference priors*

Suppose we have $Y|\theta \sim \text{Bin}(n,\theta)$, with a uniform prior $p(\theta) = 1$, $0 \le \theta \le 1$. Therefore,

$$l(\theta|y) \propto \theta^y (1-\theta)^{n-y}.$$

The posterior is

$$p(\theta|y) \propto \theta^y (1-\theta)^{n-y} \propto l(\theta|y),$$

which is the kernel of a beta distribution with parameters $y+1$ and $n-y+1$, such that, $\theta|y \sim \text{Beta}(y+1, n-y+1)$.

5.7.3 Transformations

As seen in Section 5.6, prior and posterior distributions are not invariant to transformations of parameters. If we use the transformation, $\phi = \theta^{-1}$ then a uniform prior for θ is equivalent to using $p_\phi(\phi) = \frac{1}{\phi^2}$, $1 < \phi < \infty$. Here, $p_\theta(\theta)$ represents the situation where there is no knowledge about θ; in this case, it seems reasonable to assume that there is equally no knowledge about ϕ. However, the prior for ϕ is informative.

In practice, lack of knowledge about θ might not be too much of a problem as long as there is sufficient data to give greater weight to the likelihood. This will mean there is less influence of the prior in the posterior, meaning that the posterior $p_\theta(g^{-1}(\phi)|\mathbf{y})$ will not differ greatly from $p_\phi(\phi|\mathbf{y})$.

5.7.4 Jeffreys prior

Jeffreys prior is a choice of prior based on the amount of information contained in the data, as captured by the Fisher Information matrix $I(\theta|\mathbf{y}) = -E_{y|\theta}\left[\frac{\partial^2}{\partial\theta^2} \log l(\theta|\mathbf{y})\right] =$

$-E_{y|\theta}\left[\left(\frac{\partial}{\partial\theta}\log l(\theta|\mathbf{y})\right)^2\right]$, where the expectation is with respect to the data $\mathbf{y}|\theta$. It takes the form $p_\theta(\theta) \propto [I(\theta|\mathbf{y})]^{1/2}$ and is often used as a reference prior, as it has the property of invariance under parameterization.

5.7.5 Improper priors

A density is *proper* if it integrates to one. Priors that do not have a finite integral, that is priors that are not real densities, are known as *improper* priors. Reference priors often lead to improper priors, but even when this is the case, the posterior may still be proper. A posterior density will always be proper if the prior density is proper.

> **Example 5.5.** *A reference prior for the probability of success of a Binomial distribution*
>
> Using the improper prior, $p(\theta) \propto \theta^{-1}(1-\theta)^{-1}$, as a reference prior for the probability of success θ in Binomial data leads to a posterior of the form $p(\theta|\mathbf{y}) \propto \theta^{y-1}(1-\theta)^{n-y-1}$. This is the kernel of a Beta distribution; $\theta|\mathbf{y} \sim$ Beta$(y, n-y)$; but in the case of either $y = 0$ or $y = n$, this will be an improper posterior.

5.7.6 Joint priors

In all but the simplest examples, there will be more than one unknown quantity, which means that a *joint prior distribution* will have to be specified leading to a *joint posterior distribution*. Considering now a vector of unknown parameters, θ, then a joint distribution $p(\theta)$ is combined with the data to obtain the joint posterior distribution: $p(\theta|\mathbf{y}) \propto l(\theta|\mathbf{y})p(\theta)$. Conjugate priors are more difficult to work with for more than one parameter, as they are not generally independent.

> **Example 5.6.** *Normal data with unknown mean and variance*
>
> If data $Y_i; i = 1, \ldots, n$, is normally distributed with, $Y_i|\mu, \phi \sim N(\mu, \phi)$ then the unknown parameters will be $\theta = (\mu, \phi)^T$. A joint distribution is required for both μ and ϕ and choosing an appropriate joint distribution may not be entirely straightforward. Here we consider the non-informative (improper) prior, $p(\mu, \phi) \propto \frac{1}{\phi}$, which assigns reference priors for both μ and ϕ and assumes independence between the two.
>
> The likelihood is $l(\mu, \phi|\mathbf{y}) \propto \phi^{-n/2} \exp\left\{-\frac{1}{2\phi}\left(S + n(\bar{y}-\mu)^2\right)\right\}$ where $\bar{y} = \frac{1}{n}\sum_{i=1}^n y_i$ or $S = \sum_{i=1}^n (y_i - \bar{y})^2$ are sufficient statistics. The posterior will be $p(\mu, \phi|\mathbf{y}) \propto \phi^{-n/2-1} \exp\left\{-\frac{1}{2\phi}\left(S + n(\bar{y}-\mu)^2\right)\right\}$, which is sometimes referred to as the Normal-Inverse-Gamma distribution.

5.7.7   Nuisance parameters

The set of unknown parameters in a model may include some that are not of primary interest and could be considered nuisance parameters. When this is the case, the joint posterior distribution need only include the parameters of interest and not the nuisance parameters. This will be the *marginal posterior distribution* for the parameters of interest.

Consider a parameter vector $\theta = (\theta_1, \theta_2)^T$ containing the parameter of interest, θ_1, and a nuisance parameter, θ_2. The marginal distribution for θ_1 will be $p(\theta_1|\mathbf{y}) = \int p(\theta|\mathbf{y}) \, d\theta_2$.

> **Example 5.7.** *Marginal distribution for normal data with unknown mean and variance*
>
> If data Y_i; $i = 1,\ldots,n$, are normally distributed with $Y_i|\mu,\phi \sim N(\mu,\phi)$, and prior distribution $p(\mu,\phi) \propto \frac{1}{\phi}$ then, as seen in Example 5.6, the full joint posterior is $p(\mu,\phi|\mathbf{y}) \propto \phi^{-n/2-1}\exp\left\{-\frac{1}{2\phi}\left(S+n(\bar{y}-\mu)^2\right)\right\}$. If interest is only in μ, then ϕ is integrated out of the joint posterior distribution, $p(\mu|\mathbf{y}) \propto \int_0^\infty \phi^{-n/2-1}\exp\left\{-\frac{1}{2\phi}\left(S+n(\bar{y}-\mu)^2\right)\right\}d\phi$. It can be shown that the marginal posterior distribution of μ follows a Student-t distribution, with $n-1$ degrees of freedom, location $\bar{y}$ and scale S/n, similarly, $\mu|\mathbf{y} \sim t_{n-1}(\bar{y},S/n)$. Note that if a $100(1-\alpha)\%$ posterior credible interval is computed for $\mu|\mathbf{y}$, it will have limits $\left(\bar{y}-t_{\alpha/2,n-1}\frac{\sqrt{S}}{n}, \bar{y}+t_{\alpha/2,n-1}\frac{\sqrt{S}}{n}\right)$, where $t_{\alpha/2,n-1}$ is the $\alpha/2$ quantile of the Student-t distribution with $n-1$ degrees of freedom. Although this interval has the same numerical limits as a $100(1-\alpha)\%$ confidence interval for the mean of a normal distribution when the variance is unknown, their interpretations differ. The Bayesian posterior credible interval is interpreted as the posterior *probability of θ* lying within the interval above.

5.8   Summary

This chapter introduces the Bayesian approach, which provides a natural framework for dealing with uncertainty and also for fitting the models that will be encountered later in the book. The reader will have gained an understanding of the following topics:

- The use of prior distributions to capture beliefs before data are observed;
- The combination of prior beliefs and information from data to obtain posterior beliefs;
- The manipulation of prior distributions with likelihoods to formulate posterior distributions and why conjugate priors are useful in this regard;
- The difference between informative and non-informative priors;
- The use of the posterior distribution for inference and methods for calculating summary measures.

5.9 Exercises

Exercise 5.1. For each of the following distributions, write down the probability density function and find the kernel:

(i) $Y|\theta \sim \text{Po}(\theta)$;

(ii) $X|\theta,b \sim \text{Beta}(b\theta,b)$;

(iii) $\theta|a,b,y \sim \text{Gamma}(a+y+1,b-3y)$;

(iv) $\phi|\mu,\bar{x},\tau \sim N(\tau\mu+(1-\tau)\bar{x},\bar{x}^2\tau^{-2})$.

Exercise 5.2. Let $Y_i,\ldots,Y_n$ be a sample of data. For each of the following distributions for Y_i, find the conjugate prior distribution and the corresponding posterior distribution.

(i) $Y_i|\theta \sim \text{Bern}(\theta)$;

(ii) $Y_i|\theta \sim \text{Po}(\theta)$;

(iii) $Y_i|\theta \sim N(\theta,\sigma^2)$, with σ^2 known;

(iv) $Y_i|\phi \sim N(\mu,\phi)$, with μ known.

Exercise 5.3. Suppose that Y_i are n exchangeable Normal random variables, with mean θ and known variance σ^2. We are interested in inference about the mean θ. Consider the prior distribution $\theta \sim N(\theta_0,\sigma_0^2)$ for known constants θ_0,σ_0^2.

Suppose we wish to make predictions about a future observation Z. Show that the predictive distribution is

$$z|\mathbf{y} \sim N\left(w\bar{y}+(1-w)\theta_0,\sigma^2+\frac{w\sigma^2}{n}\right).$$

Exercise 5.4. Suppose $X|\mu,\phi \sim N(\mu,\phi)$ and $Y|\mu,\delta \sim N(\mu+\delta,\phi)$, where ϕ is known, and X and Y are conditionally independent.

(i) Find the joint distribution of X and Y.

(ii) Consider the improper, non-informative joint prior distribution:

$$p(\mu,\delta) \propto 1.$$

Find the joint posterior distribution. Are $\mu|x,y$ and $\delta|x,y$ independent?

(iii) Find the marginal posterior distribution $p(\delta|x,y)$.

(iv) Suppose a future observation z is given by $z|\mu,\delta \sim N(\mu-\delta,\phi)$. Find the predictive distribution $p(z|x,y)$.

Jeffreys' prior takes the form $p_\theta(\theta) \propto [I(\theta|\mathbf{y})]^{1/2}$ where I is the Fisher's information. Considering the parameterization $\phi = g(\theta)$,

(i) show that the information contained in the data, $I(\phi|y)$ about ϕ is $\left(\frac{\partial\theta}{\partial\phi}\right)^2 \times I(\theta|\mathbf{y})$

(ii) show that the Jeffreys' prior is therefore invariant to parameterization, that is the Jeffreys' prior for ϕ is the same as that for θ.

Exercise 5.5. Let Y_i, $i=1,\ldots,n$, be exchangeable Poisson random variables, with mean θ. Consider a prior distribution $\theta \sim \text{Gamma}(a,b)$.

(i) Find the posterior distribution $p(\theta|\mathbf{y})$.

(ii) Show that the posterior mean can be written as a weighted average of the prior mean, θ_0, and the maximum likelihood estimator $\hat{\theta} = S_n/n$, where $S_n = Y_1 + \cdots + Y_n$ is the sum.

(iii) Let z be a future (unobserved) observation. Find the mean and variance of the predictive distribution $z|\mathbf{y}$.

(iv) The data in the table below are the number of cases of a disease in a specified area between 2001 and 2010.

2001	2002	2003	2004	2005	2006	2007	2008	2009	2010
213	189	222	231	199	245	220	299	289	267

Suppose our prior beliefs about cases of the disease in this area can be expressed as $\theta \sim \text{Gamma}(375, 1.5)$. Let z be the number of cases in 2011. Assuming

$$p(z|\mathbf{y}) \sim_{\text{approx}} N\left(E[z|\mathbf{y}], \text{var}(z|\mathbf{y})\right),$$

find an approximate 95% predictive interval for the number of cases in 2011.

Exercise 5.6. Suppose that $Y_i|\phi \sim N(\mu, \phi)$, $i = 1, \ldots, n$, where μ is known, and the aim is to estimate ϕ.

(i) Show that $S = \sum_i (y_i - \mu)^2$ is a sufficient statistic for ϕ.

(ii) Consider an inverse-gamma prior distribution for ϕ:

$$p(\phi) = \frac{b^a}{\Gamma(a)} \phi^{-(a+1)} \exp(-b/\phi).$$

Show that this corresponds to a gamma distribution for τ, where $\tau = 1/\phi$, the *precision* of y.

(iii) Find the posterior distribution of $\phi|\mathbf{y}$.

## Chapter 6

Approaches to Bayesian computation

6.1 Overview

In stylized problems, conjugate prior distributions are available that allow for analytical solutions to finding posterior distributions (see for example Gelman et al. (2013)). However, in most practical situations such conjugacy is either not available or overly restrictive and in order to evaluate the posterior model probabilities there are several computational matters that have to be considered. There is therefore a need to compute, or estimate, integrals of the form $p(y) = \int p(y|\theta)p(\theta)d\theta$.

6.2 Analytical approximations

One approach is to use an analytic approximation such as Laplace's, which is based on the Taylor series expansion of a real valued function $f(u)$

$$\int e^{f(u)}du \approx (2p)^{r/2}|H|^{1/2}\exp\{f(u^*)\}, \tag{6.1}$$

where r is the dimension of the vector u, u^* is the value of u at which f attains its maximum and H is minus the inverse Hessian information of f evaluated at u^*. We return to the subject of Laplace approximations in more detail when we discuss Integrated Nested Laplace approximations (INLA) in Section 6.7.

> **Example 6.1.** *Using a normal approximation for a posterior distribution*
>
> If $p(\theta|\mathbf{y})$ is unimodal and roughly symmetric, we may approximate it by a multivariate normal distribution. In general cases where the posterior is not in a tractable form, finding the mean and variance of the posterior may be non-trivial. In such cases, we may consider a Taylor expansion of $\log p(\theta|\mathbf{y})$ about the mode $\widetilde{\theta}$.
>
> We begin by recalling the one-dimensional Taylor series expansion for a function $g(x)$ about x_0 expressed in terms of its derivatives $g^{(j)}$, $j = 0, 1, \ldots$.
>
> $$g(x) = g(x_0) + (x - x_0)g'(x_0) + \ldots + \frac{(x - x_0)^r}{r!}g^{(r)}(x_0) + \ldots .$$

DOI: 10.1201/9781003352655-6

Then we apply this expansion by letting $x = \theta$, $x_0 = \widetilde{\theta}$ and $g(x) = \log p(\theta|\mathbf{y})$, so that

$$
\begin{aligned}
\log p(\theta|\mathbf{y}) &\approx \log p(\widetilde{\theta}|\mathbf{y}) + (\theta - \widetilde{\theta})\left[\frac{d}{d\theta}\log p(\theta|\mathbf{y})\right]_{\theta=\widetilde{\theta}} \\
&+ \frac{1}{2}(\theta - \widetilde{\theta})^2\left[\frac{d^2}{d\theta^2}\log p(\theta|\mathbf{y})\right]_{\theta=\widetilde{\theta}} \\
&= \log p(\widetilde{\theta}|\mathbf{y}) + \frac{1}{2}(\theta - \widetilde{\theta})^2\left[\frac{d^2}{d\theta^2}\log p(\theta|\mathbf{y})\right]_{\theta=\widetilde{\theta}} \\
&\propto \frac{1}{2}(\theta - \widetilde{\theta})^2\left[\frac{d^2}{d\theta^2}\log p(\theta|\mathbf{y})\right]_{\theta=\widetilde{\theta}} \\
p(\theta|\mathbf{y}) &\approx \exp\left\{-\frac{1}{2I^{-1}(\widetilde{\theta})}(\theta - \widetilde{\theta})^2\right\}.
\end{aligned}
$$

The remaining terms of the Taylor series will be small when θ is close to $\widetilde{\theta}$ and n is large. Under these conditions, we obtain the useful approximation

$$
\theta|\mathbf{y} \sim_{\text{approx}} N\left(\widetilde{\theta}, I^{-1}(\widetilde{\theta})\right),
$$

where $I(\theta)$ is the *observed information*:

$$
I(\theta) = -\frac{d^2}{d\theta^2}\log p(\theta|\mathbf{y}).
$$

More generally, we can use a multivariate Taylor series expansion to get

$$
\theta|\mathbf{y} \sim_{\text{approx}} N\left(\widetilde{\theta}, I^{-1}(\widetilde{\theta})\right).
$$

6.3   Markov Chain Monte Carlo (MCMC)

Often, posterior densities may be difficult or impossible to integrate explicitly, particularly when we have a complex model with many parameters. An alternative approach, which avoids the problems of integration, is to use simulation techniques where a random sample from the posterior distribution is used to estimate $E_{\theta|\mathbf{y}}[g(\theta)] = \int g(\theta)p(\theta|\mathbf{y})d\theta$ for some function g. In this situation, numerous samples are drawn from $p(\theta|y)$, which can be used to estimate quantities of interest such as the posterior mean. These samples can be generated using a number of techniques including *rejection sampling*, *importance sampling* and *adaptive rejection sampling*. For further details about these direct sampling methods, see Ripley and Corporation (1987); Gilks, Richardson, and Spiegelhalter (1996); Givens and Hoeting (2013).

Markov Chain Monte Carlo (MCMC) provides another approach to obtaining samples from the required posterior distributions and is based on the premise that it is possible to construct a Markov chain , $\theta^1, \theta^2, \theta^3...$, whose stationary distribution is the joint posterior $p(\theta|y)$ that is of interest. This again avoids the problems of integration and may be used in situations where direct simulation is not feasible. MCMC is used extensively to perform inference in Bayesian analyzes. In this section, we give a brief review of MCMC techniques and their use. For more comprehensive treatments, see Gilks et al. (1996); Gelman et al. (2013); Gamerman and Lopes (2006).

We now give a brief review of two methods for obtaining samples from the posterior distribution using MCMC: (i) Metropolis-Hastings algorithm (Metropolis, Rosenbluth, Rosenbluth, Teller, and Teller, 1953; Hastings, 1970) and (ii) the Gibbs sampler (A. F. M. Smith and Roberts, 1993).

6.3.1 Metropolis-Hastings algorithm

Starting with an initial value θ^0, a sequence, $\theta^{(k)}$, $k = 1, ..., K$ is generated. At each stage, a 'candidate' value, θ^*, is drawn from a *proposal distribution*, and the ratio of the (unnormalized) posterior probabilities under each of the values calculated. The current candidate is then either accepted or rejected, where in the former case it becomes the next value in the chain. If it is rejected, the chain stays at the current value and the algorithm moves to the next iteration.

1. Arbitrarily draw a starting point θ^0 for the Markov chain, ensuring that its posterior probability $p(\theta^0|y)$ is positive.

2. At each iteration k, for $k = 1, ..., K$, generate a candidate θ^* from a proposal distribution $q(\theta^*|\theta^{k-1})$, that may or may not be based on the current value, θ^{k-1}, of the Markov chain. The candidate value is then accepted with probability r, given by

$$r = min\left\{ \frac{p(\theta^*|y)q(\theta^*|\theta^{k-1})}{p(\theta^{k-1}|y)q(\theta^{k-1}|\theta^*)}, 1 \right\}.$$

If the candidate value is accepted, then otherwise the chain does not move and $\theta^k = \theta^{k-1}$

For illustration, consider an initial value θ^0, with 'candidate' value, θ^*, drawn from a normal (proposal) distribution with mean θ^0 and variance b^2. The ratio of the (unnormalized) posterior probabilities under each of the values is calculated. The minimum of that ratio and 1 is then taken. If a random sample is then taken from a Uniform distribution, $U \sim (0,1)$ and $U < r$, $\theta^1 = \theta^*$, the value sampled from the Normal distribution, otherwise let $\theta^1 = \theta^0$, the original value. When this step is repeated N times, by drawing each of the candidate variables from $N(\theta^1, b^2), N(\theta^2, b^2), ...$ etc. then the resulting sample $\theta^0, \theta^1, .., \theta^N$ will approximate a random sample from the posterior distribution.

3. Repeat step 2 until the sequence of drawn samples reaches convergence.
   Since the proposal density need only be proportional to the interested density rather than exactly equal to it, the Metropolis-Hastings algorithm presents a relatively straightforward and efficient way of simulating from any unspecified probability distribution.

MCMC can be complex to implement, and the results can be affected by the choice of starting values. Although the starting point should not impact the stationary distribution when chains are *mixing* well, that is, covering all possibilities in the parameter space, it may need to be chosen carefully for slowly mixing chains which can often stick in a small area of the parameter space for a long time.

The choice of proposal distribution can have a large impact on the convergence and acceptance rate of the Metropolis-Hastings algorithm. Acceptance rates are significantly influenced by the variance of proposal distribution. A 'cautious' proposal distribution with relatively small variance will generate small steps, that is, candidate values which are close to the current (accepted) value and therefore the acceptance rate will be high. Proposal distributions with large variance will result in much more variation in the candidate values and therefore may explore more of the parameter space in a shorter time, but the probability of acceptance at each step is likely to be smaller and thus more iterations of the algorithm will be required in order to reach convergence. Typically, 20–30% of acceptance rate is considered reasonable (Gelman et al., 2013).

6.3.2   Gibbs sampling

The Gibbs sampler is a special case of the Metropolis-Hasting algorithm, where the proposal distribution is the full conditional distribution of the parameter in question. This gives an acceptance probability of one, which effectively removes the accept or reject stage; hence the movement of the Markov chain is ensured.

For a vector random variable θ with joint density $p(\theta) = p(\theta_1, \theta_2, \ldots, \theta_p)$ where the full conditional distribution $p(\theta_i | \theta_{-i})$ for each parameter is known, then the Gibbs sampler algorithm works as follows:

1. Arbitrarily choose a starting point $\theta^0 = (\theta_1^0, \theta_2^0, \ldots, \theta_p^0)$;

2. Let θ^{j-1} be the value of the elements of θ at iteration $j - 1$, then for $j = 1, \ldots, L$,

    (a) sample θ_1^j from $p(\theta_1 | \theta_2^{j-1}, \ldots, \theta_p^{j-1})$;
    (b) sample θ_2^j from $p(\theta_2 | \theta_1^j, \theta_3^{j-1}, \ldots, \theta_p^{j-1})$;
    (c) sample θ_3^j from $p(\theta_3 | \theta_1^j, \theta_2^j, \theta_4^{j-1}, \ldots, \theta_p^{j-1})$;

    $\vdots$

    (d) sample θ_p^j from $p(\theta_p | \theta_1^j, \theta_2^j, \ldots, \theta_{p-1}^j)$.
3. repeat step 2. until the sequence converges.

Note that the order in which you sample the elements of θ should not affect the convergence of the sequence. Depending on the complexity of the posterior distribution, it might happen that some orders lead to faster convergence than others.

6.3.3   Hybrid Gibbs sampler

Commonly, not all the posterior full conditionals have a closed form. In these cases, the sampling proceeds by using alternative algorithms to sample from those full conditionals that do not have a closed form. Then, we say that the MCMC algorithm is a hybrid Gibbs sampler . The most common approach is to use a Metropolis-Hastings step to sample from the unknown full conditionals. Alternative approaches include the adaptive rejection sampler and slice sampler, among others. These alternative sampling algorithms will be briefly discussed in Section 6.5.

6.3.4   Block updating

In simple implementations, parameters are updated independently, as it is often easier to sample from univariate distributions, and they are more likely to be available in closed form. However, this single updating method can have very poor convergence properties, poor mixing and can be computationally slow. Knorr-Held (1999) suggests that using block updating is potentially faster with better mixing properties.

6.3.5   Hamiltonian Monte Carlo

The Hamiltonian Monte Carlo (HMC) (also known as Hybrid Monte Carlo) is an alternative algorithm to Metropolis-Hastings and Gibbs sampling. Random walk Metropolis-Hastings and Gibbs sampling algorithms can take long to explore the space of the target distribution because of their random walk behavior. The HMC is the main algorithm used in Stan, a software package that has been widely used to obtain samples from the distribution of interest and will be briefly described in Section 6.6.

   The HMC can only be used to provide samples from continuous distributions in $\mathbb{R}^p$. As described in RStan's manual (Stan Development Team, 2023), HMC uses the derivatives of the density function being sampled to generate efficient transitions spanning the posterior. It uses an approximate Hamiltonian dynamics simulation based on numerical integration, which is then corrected by performing a Metropolis acceptance step. See Gelman et al. (2013) for details on how to implement HMC.

6.3.6   Checking convergence

The chain is initialized by a starting value θ^0, and run until it has converged to its target distribution. The initial period of non-convergence is known as 'burn-in'. After this, the Markov chain will produce samples from the posterior distribution. It is important that the Markov chain has covered the entire posterior distribution, but this may be difficult to check. Although there are no methods that guarantee that after the burn-in, samples are being generated from the distribution of interest; there are different tools available that help investigate if there is evidence of convergence.

   One of the most popular approaches is to start the chains from very different values and, after a burn-in period, compare the trace-plots to check if they are exploring approximately the same region of the parameter space.

Example 6.2. *Gibbs sampling with a Poisson-Gamma model – hospital admissions for chronic obstructive pulmonary disease (COPD) for England between 2001-2010*

In this example we show the full conditional distributions for a Poisson model where the prior distribution on the rates is Gamma, that is, $y_i \mid \theta_i E_i \sim Poi(\theta_i E_i)$ where E_i is the expected number of cases in area i. In particular, let $\mathbf{y} = (y_1, ..., y_N)$ be a N-dimensional vector with observed counts on the total number of hospital admissions for chronic obstructive pulmonary disease (COPD) for England between 2001 and 2010. The expected numbers of hospital admissions by local authority were computed as described in Chapter 2, Section 2.4.

If we assign a Gamma prior to the random effects θ_i, that is, $\theta_i \sim Gamma(a, b)$ for $i = 1, ... N$, and independent exponential distributions to the hyperparameters a and b then we can find the full conditional distributions required for Gibbs sampling.

The joint posterior is proportional to

$$p(a, b, \boldsymbol{\theta} | \mathbf{y}) \quad \propto \quad \prod_{i=1}^{N} \frac{(\theta_i E_i)^{y_i}}{y_i!} \exp(-\theta_i E_i) \frac{b^a}{\Gamma(a)} \theta_i^{a-1} e^{-b\theta_i}$$
$$\times \lambda_a \exp(-\lambda_a) \lambda_b \exp(-\lambda_b),$$

and the full conditionals are:

1. Posterior full conditional for each θ_i, $i = 1, \ldots, N$:

$$p(\theta_i | \boldsymbol{\theta}_{-i}, a, b, \mathbf{y}) \propto \theta_i^{y_i + a - 1} \exp[-(E_i + b)\theta_i],$$

   which is the kernel of a Gamma distribution with parameters $y_i + a$ and $E_i + b$;

2. Posterior full conditional for b:

$$p(b | \boldsymbol{\theta}, a, \mathbf{y}) \propto b^{Na} \exp\left[-\left(\sum_{i=1}^{N} \theta_i + \lambda_b\right) b\right],$$

   which is the kernel of a Gamma distribution with parameters $Na + 1$ and $(\sum_{i=1}^{N} \theta_i + \lambda_b)$;

3. Posterior full conditional for a:

$$p(a | \boldsymbol{\theta}, b, \mathbf{y}) \propto \frac{\left(b^N \prod_{i=1}^{N} \theta_i\right)^{a-1}}{\Gamma(a)^N},$$

   which does not have a closed form. We propose to sample from $p(a | \boldsymbol{\theta}, b, \mathbf{y})$ through a random walk, Metropolis-Hastings step. As a must be strictly positive, the proposal is a log-normal distribution whose associated normal distribution has mean at the logarithm of the current value and some fixed variance, say u, that needs to be tuned.

```
#initial values
theta[1,]<-y/E
a<-rexp(1,lambda_a)
b<-rexp(1,lambda_b)
fit.y[1,]<-rpois(N,E*theta[1,])
#starting the loop from l=2
for(l in 2:L){
  for(i in 1:N)
    theta[l,i]<-rgamma(1,(y[i]+a[(l-1)]),rate=(E[i]+b
      [(l-1)]))
  b[l]<-rgamma(1,(N*a[(l-1)]+1),rate=(sum(theta[l,])+
    lambda_b))
  a[l]<-a[l-1]
  laprop<-rnorm(1,log(a[l-1]),u) #proposal in the log-
    scale
  aprop<-exp(laprop)
  num<-log(aprop)+N*(aprop*(log(b[l]))-lgamma(aprop))
      +(aprop-1)*sum(log(theta[l,]))-aprop*lambda_a
  den<-log(a[(l-1)])+N*(a[l-1]*(log(b[l]))-lgamma(a[l
    -1]))
      +(a[(l-1)]-1)*sum(log(theta[l,]))-a[(l-1)]*
        lambda_a
  ratio<-exp(num-den)
  unif<-runif(1)
  if (unif<ratio) a[l]<-aprop
  #posterior sample of the fitted values
  fit.y[l,]<-rpois(N,E*theta[l,])
}
```

See the online resources for a discussion on how to fix the variance of the proposal distribution to sample from the posterior full conditional of a.

6.4   Using samples for inference

If the Markov chain is ergodic, meaning that all of its states can be revisited with positive probability in a finite mean number of steps, then samples can be used to perform inference on the posterior distribution with assurance that the estimates will converge to the correct values as the length of the chain tends to infinity (Gamerman and Lopes, 2006). Starting at an initial value θ_0, after a period of time the Markov chain will converge. The period before convergence is known as the *burn-in* period. The length of that period will depend on the rate of convergence. Estimates of the rate of convergence are in general difficult to obtain, and determining the length of burn-in required for a specific problem may not be feasible. The most commonly used method for determining burn-in is to produce a time series plot of the values over time; this will also highlight any obvious problems such as slow mixing, and running multiple chains from different starting points.

Samples can be used to summarize the posterior distribution in terms of modes, percentiles and probabilities based on the sample. In addition, we can compute quantities derived from the posterior such as a marginal mean that can be estimated by

$$E[\theta_i|\mathbf{y}] \approx \frac{1}{K-m} \sum_{k=m+1}^{K} \theta_i^k = \bar{\theta}_i$$

where N is the number of samples omitting m, the number within the burn-in period.

We can also transform between different parameterization. For example, if the Markov chain gives samples from $p(\theta|\mathbf{y})$ but we are interested in $\phi|\mathbf{y}$, where $\theta = g(\phi)$ we can transform each value of the chain

$$\phi_k = g^{-1}(\theta_k)$$

to produce a Markov chain with samples (ϕ_k) from the distribution $p(\phi|\mathbf{y})$. These can then be used to estimate quantities of the posterior distribution of $\phi|\mathbf{y}$.

To determine how many samples we need to obtain adequate precision in the estimator, $\bar{\theta}_1$ we need to consider the variance of $\bar{\theta}_1$. This is complicated since the samples produced by MCMC techniques will be dependent samples. If the chains display slow mixing, which may arise due to high dependence in the Gibbs sampler, or low acceptance rates when using the Metropolis-Hastings algorithm, we will require larger runs. In such cases, parameterization may help (Gamerman and Lopes, 2006). While formal methods to estimate the variance have been proposed, a simple informal method is to run multiple chains of length K and compare the estimates $\bar{\theta}_1$. If they do not agree adequately, then K should be increased.

6.5   NIMBLE

We now provide a short introduction to the NIMBLE (de Valpine et al., 2017) language which can be used for specifying Bayesian models. NIMBLE is a powerful tool that allows the user to perform Markov chain Monte Carlo (MCMC) using hybrid Gibbs sampling. As summarized in the NIMBLE manual (de Valpine et al., 2022), it is a system for building and sharing analysis methods for statistical models, especially for hierarchical models and computationally-intensive methods. NIMBLE is built in R but compiles models and algorithms using C++ for speed. It is an advancement of BUGS/WinBUGS (Lunn, Jackson, Best, Thomas, and Spiegelhalter, 2012), which was the first software to allow for the implementation of MCMC methods in the same fashion as you were writing statistical models. NIMBLE requires the user to define their model but not to have to code the actual MCMC as in listing 6.2. Given a model, NIMBLE will derive the required full conditionals for hybrid Gibbs sampling and offer visual representations of the chains and the facilities to summarize the resulting samples from the posterior distributions of the parameters of interest. One of the advantages of NIMBLE is that it allows the user to write their own sampler in case it does not have an efficient algorithm to generate from certain full conditionals.

Broadly speaking, NIMBLE includes three components:

1. A system for using models written in the BUGS model language as programmable objects in R.

2. An initial library of algorithms for models written in BUGS, including basic MCMC, which can be used directly or can be customized from R before being compiled and run.

3. A language embedded in R for programming algorithms for models, both of which are compiled through C++ code and loaded into R.

The input to NIMBLE consists of

- a model describing the prior and likelihood distributions, contained within nimbleCode{};

- a list containing the observed data;

- a list of constants;

- a list containing starting values for all the unknown parameters contained within inits{}.

Example 6.3. *Fitting a Poisson regression model in NIMBLE*

In this example, we consider the Poisson log-linear model seen in Chapter 2, Section 2.7;

$$\log \mu_l = \beta_0 + \beta_1 X_l + \beta_d X_l \qquad (6.2)$$

where β_1 represents the effect of exposure and β_d is the effect of the area-level covariate.

The NIMBLE code to fit this model is as follows:

```
Example6.3Code<-nimbleCode({
  for (i in 1 : N) {
    Y[i] ~ dpois(mu[i])
    log(mu[i]) <- log(E[i])+beta0+beta1*X1[i] + betad*
      X2[i]
  }
  # Priors
  beta0 ~ dnorm (0 ,sd=100)
  beta1 ~ dnorm (0 ,sd=100)
  betad ~ dnorm (0 ,sd=100)
  # Functions of interest:
  base <- exp(beta0)
  RR <- exp(beta1)
})
```

The following code shows how to run the code above for 22,000 iterations, with a burnin of 2,000 iterations.

```
ex.const<-list(N=393, E = data$exp_lungc65pls,
    X1 = as.vector(scale(data$k3)),
    X2 = as.vector(scale(data$k2)))

ex.data<-list(Y = data$lungc65pls)

# Function to generate initial values
inits<-function() list(beta0=rnorm(1),beta1=rnorm(1),
    betad=rnorm(1))

#parameters to monitor
params<-c("beta0","beta1","betad","base","RR")

samples <- nimbleMCMC(
  code = Example5.3Code,
  constants = ex.data, ## provide the combined data &
      constants as constants
  inits = inits,
  monitors = params,
  niter = 22000,
  nburnin = 2000,
  thin = 10,WAIC=TRUE,nchains=2,
  samplesAsCodaMCMC = TRUE)
```

The result is that samples will be drawn from the posterior distributions of the parameters of interest, β_0, β_1 and β_d and also of the functions of those parameters, the underlying mortality rate over all the areas (the exponent of the intercept), $base = \exp(\beta_0)$, and the relative risk associated with differences in air pollution, the exponent of the estimated coefficient associated with X, $RR = \exp(\beta_1)$. See the online resources for a full analysis of this example.

6.6 RStan

RStan is a package in R which works as an interface to Stan. As described in the manual, Stan is a library written in C++ for Bayesian inference using the No-U-Turn sampler (a variant of Hamiltonian Monte Carlo) or frequentist inference via optimization (Stan Development Team, 2023). We refer the reader to the RStan manual (Stan Development Team, 2023) to learn how to install the package RStan as it depends on several other R packages.

As Stan is written in C++, it requires that every quantity used in the program must be declared. Besides only using the HMC and NUTS samplers to obtain samples from the target distribution, this is another difference between NIMBLE and RStan.

A Stan code is divided into different blocks defined by keywords; the commands of a block must be within {}. Usually, the blocks data, parameters and model are always included in a Stan code. If one needs to sample from functions

of parameters, these functions are defined in the `transformed parameters` block.
The efficiency of the sampler is related with where the quantities are defined. For
example, assume one is fitting a model to longitudinal data where the index i refers
to the sampling unit and j to the replicate within unit i; assume further that a unit
random effect, θ_i, is included in the model and its prior follows a normal distribution centered at μ with variance τ^2. In this case, it is more efficient to define a
vector `theta` in the `transformed parameters` block and write `theta=mu+eta`
within the `transformed parameters` block. In this case, `eta` is defined in the
`parameters` block and its prior is defined as a standard normal distribution in the
`model` block, `mu` and `tau2` are also defined in the `parameters` block. The online
resources provide codes in Stan for the examples that also have code in Nimble. We
suggest the reader runs both codes as there are cases in which the `Stan` code will
reach convergence faster, requiring a smaller number of iterations of the MCMC.
Also, we encourage the reader to follow the online Stan documentation and follow
the latest updates.

Example 6.4. *Fitting a Poisson regression model in RStan*

Here, we describe how to fit the model in Example 6.3 using `RStan`. The
following list describes the `Stan` code. Usually, this is saved as a separate file
with a `stan` extension.

```
//data block
data {
  int<lower=0> N;
  vector[N] E; // expected cases
  vector[N] X1; // covariate X1
  vector[N] X2; // covariate X2
  int Y[N] ;
}
//parameters block
parameters {
  real beta0;
  real beta1;
  real beta2;
}
// transformed parameters block
transformed parameters{
  real base = exp(beta0);
  real RR = exp(beta1);
}
```

```
// model block
model {
  vector [N] mu;

  for (i in 1:N){
    mu[i] = log(E[i])+ beta0 + beta1*X1[i] + beta2*X2[
        i];
    Y[i] ~ poisson_log(mu[i]);
  }

  beta0 ~ normal(0 , 100);
  beta1 ~ normal(0 , 100);
  beta2 ~ normal(0 , 100);
}
```

The following listing describes the steps to run the code above. The online resources discuss the results of this analysis using RStan.

```
data <- read.csv("data/DataExample63.csv", sep = ",")

stan_data <- list(
  N = nrow(data),
  E = data$exp_lungc65pls,
  X1 = as.vector(scale(data$k3)),
  X2 = as.vector(scale(data$k2)),
  Y = data$lungc65pls
)

Example6_4_Stan  <- stan(
  file = "functions/Example6_4.stan",
  data = stan_data,
  warmup = 5000,
  iter = 10000,
  chains = 3,
  include = TRUE
)
```

6.7   INLA

If we have a model that can be expressed in terms of a Latent Gaussian Model (LGM) then we can take advantage of methods based on Laplace approximations that offering efficient computation when performing Bayesian inference. Bayesian inference using Integrated nested Laplace approximations (INLA), as proposed in Rue et al. (2009), can be implemented in the R-INLA software (Rue, Martino, and Lindgren, 2012).

6.7.1 Latent Gaussian models

Given $\eta_s = g(E(Y_s))$, where $g(\cdot)$ is a link function,

$$\eta_s = \beta_0 + \sum_{p=1}^{P} \beta_p X_{qs} + \sum_{q=1}^{Q} f_q(Z_{qs})$$

where β_0 is an overall intercept term, the set of β_p $(p = 1, \ldots, P)$ are coefficients associated with covariates, X; the fixed effects. The set of functions, $f_1(\cdot), \ldots, f_Q(\cdot)$ represent random effects, with the form of the function being determined by the model. For example, a hierarchical model may have $f_1(\cdot) \sim N(0, \sigma_f^2)$, with a distribution defined for σ_f^2, whereas for standard regression, $f(\cdot) \equiv 0$, leaving just fixed effects.

The set of unknown parameters, θ, will include both the coefficients of the model shown above, and the parameters required for the functions, that is $\theta = (\beta_p, f_q)$. The overall set of parameters, $\psi = (\psi_1, \psi_2)$, also contains $\psi_1 = (\sigma_\varepsilon^2)$, which relates to the variance of the measurement error in the data.

Assigning a Gaussian distribution to the parameters in θ, $\theta | \psi \sim MVN(0|\Sigma(\psi_2))$ will result in an LGM. The computation required to perform inference will be largely determined by the characteristics of the covariance matrix, $\Sigma(\psi_2)$, which will often be dense, that is, it will have many entries that are non-zero, leading to a high computational burden when performing the matrix inversions that will be required to perform inference. If $\theta | \psi_2$ can be expressed in terms of a Gaussian Markov random field (GMRF), then it may be possible to take advantage of methods that reduce computation when performing Bayesian analysis on models of this type ((Rue and Held, 2005)). Using a GMRF means that typically the inverse of the covariance matrix, $Q = \Sigma^{-1}$ will be sparse (i.e. more zero entries) due to the conditional independence between sets of parameters in which $\theta_l \perp\!\!\!\perp \theta_m | \theta_{-lm} \iff Q_{lm} = 0$ (where $-lm$ denotes the vector of θ with elements l and m removed) (Rue and Held, 2005).

6.7.2 Integrated Laplace approximations

Estimation of the (marginal) distributions of the model parameters and hyperparameters of a LGM will require evaluation of the following integrals:

$$p(\theta_j | Y) = \int p(\theta_j | Y, \psi) p(\psi | Y) d\psi$$

$$p(\psi_k | Y) = \int p(\psi | Y) d\psi_{-k} \tag{6.3}$$

In all but the most stylized cases, these will not be analytically tractable. Samples from these distributions could be obtained using Markov chain Monte Carlo (MCMC) methods, but there may be issues when fitting LGMs using MCMC, as described in (Rue et al., 2009), and the computational burden may be excessive, especially large numbers of predictions are required. Here, approximate Bayesian inference is performed using INLA. It is noted that the dimension of θ is much larger than the dimension of ψ and this will help in the implementation of the model as the computational burden increases linearly with the dimension of θ but exponentially with the dimension of ψ.

The aim is to find approximations for the distributions shown in Equation 6.3. For the hyperparameters, the posterior of ψ given Y can be written as

$$
\begin{aligned}
p(\psi|Y) &= \frac{p(\theta,\psi|Y)}{p(\theta|\psi,Y)} \\
&\propto \frac{p(Y|\theta)p(\theta|\psi)p(\psi)}{p(\theta|\psi,Y)} \\
&\approx \left. \frac{p(Y|\theta)p(\theta|\psi)p(\psi)}{\tilde{p}(\theta|\psi,Y)} \right|_{\theta=\hat{\theta}(\psi)} \\
&= \tilde{p}(\psi|Y) .
\end{aligned}
$$

Here, a Laplace approximation (LA) is used in the denominator for $\tilde{p}(\theta|\psi,Y)$. For univariate θ with an integral of the form $\int e^{g(\theta)}$, the LA takes the form $g(\theta) \sim N(\hat{\theta}(\psi), \hat{\sigma}^2)$, where $\hat{\theta}(\psi)$ is the modal value of θ for specific values of the hyperparameters, ψ and $\hat{\sigma}^2 = \left\{ \frac{d^2 \log g(\theta)}{d\theta^2} \right\}^{-1}$.

The mode of $\tilde{p}(\psi|Y)$ can be found numerically by Newton-type algorithms. Around the mode, the distribution, $\log \tilde{p}(\psi|Y)$, is evaluated over a grid of H points, ψ_h^*, each with associated integration weight Δ_h. For each point on the grid, the marginal posterior, $\tilde{p}(\psi_h^*|Y)$ is obtained from which approximations to the marginal distributions, $\tilde{p}(\psi|Y)$, can be found using numerical integration.

For the individual model parameters, θ_j,

$$
\begin{aligned}
p(\theta_j|Y) &= \frac{p((\theta_j,\theta_{-j}),\psi|Y)}{p(\theta_{-j}|\theta_j,\psi,Y)} \\
&\propto \frac{p(Y|\theta)p(\theta|\psi)p(\psi)}{p(\theta_{-j}|\theta_j,\psi,Y)} \\
&\approx \left. \frac{p(Y|\theta)p(\theta|\psi)p(\psi)}{\tilde{p}(\theta_{-j}|\theta_j,\psi,Y)} \right|_{\theta_{-j}=\hat{\theta}_{-j}(\theta_j,\psi)} \\
&= \tilde{p}(\theta_j|\psi,Y) .
\end{aligned}
$$

For an LGM, $(\theta_{-j}|\theta_j,\psi,Y)$ will be approximately Gaussian. There are a number of ways of constructing the approximation in the denominator, including a simple Gaussian approximation, which will be computationally attractive but may be inaccurate. Alternatively, an LA would be highly accurate but computationally expensive. R-INLA uses a computationally efficient method, a simplified LA, that consists of performing a Taylor expansion around the LA of $\tilde{p}(\theta_j|\psi,Y)$, aiming to 'correct' the Gaussian approximation for location and skewness (Rue et al., 2009).

The marginal posteriors, $\tilde{p}(\psi_h^*|Y)$, evaluated at each of the points ψ_h^*, are used to obtain the conditional posteriors, $\tilde{p}(\theta_j|\psi_h^*,Y)$, on a grid of values for θ_j. The marginal posteriors, $\tilde{p}(\theta_j|Y)$, are then found by numerical integration: $\tilde{p}(\theta_j|Y) = \sum_h^H \tilde{p}(\theta_j|\psi_h^*, Y)\tilde{p}(\psi_h^*|Y)\Delta_h$, with the integration weights, Δ_h, being equal when the grid takes the form of a regular lattice.

6.7.3   R-INLA

There are three main components when fitting a model using R-INLA:

1. The data.

2. Defining the model formula.

3. The call to the INLA program.

   The basic syntax of running models in R-INLA is very similar in appearance to that of glm and takes the general form formula, data, family but with the addition of the specification of the nature of the random effects, f(). For the latter component, common examples include f(i, model="iid") (independent), f(i, model="rw") (random walk of order one) and f(i, model="ar") (autoregressive of order p). .

   The class of models that can be expressed in the form of an LGM, and thus can be used with R-INLA, is very large and includes, amongst others, the following:

- Dynamic linear models.

- Stochastic volatility models.

- Generalized linear (mixed) models.

- Generalized additive (mixed) models.

- Spline smoothing.

- Semi-parametric regression.

- Disease mapping.

- Log-Gaussian Cox processes.

- Model-based geostatistics.

- Spatio-temporal models.

- Survival analysis.

   Further details on R-INLA, including the latent process models that can be accommodated, can be found on the R-INLA website: http://www.R-INLA.org. In Chapters 9, 10 and 11 we show how R-INLA can be used to provide a computationally efficient way of implementing complex Bayesian hierarchical models.

Example 6.5. *Fitting a Poisson-lognormal regression model in R-INLA*

The Poisson log-linear model seen in Chapter 2, Example 2.8 can be extended to incorporate random effects (see Chapter 7, Section 7.3 for further details). An extension of the standard Poisson model shown in Equation 2.11 to include log-normal random effects in the linear predictor will allow for over-dispersion, as described in Chapter 2, Section 2.7.2. Using log-normal random effects gives the model,

$$\log \mu_i = \beta_0 + \beta_{0i} + \beta_1 X_i + \beta_d X_i, \tag{6.4}$$

where β_1 represents the effect of exposure, β_d is the effect of the area-level covariate and β_{0i} denotes the random effect for area i. The syntax of the R-INLA code to fit this model is very similar to that of a standard glm in R:

```
formula = Y ~ X1+X2 + f(i, model="iid")
model   = inla(formula, family="poisson", data=data)

Call:
"inla(formula = formula, family = "poisson", data =
    data)"

Time used:
 Pre-processing      Running inla Post-processing
              Total
       0.278389          0.286911            0.125699
             0.690999

Integration Strategy: Central Composite Design

Model contains 1 hyperparameters
The model contains 3 fixed effect (including a
    possible intercept)

Likelihood model: poisson

The model has 1 random effects:
1.'i' is a IID model
```

The result is similar to that obtained when using a standard glm, although now there are additional details related to the random effects:

```
summary(model)
Call:
"inla(formula = formula, family = "poisson", data =
    data)"

Time used:
 Pre-processing      Running inla Post-processing
              Total
        0.2784            0.2869             0.1257
              0.6910

Fixed effects:
                mean     sd 0.025quant 0.5quant 0.975
                    quant
```

```
(Intercept) 2.4960 0.0713    2.3553    2.4962       2.6355
X1          0.1187 0.0310    0.0578    0.1186       0.1796
X2          0.0578 0.0074    0.0433    0.0578       0.0722

Random effects:
Name     Model
 i    IID model

Model hyperparameters:
                     mean      sd 0.025quant  0.5quant  0.975
                        quant
Precision for i 3.784 0.3548            3.131     3.769
    4.525

Expected number of effective parameters(std dev):
    321.42(3.926)
Number of equivalent replicates : 1.223

Marginal Likelihood:   -1513.92
```

6.8 Summary

This chapter describes methods for implementing Bayesian models when their complexity means that simple, analytic solutions may not be available. The reader will have gained an understanding of the following topics:

- Analytical approximations to the posterior distribution;
- The use of samples from a posterior distribution for inference and Monte Carlo integration;
- Methods for direct sampling such as importance and rejection sampling;
- Markov Chain Monte Carlo (MCMC) and methods for obtaining samples from the required posterior distribution including Metropolis-Hastings and Gibbs algorithms;
- The use of NIMBLE and RStan packages to fit Bayesian models using Gibbs sampling;
- Integrated Nested Laplace Approximations (INLA) as a method for performing efficient Bayesian inference including the use of R-INLA to implement a wide variety of latent Gaussian models.

6.9 Exercises

Exercise 6.1. Suppose $X|\mu \sim N(\mu, \phi)$ and $Y|\mu, \delta \sim N(\mu + \delta, \phi)$ from Question 5.4 in Chapter 5, where ϕ is known, and consider the improper non-informative joint prior distribution, $p(\mu, \delta) \propto 1$.

(i) Describe how the Gibbs sampler may be used to sample from the posterior distribution, deriving all required conditional distributions.

(ii) Suppose we have samples from the Gibbs sampler $\left\{\mu^{(t)}, \delta^{(t)}\right\}$, $t = 0, \ldots N$, where N is large. Explain how these samples may be used to estimate the marginal mean, $E[\delta|x, y]$.

Exercise 6.2. The *independence sampler* is the Metropolis-Hastings algorithm with proposal distribution

$$q(\theta^*|\theta_{t-1}) = q(\theta^*)$$

(i) Describe the Metropolis-Hastings algorithm for this transition probability.

(ii) Show that if $q(\theta)$ is proportional to the required posterior distribution, $p(\theta|\mathbf{y})$ then the Metropolis algorithm reduces to simple Monte Carlo sampling.

(iii) Suppose we take $q(\theta) = p(\theta)$, the prior distribution. Show that the acceptance probability depends only on the ratio of likelihoods. Under what circumstances will be using the prior distribution as the proposal distribution be a good choice?

Exercise 6.3. In Example 6.2 change the gamma prior for θ_i for a lognormal prior whose associated normal distribution has unknown mean μ and variance σ^2. Derive the full conditional distributions for the parameter vector of this model.

Exercise 6.4. The exercise involves performing hybrid Gibbs sampling where not all full conditionals are from a standard distribution.

(i) Based on the full conditional distributions for the Poisson-lognormal model derived in Exercise 6.3, write a Gibbs sampler in R to perform inference using this model.

(ii) Test your code using simulated data and then use it to fit the model to the data on COPD hospital admissions which are included in the online resources and are the basis of Figure 1.2.

(iii) Fit the same model in NIMBLE and compare the results with those obtained when using your Gibbs sampler. Are the results the same?

Exercise 6.5. Consider the extension to the Poisson-lognormal model shown in Example 6.5 with log-normal random effects assigned to each of the areas, for example

$$Y_l \sim Poisson(\mu_l) for \ l = 1, \ldots, N_L$$
$$\beta_{0l} \sim N(0, \sigma_{\beta_0}^2),$$

(i) Write down the full conditional distributions of this model and a hybrid Gibbs sampler in R to perform inference. Fit the model to the black smoke data which are included in the online resources.

(ii) Fit this model in NIMBLE and compare the results with those obtained from your R code.

(iii) Produce a histogram of the area-level random effects. What does this tell you about the heterogeneity of baseline risks in this example?

Chapter 7

Strategies for modeling

7.1 Overview

The most common reason for performing a regression analysis in epidemiology is to obtain estimates of the coefficients associated with the variables of interest, for example, the effect of an increase in particulate matter air pollution on the risk of respiratory death. In order to perform such analyzes, there will be a need for accurate estimates of exposures on which to base the associations with health. Often, there will be locations and periods of time for which such data will not be available. This may be due to a fault in monitoring equipment or may be due to design. In many epidemiological studies, the locations and times of exposure measurements and health assessments do not match, in part because the health and exposure data will have arisen from completely different data sources and not as the result of a carefully designed study. This is termed the 'change of support problem' (Gelfand, Zhu, and Carlin, 2001). In such cases, a direct comparison of the exposure and health outcome is often not possible without an underlying model to align the two in the spatial and temporal domains. In this chapter we consider how predictions from exposure models, which are covered in detail in Chapters 10, 11 and 12 can be used in models for estimating health risks.

In developing a model intended for estimating parameters, for example, risks to health, the choice of which variables are included or eliminated is of great importance. If several of the variables are highly correlated, which is likely to be the case when using several different pollutants and particularly so when dealing with different lagged values of variables, including a variable which is highly correlated with the one of interest, may dramatically alter the estimate of its effect or possibly even lead to the variable of interest being excluded from the model. In terms of interpretation and drawing conclusions, there is an obvious desire to have a relatively simple model that nevertheless includes all the important variables, but there are also important theoretical reasons for eliminating irrelevant variables from the model. The effect that this can have on selection procedures, both for explanatory variables but also for models themselves, is explored. In this chapter, we consider the effects of covariates and model selection, including those within the Bayesian setting in which the choice of the models themselves is part of the overall inferential process.

DOI: 10.1201/9781003352655-7

7.2   Contrasts

Variability in a process, Y, may be partially accounted for by a set of covariates, X. Covariates may be

- spatial contrasts – constant over time but vary over space;
- temporal contrasts – constant over space but vary over time;
- spatio-temporal contrasts – vary over both space and time.

The variability that creates uncertainty in a process is also responsible for creating the 'contrasts', which lie at the heart of statistical inference. In order to best determine relations between a response and a predictor, it is important to ensure strong contrasts in the levels of the predictors. In spatial sampling, this might involve putting 1/2 the observations in a (quasi-) control region to measure background levels where exposures are small, with the other 1/2 being located where exposures are large.

Example 7.1. *Contrasts in a linear model*

Suppose we have a covariate, $X_s \in [a,b]$, which varies over space and

$$Y_s = \alpha + \beta X_s + v_s, s = 1, 2, \ldots, N_S,$$

with the X's being fixed and $v_s \sim$ i.i.d.$N(0, \sigma_v^2)$. How should the x's be chosen to best estimate β?

The solution is simple in this case. Given observations y_s of Y_s, we have the standard formula $\hat{\beta} = \sum_s^{N_S} y_s [x_s - \bar{x}] / \sum_s [x_s - \bar{x}]^2$.

$$Var(\hat{\beta}) = \frac{\sigma^2}{\sum_i [x_i - \bar{x}]^2}. \tag{7.1}$$

Therefore, putting $N/2$ of the observation's x's at a and the other $N/2$ at b minimizes the standard error of estimation.

Of course, this solution would not be robust against model misspecification. If, for example, the model were actually parabolic, this design would fail.

Example 7.2. *Spatial network design and organisms on the sea floor*

The principle of obtaining strong contrasts underlies the spatial sampling design proposed to determine changes in the concentrations of benthic organisms in the sea floor of the north slopes of Alaska before and after the start-up of exploratory drilling for petroleum (Schumacher and Zidek, 1993). There was concern about the effects of toxic trace elements in the drilling mud that was to be discharged into the sea when drilling commenced. That concern was more about human welfare rather than health; the benthic organisms lay at the bottom of a food chain, the top end of which was the bowhead whale, a staple food of the Inuit people who lived there. There is an extensive literature on the optimal design of experiments for model fitting (Müller, 2007; Zidek and Zimmerman, 2019) which is discussed in Chapter 14.

7.3 Hierarchical models

Many epidemiological studies involve data that inherently have a hierarchical structure, for example when assessing the differences in mortality rates across hospitals for a particular procedure, data may be measured both at the hospital 'level' (e.g. size, specialty) and on individual patients within the hospitals (e.g. age, gender). An introduction to the need for hierarchical models and the implementation of the linear case are given in Goldstein (1987), Sullivan, Dukes, and Losina (1999) and Burton, Gurrin, and Sly (1998). In this section, a simple regression example is presented leading to a discussion of *Generalized Linear Mixed Models* (GLMM) (Breslow and Clayton, 1993), which are an extension of GLMs that allows the inclusion of random effects. Hierarchical models are also known as multi-level models and may be fitted using likelihood methods, but are naturally viewed from a Bayesian perspective.

Hierarchical models offer a convenient way of handling the different levels of correlation that may be present between outcomes in longitudinal studies where repeated measurements, j, may be made on a set of subjects, i. They provide a framework for incorporating the correlation that may be present between measurements made at different times but on the same individual. A comprehensive introduction to the subject of analyzing longitudinal data of this type can be found in P. J. Diggle, Heagerty, Liang, and Zeger (2002). For example, the first or top level of the model might relate the outcome on an individual i to a set of level 1 covariates

$$Y_{ij} = \beta_0 + \beta X_{ij} + \varepsilon_{ij}. \tag{7.2}$$

In a naive pooled analysis, the ε_{ij}'s would be considered *i.i.d* $N(0, \sigma^2)$. However, as each of the i sets of j readings made on each individual are likely to be correlated outcomes, this assumption is unlikely to be tenable. One approach would be to fit a different intercept term for each individual (a fixed effect), but this requires the ratio of J to I to be suitably large.

Alternatively, a random effect can be fitted, referring to the fact that the regression coefficients can vary from individual to individual. This alternative to fitting a separate intercept for each individual, i, assumes that there exists an overall intercept (β_0) for the whole population and that a separate intercept β_{0i} for each individual comes from a distribution with expectation β_0 and a suitable variance. For example, $\beta_{0i} \sim N(\beta_0, \sigma_{\beta_0}^2)$ or $u_i = \beta_{0i} - \beta_0 \sim N(0, \sigma_{\beta_0}^2)$. Model (7.2) can therefore be expressed as

$$Y_{ij} = \alpha_0 + u_i + \beta X_{ij} + \varepsilon_{ij}, \tag{7.3}$$

with $E[\varepsilon_{ij}] = 0, Var(\varepsilon_{ij}) = \sigma_e^2, Cov(\varepsilon_{ij}, \varepsilon_{ik}) = 0$ and $E[u_i] = 0, Var(u_i) = \sigma_u^2,$ $Cov(u_i, u_l) = 0, \forall i \neq l$. The variance of Y_{ij} is, thus $\sigma_e^2 + \sigma_u^2$, where the variance between Y_{ij} within a single individual is σ_u^2. The intra-subject correlation coefficient is therefore $\sigma_u^2/(\sigma_u^2 + \sigma_e^2)$. Given estimates of σ_u^2 and σ_e^2, the *exchangeable* correlation structure means that every observation within an individual is equally correlated with every other observation in that individual, that is $\rho_{jj} = 1, \rho_{jk} = \rho \; j \neq k$, the infraclass correlation coefficient.

In non-hierarchical models, tests of statistical significance are associated with the addition (or deletion) of one or more parameters and the likelihood ratio test (see Chapter 2, Section 2.5.3). However, when drawing inference about random parameters, the usual null hypothesis, that a single variance is zero, will violate one of the standard regularity conditions needed to ensure that the asymptotic distribution of the test statistic is χ^2. In such cases, a standard χ^2 test will underestimate the significance of an observed departure from the null hypothesis (Laird and Ware, 1982).

7.3.1   Cluster effects

Often in environmental epidemiology, samples are collected using a multi-stage sampling design, where the first stage is the selection of a random subset of large areas and the second stage the selection of smaller areas within them. The sample will therefore contain cluster effects; items from the same areas (clusters) will be more alike than items from different clusters. There is then the possibility of inducing correlation across space and hence reducing the effective sample size. In the extreme case where all the items in a cluster are identical, the information will be the same as the information obtained from a single item. If this effect is ignored and the assumption is made that the items are drawn independently, then inferences will be flawed, and the uncertainty associated with estimates will be under-represented, resulting in the error bands on estimates being too narrow. An expected $\alpha = 0.05$ level test of significance will in reality be much larger.

Example 7.3. *The effect of clusters on modeling*
Let Y_s be the measured response with realizations indexed over space, $s = 1, \ldots, N_S$. Interest lies in the association between a variable of interest, X_s, that is, an exposure and Y_s. The data are collected in spatial clusters $i, 1, \ldots I$ with random cluster effects β_{0i}. The following model relates the Y to X:

$$Y_{si} = \beta_0 + \beta_{0i} + \beta X_{si} + \varepsilon_{si} \qquad (7.4)$$
$$= \beta_0 + \beta x_{si} + \varepsilon_{si}^*, \qquad (7.5)$$

where $\varepsilon_{si} \sim$ i.i.d.$N(0, \sigma^2)$ and $\beta_{0i} \sim$ i.i.d. $N(0, \sigma_{\beta_0}^2)$.

It can be seen in Equation (7.5) that $\varepsilon_{si}^* \sim$ i.i.d. $N(0, \sigma_{\beta_0}^2 + \sigma^2)$. The random cluster effects are now hidden in the so-called error term, ε_{si}^* with the result that the residual variance is inflated and the effect of X will be masked. We can see that if the cluster-effect exceeds the effect of X, then the relative lack of variation in the X_s would mean a lack of power to detect a relationship between X and Y. Equation (7.5) shows the naive model that ignores the cluster effect, which will be 'hidden' in ε_{si}^*. This will inflate the residual sum of squares and the significance level of the test will be increased.

Cluster effects can also induce temporal autocorrelation, and if such an effect were strong, there would be little incremental information in the data obtained over time. In such a case, little information would be lost by taking averages of the process and the measurements generated over time, $\bar{Y}_{s.} = \beta_{0s.}^* + \bar{\varepsilon}_{s.}^*$, where Y_{st} and ε_{st} are now indexed by space and time and β_{0s}^* are the associated cluster (random) effects. In this situation, it will only be the spatial variation in $\bar{X}$ that provides the contrasts in X and this would have to be substantial for a significant effect to be seen.

Problems with this approach arise when β_{0i} and X_s are aligned and correlated over space, causing confounding. If their variations were roughly equal then the resulting co-linearity would lead to the information in the sample being split between the two effects, leading to the possibility that neither would prove to be significant, meaning important risk factors may be masked. This may occur even if β were large.

Overall, the confounding of the effects of the variable of interest in cluster effects generally leads to a set of undesirable effects. These concerns may suggest that an alternative to averaging over time may be preferable, for example based on similar principles to the paired t-test, we may use $Y_s' = Y_{s'} - Y_s = \beta(x_{s'} - x_s) + (\varepsilon_{s'} - \varepsilon_s)$, which eliminates cluster effects and thus autocorrelation.

7.4   Generalized linear mixed models

Generalized linear mixed models (GLMMs) are essentially GLMs (see Chapter 2, Section 2.5) that include one or more random effects. Conditional on random effects, b_i, the Y_i are assumed independent, with expectation, $E(Y_i|b_i) = \mu_i = g^{-1}(\gamma_i) = g^{-1}(X_i\beta + z_ib_i)$ and variance, $VAR(Y_i|b) = \sigma^2 = a(\phi)v(\mu_i)$. The likelihood for N subjects, each with N_j measurements will thus be

$$L(\beta,b,\sigma^2|Y) \propto \prod_{i=1}^{N}\prod_{j=1}^{n_j} p(Y_{ij}|\beta,b_i,\sigma^2). \qquad (7.6)$$

If the random effects are assumed to be normally distributed, $b = (b_1, b_2, \cdots, b_N)' \sim N(0, D)$, then within subject correlation can be taken into account whilst allowing each subject to have a unique covariance structure. The correlation structure can be defined using the covariance, D (rather than simply using $\sigma^2 I$). In a Bayesian setting, where the covariance matrix will be assigned a prior distribution, D^{-1} is often assumed to have a Wishart prior, this being conjugate to the multivariate normal distribution.

Frequentist approach

The parameters of the distribution of the random effect are known as *hyperparameters*, θ, and must also be estimated from the data. In the case of linear regression, the parameters, β, ϕ and θ can be estimated by maximum likelihood using iterative generalized least squares (Goldstein, 1987). In the more general case, the usual strategy is to attempt to estimate the parameters by using the integrated likelihood, details of which can be found in Laird and Ware (1982) and P. J. Diggle et al. (2002),

$$p(Y|\beta,\phi,\theta) \propto \int p(Y|\beta,b,\phi)p(b|\theta)db. \qquad (7.7)$$

In general, $\hat{b} = E(b|\hat{\theta},\hat{\beta},\hat{\phi})$, using the MLEs obtained from Equation (7.7). Whilst this approach is feasible for Normal models, the computations are intractable in other cases, although they can be approximated. Breslow and Clayton (1993) review approaches to approximate these calculations, including penalized quasi-likelihood, which is estimated using a variation of the iteratively reweighted least squares calculations used for GLMs (see Chapter 2, Section 2.5).

   The problem with this approach, however, is that the underlying uncertainty in $\hat{\beta}, \hat{\phi}$ and $\hat{\theta}$ is not acknowledged.

Bayesian approach

In assigning the prior distributions of the hyperparameters, θ, the Bayesian approach provides a natural framework for dealing with hierarchical models, incorporating the uncertainty in the estimates of the parameters. For illustration, the set of level one (non-hyper) parameters are denoted simply by β (omitting σ^2/ϕ for clarity), in which case the appropriate Bayesian posterior distribution is the vector (θ,β), with joint prior distribution, $p(\theta,\beta) = p(\theta)p(\beta|\theta)$. The joint posterior distribution is then $p(\theta,\beta|y) \propto p(y|\beta)p(\theta,\beta)$. The hyperparameters can be estimated by obtaining the marginal posterior distribution , $p(\theta|y)$, which involves integrating the joint posterior distribution, $p(\theta|y) = \int p(\beta,\theta|y)d\beta$.

7.5   Bayesian hierarchical models

Bayesian hierarchical models are an extremely useful and flexible framework in which to model complex relationships and dependencies in data, and they are used extensively throughout the book. In the hierarchy we consider, there are three levels;

(i) *The observation, or measurement, level;* $Y|Z,X_1,\theta_1$.
   Data, Y, are assumed to arise from an underlying process, Z, which is unobservable but from which measurements can be taken, possibly with error, at locations in space and time. Measurements may also be available for covariates, X_1. Here θ_1 is the set of parameters for this model and may include, for example, regression coefficients and error variances.

(ii) *The underlying process level; $Z|X_2, \theta_2$.*

The process Z drives the measurements seen at the observation level and represents the true underlying level of the outcome. It may be, for example, a spatio-temporal process representing an environmental hazard. Measurements may also be available for covariates at this level, X_2. Here θ_2 is the set of parameters for this level of the model.

(iii) *The parameter level; $\theta = (\theta_1, \theta_2)$.*

In this book we advocate a Bayesian approach and so there will be an additional level at which distributions are assigned to all unknown quantities. This contains models for all the parameters in the observation and process level and may control things such as the variability and strength of any spatio-temporal relationships.

Here, the notation $Y|X$ means that the distribution of Y is conditional on X.

This book involves models for both health counts and exposures, and each of these can be framed in the context of a hierarchical model. To avoid ambiguity between the two, we use $Y^{(1)}$, $X^{(1)}$, $Z^{(1)}$, $\theta^{(1)}$ for health models and $Y^{(2)}$, $X^{(2)}$, $Z^{(2)}$, $\theta^{(2)}$ for exposure models.

When health or exposure models are considered separately, the $Y^{()}$ notation is dropped for clarity of exposition. Also, it is noted that we do not generally consider cases where health counts from routinely available data sources may not be an accurate reflection of the underlying health of the population at risk, that is, it is assumed that $Y^{(1)} = Z^{(1)}$. In practice this might not be an entirely accurate assumption due to misclassification, migration or data anomalies.

7.6 Linking exposure and health models

In order to perform health analysis there will be a need for accurate estimates of exposures during periods and in locations where there is missing data, either by design, for example where a monitor is not located or in operation, or due to shorter periods where measurements are not available. In addition, in many epidemiological studies, the locations and times of exposure measurements and health assessments do not match, in part because the health and exposure data will have arisen from completely different data sources and not as the result of a carefully designed study; termed the 'change of support problem' by Gelfand et al. (2001). Hence, a direct comparison of the exposure and health outcome is often not possible without an underlying model to align the two in the spatial and temporal domains (Gryparis, Paciorek, Zeka, Schwartz, and Coull, 2009; Peng and Bell, 2010).

A few studies have used spatio-temporal modeling within such health studies, largely due to the health data being available at a lower geographical temporal resolution than the exposure data (J. Zidek, White, Sun, Burnett, and Le, 1998; L. Zhu, Carlin, and Gelfand, 2003; Fuentes, Song, Ghosh, Holland, and Davis, 2006; D. Lee and Shaddick, 2010) meaning pollution concentrations were not available in each spatial unit. These studies are ecological in nature, being based on spatially aggregated health and exposure data modeled at the same resolution. As such, there is the potential for ecological bias; assuming that associations observed at the level of the area hold for the individuals within the areas can lead to the so-called ecological fallacy. Ecological bias can manifest itself in a variety of ways, and in this case bias in the resulting health risks may occur due to the aggregation of a non-linear model. For more details of the issues related to ecological studies and ecological bias, see Chapter 13.

More commonly, simple methods for handling missing values are used, including simply discarding them from the analysis or replacing them by a specific single value, for example the overall mean. By discarding missing values, we may lose useful information and may in fact introduce bias. By replacing missing values by a single value, for example the posterior mean from an exposure model, important features of the data and the intrinsic variability in using a summary value may be ignored.

Environmental exposure data are generally obtained from N_S fixed site monitors, S, located within the spatial domain, $\mathscr{S}$. The set of monitoring sites are collectively denoted by $S = \{s_1,\ldots,s_{N_S}\}$, where $s_l = (a_l, b_l) \in \mathscr{R}^2$. However, health data are commonly available only at aggregated level for administrative areas, $A_l, l = 1,\ldots,N_L$ and therefore a suitable summary of the concentrations in an area for a particular time period is required. Using the notation described in Chapter 1, Section 7.5, the true values are denoted by $Z^{(2)}$ where the $^{(2)}$ indicates that they are measurements of exposures rather than $^{(1)}$ which would indicate health outcomes. The true mean exposure in a health area, A_l is given by

$$\bar{Z}_l^{(2)} = \int_{s \in A_l} M_s Z_s^{(2)} ds, \qquad (7.8)$$

where $Z_s^{(2)}$ is the true level of exposure at all possible locations s in A_l and M_s is the population density such that $\int_{s \in A_l} M_s ds = 1$. However, the information required to compute the integral will be unavailable. Therefore, there is a need to approximate this, with the simplest and most commonly used approach being to take the average of the observed measurements from actual monitoring sites located within the health area,

$$\bar{y}_l^{(2)} = \frac{1}{N_{A_l}} \sum_{s \in A_l} y_s^{(2)}, \qquad (7.9)$$

where N_{A_l} is the number of monitoring sites located within the area A_l.

There may be situations where the assumption that the average of measured values will be a suitable representation of the (average of the) true concentrations may not be tenable, that is $\bar{y}_l^{(2)} \neq \bar{Z}_l^{(2)}$. If this is the case, then bias may potentially occur in the estimation of the effects of pollution, with the magnitude being largely dependent on two characteristics of the underlying pollution surface:

- **Spatial variation**
  If the underlying surface exhibits substantial spatial variation, the measurements at the monitor locations may not be a representative sample of the pollution concentrations throughout $\mathscr{S}$. This is because the number of monitor locations is likely to be small, unequally spaced throughout the study region and may be located for specific reasons (for example at a well-known pollution hot spot), meaning that averaging the values at these sites may not produce a good estimate of Z.

- **Measurement error**
  The ambient monitors are known to measure with error (DETR, 1998), meaning that $Y^{(2)}$ may be a biased estimate of $Z^{(2)}$. Details of the effects of measurement error can be seen in Chapter 8, Section 8.3.

If both these factors are negligible, then the pollution surface across $\mathscr{R}$ will be relatively flat and the observed monitoring data is likely to provide an adequate representation of the pollution surface, meaning that the simple average $Y^{(2)}$ will be an unbiased estimate of the true (unobserved) average over Z. However, if that is not the case, then this naive approach can induce bias and underestimate uncertainty (Director and Bornn, 2015).

7.6.1 Two-stage approaches

Much of the material in this book advocates a Bayesian approach to modeling environmental exposures in space and time. An introduction to the Bayesian approach is given in Chapter 5 and methods of implementation in Chapter 6. In a fully Bayesian framework, estimation of health and exposure models, including prediction at locations where data is not available, is performed simultaneously. The uncertainty in estimating the coefficients of the exposure model is therefore acknowledged and 'fed through' the model to the predictions and further to the estimation of the coefficients in the health model. Often the exposure models are fit separately from the health model, removing the dependence between $Y^{(2)}$ and $Y^{(1)}$, in order to ease the computational burden in running a combined model, an approach that has also been adopted in Carlin, Xia, Devine, Tolbert, and Mulholland (1999) and L. Zhu et al. (2003).

There are likely to be computational considerations associated with jointly fitting the health and exposure models, especially if the latter uses large amounts of data over space and time. When the exposure model is complicated or when one is interested in running multiple candidate epidemiological models with different sets of covariates either for a single outcome or multiple outcomes, a single model is not going to provide an efficient method of investigation.

Often the exposure models are fit separately from the health model, removing the dependence of $Z^{(2)}$ on $Y^{(1)}$. The joint model is therefore decomposed into separate health and exposure components. The exposure component is of the form:

$$[Z^{(2)}|\theta^{(2)},Y^{(2)}] \propto [Y^{(2)}|Z^{(2)},\theta^{(2)}][\theta^{(2)}],$$

and the health component of the form

$$[\theta^{(1)}|Z^{(2)},Y^{(1)}] \propto [Y^{(1)}|Z^{(2)},\theta^{(1)}][\theta^{(1)}],$$

noting that the first-term exposure model is different from, $[Z^{(2)}|\theta^{(2)},Y^{(2)},Y^{(1)}]$ which would be used in a fully Bayesian analysis. This is often done in order to ease the computational burden in running a combined model, and that has been adopted in a number of cases, for example, Carlin et al. (1999), L. Zhu et al. (2003), Lee and

Shaddick (2010), Chang, Peng, and Dominici (2011) and Peng and Bell (2010). This *two-stage approach* has the advantage that the exposure model, which is likely to be the most computationally demanding, does not have to be refit when running multiple health effect analyzes. Two stage approaches separate the exposure and health components whilst still allowing uncertainty from the exposure modeling to be incorporated into the health model (Chang et al., 2011; Peng and Bell, 2010; Lee and Shaddick, 2010).

There are other reasons why fitting a joint model may be unappealing; it is not intended that the health counts should inform the estimation of the exposures, which should be based on data from the monitored concentrations. It is possible to 'cut' feedback between the stages within MCMC, for example in WinBUGS (Lunn, Thomas, Best, and Spiegelhalter, 2000), however the result is that the posteriors may not be proper probability distributions (Plummer, 2014). Liu, Bayarri, and Berger (2009) consider that the overall model consists of a number of distinct components, which are called modules. And they define modularization as the technique that keeps modules partly separated in a Bayesian analysis. Jacob, Murray, Holmes, and Robert (2017) investigate why modular approaches might be preferable to the full model in misspecified settings

7.6.2 Multiple imputation

One approach to performing a two-stage analysis is to use multiple imputation (Little and Rubin, 2014). This allows the uncertainty in predictions to be represented by using a set of plausible values for the exposures, which comprise samples from the posterior distributions of the predictions at the required locations in space and time. Taking D multiple (joint) samples from the posteriors results in D multiple datasets that are repeatedly used in the health model, $(Y^{(1)}|Z^{(1)})$.

Repeatedly running the health model results in an estimate of the log relative risk, β_1, and associated standard error for each dataset. These are then combined to give an overall estimate of relative risk, together with a combined standard error that can be used to calculate confidence intervals (Little and Rubin, 2014). Assume β_{1d} is the estimate obtained from the data set $d = 1, 2, ..., D$ and $\sigma_{\beta d}$ is the standard error associated with β_d. The overall estimate is the average of the individual estimates,

$$\bar{\beta} = \frac{1}{D} \sum_{d=1}^{D} \beta_d. \tag{7.10}$$

The overall estimate of the standard error will be a function of a combination of within-imputation variance and between-imputation variance. The first of these is given as

$$\sigma_{w\beta}^2 = \frac{1}{D} \sum_{d=1}^{D} \sigma_{\beta d}^2,$$

and the between-imputation variance by

$$\sigma_{b\beta}^2 = \frac{1}{D-1}\sum_{d=1}^{D}(\beta_d - \bar{\beta})^2.$$

The total variance is therefore

$$\sigma^2 = \sigma_{w\beta}^2 + (1+\frac{1}{D})\sigma_{b\beta}^2.$$

Confidence intervals are obtained using quantiles of the t-distribution with degrees of freedom

$$df = (D-1)\left(1+\frac{D\sigma_{w\beta}^2}{(D+1)\sigma_{b\beta}^2}\right)^2.$$

This requires the ability to draw joint samples from the posterior distributions of the predictions from the exposure model which is straightforward when using MCMC. It is also possible in the R-INLA package using the function inla.posterior.sample. In computing the approximation to the required distributions, $\tilde{p}(\theta|\mathbf{y})\,\tilde{p}(z_i|\theta,\mathbf{y})$, R-INLA uses numerical integration based on interpolation between a number of chosen 'integration points' (Rue et al., 2009). Taking $\tilde{p}(z_i|\theta,\mathbf{y})$ as an example, the integration points are selected from a set of candidate points on a grid. After exploring $\log(\tilde{p}(z_i|\theta,\mathbf{y}))$ to find the mode, a point is selected if the difference between $\log(\tilde{p}(z_i|\theta,\mathbf{y}))$ evaluated at that point and the value evaluated at the mode is greater than a prespecified constant. Apart from the integration based on this procedure for finding approximations to the marginal distributions as described in Chapter 6, Section 6.7, the information stored about the distribution at these integration points can be kept. This allows the function inla.posterior.sample to be used after the main INLA run. Joint samples from the posteriors can be obtained by sampling from Gaussian approximations at the integration points for all the parameters, including predictions from the exposure model. A combined analysis of these datasets is then performed. This results in valid statistical inferences that properly reflect the uncertainty due to missing values.

7.7   Model selection and comparison

In constructing a regression model, decisions will have to be made on which variables should be included, and what form they should take, that is, should they be transformed or categorized. The choice of variables and the methods used may, in part, be determined by the reasoning behind the regression analysis, whether for estimation or prediction.

7.7.1   Effect of selection on properties of estimators

This section concentrates on the important subject of subset selection, the choice of which variables to include in the regression equation, and the effect this has on the inferential process.

In choosing which models should be considered, it is important that they have some plausibility outside the realms of statistical significance. Careful consideration of prior information is advocated by Rothman and Greenland (1998), although it is acknowledged that in most cases the prior knowledge available is likely to be too limited to provide much guidance in model selection. Chapter 5 describes how, in a Bayesian setting, if such information were available, it could be directly incorporated into the analysis. They suggest the selection procedure should start with a *credible model*, which would be considered 'compatible with available information' and give the example of modeling cancer rates, where such a model would include age and sex. Variables are then added to the starting model, their importance and thus whether they are retained, being assessed, based on their contribution to the fit of the model to the data. There are many techniques for automatically selecting variables to be included in a model, and a selection of these are described in Section 7.7.2, but the danger in using these so-called 'black box' routines is that a known confounder may be excluded from the model, possibly in favor of a variable with no biological plausibility. In addition to a credible starting model, the final model should also not conflict with prior information. The choice of which other variables are included can have a significant effect on the interpretation of the effect of the variables of interest, although if the model is to be used only for prediction there is more tolerance to the choice of variables, a point emphasized by Clayton and Hills (1993).

In this section, the effect of variable selection on the results of the regression equation are explored. It should be noted that the theoretical effects described hold for cases when the selection is not based on information from the current data, which is often not the case. In order to completely eliminate the effect of bias caused by the selection of variables, completely independent data sets would be required for (i) the selection of the model and for (ii) the estimation of the regression coefficients. However, this is unlikely to be an efficient approach in practice, as less information will be available for the actual estimation of the parameters.

For illustration, the effects of variable selection are demonstrated using linear regression, although the concepts generalize to other forms which may be better suited to an epidemiological investigation, such as Poisson regression.

Given a response variable, Y, with a single possible explanatory variable, X, to which a linear regression of the form $E(Y|X) = \alpha + \beta X$ is fitted, then an unbiased estimate, $\hat{\beta}$ of β can be found and then tested to see whether it is significantly different from zero. If it is then β is included in the equation, if not then it is dropped. Using this procedure means the estimate $\hat{\beta}$ will no longer be unbiased for β, as it depends on decisions made based on the data. If β is included in the model, rather than just fitting the intercept term, then the expectation of $\hat{\beta}$ should be written

$$E(\hat{\beta}|\hat{\beta} \text{ is significantly different from } 0),$$

which will not be equal to β. Chatfield (1995) describes a *pre-test estimator* which also considers *not* fitting the line, when $\beta = 0$, in order to give the unconditional estimate of $\hat{\beta}_{PT}$

$$\hat{\beta}_{PT} = \begin{cases} \hat{\beta}, & \text{if } \hat{\beta} \text{ is significant,} \\ 0, & \text{otherwise,} \end{cases}$$

from which it is obvious that $E(\hat{\beta}_{PT})$ is not generally equal to the unconditional estimator, $E(\hat{\beta})$. The effect of variable selection is investigated more fully later in this section, but briefly, Chatfield advises that (i) least squares theory does not apply when the same data are used to formulate and fit a model, and (ii) the analyst must always be clear exactly what any inference is conditioned on.

In order to investigate further the effects of variable selection on the estimates of the parameters and prediction, consider a linear model with n observations, each with a response variable Y and a set of p possible covariates $X_1, ..., X_p$. The full model, but not necessarily the 'true' underlying model, is obtained by fitting all the available variables,

$$Y_l = \beta_0 + \sum_{j=1}^{p} \beta_j X_{lj} + \varepsilon_l. \tag{7.11}$$

Here, the residual terms, ε_l, are assumed independently and identically distributed, and in the case of Normal linear regression are such that $\varepsilon_l \sim N(0, \sigma^2)$.

The full model is expressed in matrix notation as

$$\mathbf{Y} = \mathbf{X}\beta + \varepsilon, \tag{7.12}$$

where $\mathbf{Y}$ is the vector (of length n) of observed responses, $\mathbf{X}$ the full design matrix dimension $n \times (p+1)$, containing all the p variables for which information is available together with a column representing the intercept term (which is assumed to be included in all the models), β is the $p+1$ vector of unknown regression coefficients and ε the n vector representing the random component.

With p potential covariates, by considering all the possible models that comprise combinations of each of them being included/excluded, there will be $m = 2^p$ possible models, M_k ($k = 1, ..., m$). Assume that model, M_k, contains r_k regressors, so that $p + 1 - r_k$ have been omitted. For model, M_k, let $\mathbf{X}_k$ and β^k represent the design matrix and parameter vector respectively and $\mathbf{X}'_k$ and $\beta^{k'}$ the complement, so that $\mathbf{X}_k = (\mathbf{X}_k, \mathbf{X}'_k)$ and $\beta^T = \{(\beta^k)', (\beta^{k'})'\}$.

A natural ordering is used, so that $k = 1$ represents the null model containing just the intercept term with design matrix $\mathbf{X}_1 = \mathbf{1}_n$, a n vector of one's. The full model is represented by $\mathbf{X}_m = \mathbf{X}$, the complete $(n \times (p+1))$ design matrix containing all the variables.

Example 7.4. *Possible design matrices when using two covariates*

To clarify this notation, an example with two possible covariates, X_1 and X_2, is considered. Here, $p = 2$ and therefore, the total number of possible models is $m = 2^2 = 4$. The full design matrix, X can be written as $[\mathbf{1}_n, X_1, X_2]$, which is equivalent to X_4. The four possible models are shown in Table 7.1.

Table 7.1: Possible design matrices and corresponding regression coefficients when using combinations of two covariates.

Model, k	$\mathbf{X}_k$	r_k	β^k	$\mathbf{X}_{k'}$	$p+1-r_k$	$\beta^{k'}$
1	$[\mathbf{1}_n]$	1	β_0^1	$[X_1, X_2]$	2	$(\beta_1^1, \beta_2^1)'$
2	$[\mathbf{1}_n, X_1]$	2	$(\beta_0^2, \beta_1^2)'$	X_2	1	β_2^2
3	$[\mathbf{1}_n, X_2]$	2	$(\beta_0^3, \beta_2^3)'$	X_1	1	β_1^3
4	$[\mathbf{1}_n, X_1, X_2]$	3	$(\beta_0^4, \beta_1^4, \beta_2^4)'$	–	0	–

As discussed above, from maximum likelihood theory, if the full model is correct then the expected value of $\hat{\beta}$ is equal to the true value of β, however, if the model includes variables that are extraneous then this is no longer true. If the true model is $Y = \mathbf{X}_k \beta^k + \varepsilon$ but the full model is fitted, then the expected value and variance of $\hat{\beta}$ will be as follows:

$$E(\hat{\beta}_k) = \hat{\beta}_k + (\mathbf{X}_k' \mathbf{X}_k)^{-1} (\mathbf{X}_k' \mathbf{X}_{k'}) \hat{\beta}_{k'}$$

$$= \beta^k + A\beta^{k'} \tag{7.13}$$

$$= true\ value\ +\ bias\ term,$$

$$VAR(\hat{\beta}^k) = (\mathbf{X}_k' \mathbf{X}_{k'})^{-1} \sigma^2, \tag{7.14}$$

where $\mathbf{A} = (\mathbf{X}_k' \mathbf{X}_k)^{-1} (\mathbf{X}_k' \mathbf{X}_{k'})$.

This shows the bias in the regression coefficients that can be expected if the extraneous variables contained in $\mathbf{X}_{k'}$ are included in the model. This bias will exist unless (i) $\beta_k = 0$, the true coefficients of the additional variables are actually zero and thus the variable has no effect on the response or (ii) $\mathbf{X}_k' \mathbf{X}_{k'} = 0$, there is no correlation between the two sets of variables meaning that the inclusion of non-important variables will not have an effect on the explanatory power (and the estimates) of the variables of interest. This is often a product of design in a controlled experiment, as in the case of randomized trials where randomization is used to allow the investigator to separate the effects of different covariates, but is unlikely to be the case in observational studies.

It can be shown that the components of $\hat{\beta}^k$ will generally have less variation than those from the full model, $\hat{\beta}$. This means that the precision of the estimates can be reduced by using a subset model, even if the terms excluded are not completely extraneous, that is, do not have a true coefficient of zero. It can also be shown that the estimate of the variance, $\hat{\sigma}_k$, will generally be biased upwards.

The reason that this result is not taken to the extreme case, where just the intercept would be fit and thus predict the same value irrespective of the values of the covariates, is because of the bias that is introduced when important variables are ignored. As variables are added to the model, the usual trade-off between reducing the bias and increasing the variance has to be considered. This bias term can also be expressed in terms of the mean square error (MSE) of the estimates $\hat{\beta}$, where

$$
\begin{aligned}
MSE(\hat{\beta}) &= E(\hat{\beta}^k - \beta^k)(\hat{\beta}^k - \beta^k)' \\
&= (\mathbf{X}'_k\mathbf{X}_k)^{-1}\sigma^2 + A\beta_{k'}\beta'_{k'}A' \qquad (7.15) \\
&= variance + (bias)^2.
\end{aligned}
$$

If a variable is included that has no effect on the response then the variance will be increased without a decrease in the bias. If a variable has a small effect on the response, then the reduction in bias has to be weighed against the increase in variance.

The bias in the regression estimates and the change in the variability associated with variable selection will have an associated effect on any predicted values generated from the regression equation. If a set of explanatory variables is considered $x' = (\mathbf{X}'_k\mathbf{x}^*_{k'})$ (comprising values for both the important and extraneous variables) then the full model will produce response, $\hat{Y} = x'\beta$, with mean $x'\hat{\beta}$ and prediction variance,

$$
\mathrm{VAR}(\hat{Y}) = \sigma^2(\mathbf{x}'(\mathbf{X}'\mathbf{X})^{-1}\mathbf{x}). \qquad (7.16)
$$

As the point predictions are essentially based on the individual estimates, the variances decrease as terms are excluded from the model.

7.7.2 Stepwise selection procedures

Procedures have been developed which aim to identify good (though not necessarily the best) subset of possible models. They are based upon changes in deviance between nested models which, as described in Chapter 2, Section 2.5.3, can be tested to assess differences in model fit. Generally, these approaches, often referred to as *stepwise regression procedures*, aim to use less computation than would be necessary if all the possible regressions were performed and examined.

Dependent on the method, subset models are identified sequentially by adding or deleting variables, three commonly used stepwise methods are described here. These methods are in no way guaranteed to find the 'best' or even the same subset of variables.

Forward selection of variables adds one variable at a time to the previously chosen subset. At the beginning of the process, the first variable chosen is that which accounts for the largest amount of variation in the dependent variable, that is, the variable having the highest correlation with Y. At each successive step, each of the remaining variables are added one at a time to the model, and that which results in the largest reduction in the residual sum of squares is retained. This will be the variable with the highest correlation with the *residuals* from the current model. A stopping rule is needed to terminate the process or it would continue until all the variables have been included.

If RSS_k denotes the residual sum of squares with r_k variables in the model and if the smallest RSS which can be obtained by adding another variable is RSS_q, for new model, M_q, then

$$R = \frac{RSS_k - RSS_q}{RSS_q/(n - r_k - 2)} \qquad (7.17)$$

is calculated and compared to a 'F-to-enter' value, F_e, that is, if R is greater than F_e, then the variable is added to the selected set.

Backward elimination is similar but starts with the full model and then chooses a variable to delete at each step according to which would result in the smallest increase in the residual sum of squares (the variable with the smallest partial sum of squares). Again, a stopping rule is needed or the process will continue until all the variables have been deleted.

Let RSS_k denote the residual sum of squares with r_k variables in the model, and let RSS_t be the smallest that can be obtained by deleting any variable resulting in the model M_t. Then let

$$R = \frac{RSS_t - RSS_k}{RSS_k/(n - r_k - 1)} \qquad (7.18)$$

be calculated and compared to the 'F-to-stay' value, F_s. If R is less than F_s, then the variable is deleted from the selected set.

It should be noted that although the terms 'F-to-enter' and 'F-to-stay' suggest that the ratios, R, follow a F-distribution, this is not the case. If, after r_k variables have been entered and the next variable is chosen at random, then the assumptions required to use a F-test (that the residuals are independently, identically and normally distributed) are met. However, if the next variable is chosen to maximize, R then the distribution will not be a F-distribution. Using approximations to the distribution of R to obtain nominal 5% points for the 'F-to-enter' taken from the F-distribution have been shown to give true significance levels in excess of 50% (Draper, Guttman, and Lapczak, 1979).

Stepwise selection is a combination of the previous two approaches, neither of which takes into account the effect that adding or deleting a variable can have on the contributions of the other variables previously included in the model. A variable that has been added to the model early on may become unimportant after another, possibly highly correlated, variable has been added. This is certainly going to be the case when considering the effects of pollutants and temperature. For this reason, stepwise selection is an extension of forward selection that re-checks at each step the importance of the variables currently included in the model. If the partial sum of squares for any previously included variable(s) does not meet some predetermined criteria, then those variables are excluded from the model before the next addition step is attempted.

The stopping rules, referred to as 'F-to-stay' and 'F-to-go', are both required in stepwise selection. However, there is no reason why they should be set at the same level, indeed it might be preferable to have a more relaxed criterion for inclusion as this would force the procedure to consider larger numbers of subset models.

One criticism of these selection methods is that they imply an order of importance to the variables. This can be misleading since, for example, in forward selection, the first variable that was included is often deemed unimportant when other variables have been included. Indeed, it could be the first variable to be excluded when backwards elimination is applied. It should also be remembered that the choice of variables in the final model can be determined to a varying extent by the particular data under consideration the selection method used and the stopping rule. Unless an independent dataset is used for the selection process, the bias in the individual parameter estimates will also be affected by these factors. The more extensive the search for the model, the more chance there is that the final model might be an excellent fit to the data in question, but possibly with little other general use. By basing the inference on the results of a single model, the possibility of extreme or non-typical values in the data affecting the parameter estimates will be increased.

A danger in using these methods is that they might appear to replace the need for the investigator to obtain a genuine feel for the data, with respect to the problem under consideration, and may mask the possible effects that model assumptions and variable selection might have on the inferential process.

Example 7.5. *Model choice in studies of air pollution and health*

In studies of air pollution and health, it is common for regression models to contain a number of highly correlated pollutants in the same regression and to attempt to draw inferences about which variables were causal, or at least had the strongest relationship, from that model. Many studies have used stepwise procedures, including many highly correlated pollutants and meteorological variables in the candidate list. For example, Kinney and Ozkaynak (1991) performed multiple regression using backward selection on 5 pollutants and 3 temperature variables in Los Angeles County. After pre-whitening both the outcome (daily deaths) and the explanatory variables using moving averages, they found significant correlations only between deaths and same-day levels of the pollutants and temperature, except for ozone, for which a 1-day lag was significant. These variables were then included in the multiple regression on which backwards selection was performed, with the resulting model including same-day NO_2 and temperature, and 1-day lag O_x. The difficulties in using an automatic procedure to select between highly correlated variables have been discussed, and here there was the additional complication of the use of filtering on the data. Although this was an attempt to eliminate the problems of autocorrelation and cross correlation between the variables, the choice of which lagged variables to include in the initial model could be determined to a large extent by the exact filtering mechanism. For example, if a particular lag did not show significant correlation with the outcome after the filtering, it was not a candidate for inclusion in the initial model, even before the selection procedure was performed.

Given the problems discussed with automatic procedures of this type, the high levels of correlation between the explanatory variables and the generally low explanatory power of air pollution for mortality or morbidity, such an approach is unlikely to produce stable conclusions. The APHEA study (Katsouyanni et al., 1995) took a different approach. Initially, single pollutants models were fitted and if one or more pollutant was associated with the outcome then attempts were made to separate the effects by examining associations with one pollutant stratified by the other. There was also the advantage of having a multi-city study, in which the relative levels of the pollutants were unlikely to be the same in each city. This could help in identifying interactions that may mask the effects of some pollutants. However, the model building was performed using a log transformed outcome with the final model using Poisson regression (Katsouyanni et al., 1995).

It is not clear what effect this strategy of basing the model building and the estimation on different distributional assumptions will have. This may be done to benefit from the simplicity associated with using the Normal distribution, even if the Poisson has been stated to be more appropriate. Given the relative ease with which more appropriate models can often be used, there seems little reason to introduce this additional complication to the analysis.

7.7.3   Bayesian regularization

The area of Bayesian variable selection has experienced an enormous growth in the last decades. From a Bayesian point of view, the goal is to assign prior distributions to the coefficients that give high probability around zero. In what follows, we describe two of these prior specifications. Tadesse and Vannucci (2021) present a collection of articles that describe recent advancements on Bayesian variable selection. As outlined in the preface of Tadesse and Vannucci (2021), variable selection can be performed based on hypothesis testing or by performing penalized parameter estimation. From a Bayesian point of view, the former uses Bayes factor and posterior model probabilities, whereas the latter makes use of shrinkage priors that induce sparsity. Below, we provide two examples of continuous shrinkage priors, a class of unimodal distributions that promote shrinkage of small regression coefficients towards zero (Tadesse and Vannucci, 2021).

Lasso regression

Assume that Y_l, $l = 1, \cdots, n$ follows a linear model like in Equation (7.11) and that each β_j, $j = 1, \cdots, p$, follows an independent, double exponential prior distribution, $\beta_j \sim DE(\lambda/\sigma^2)$, such that $p(\beta_j) \propto \exp\left\{-\frac{\lambda}{2\sigma^2}|\beta_j|\right\}$. It can be shown that the maximum a posterior estimate of β_j under the double exponential prior is equal to the famous least absolute shrinkage and selection operator (lasso) estimator (Tibshrani, 1996). Note that different from the original lasso, from a Bayesian point of view, the posterior does not result in probability mass at zero. Therefore, variable selection is performed using credible intervals for the regression coefficients or by defining a selection criterion on the posterior samples (Tadesse and Vannucci, 2021).

Horseshoe prior

Carvalho, Polson, and Scott (2010) propose the following hierarchical prior for β_j in Equation (7.11)

$$\beta_j \mid \lambda_j \;\sim\; N(0, \lambda_j^2),$$
$$\lambda_j \mid \tau \;\sim\; C^+(0, \tau),$$
$$\tau \mid v \;\sim\; C^+(0, v),$$

where $C^+(0,a)$ denotes a standard half-Cauchy distribution on the positive reals with scale parameter a. To complete prior specification, v follows a Jeffrey's' prior, that is $p(v^2) \propto 1/v^2$. The name of the prior is because the half-Cauchy prior for λ_j implies a horseshoe-shaped beta$(1/2,1/2)$ prior for the shrinkage coefficient. See Carvalho et al. (2010) for details.

Example 7.6. *Variable selection in land use regression using lasso and horseshoe priors*

Land use regression (LUR) is commonly used to estimate the spatial distribution of pollutant concentrations across a densely populated region. In this example, we perform selection of land use variables in a model for concentration of levels of benzene observed across 130 monitoring sites in Montreal (Zapata-Marin et al., 2022). Benzene is a volatile organic compounds (VOC) which are organic compounds that have high vapor pressures ($\sim$10 Pa) at room temperature. Acute and chronic exposures to these chemical compounds can cause adverse health effects, for example, irritation of the eyes and upper respiratory tract, and effects on the central nervous system (Zapata-Marin et al., 2022). We have some following land use variables, for example, average NOx emissions, average daily traffic volume, proportion of buildings land use, proportion of open area land use, proportion of residential area land use, population density from 2016, proportion of roads land use. The buffer radius of these land use variables is 100 m. On the online resources, we compare a linear model using independent normal prior distributions for the coefficients of the land use variables with the lasso and horseshoe priors.

7.8   What about the p-value?

As noted in Chapter 3, reproducibility has been a hallmark of science. Statistics came to play a key role in compensating for the inevitable measurement error that arises even in well-designed lab experiments and statistics provided a solution; results from repetitions of the experiment could be considered in agreement with a hypothesis if they were not *significantly* different from what one would expect to see under that hypothesis. To ensure objectivity, that meant extracting the evidence provided by the experiment and testing the (null) hypothesis (H_0) of no difference.

For reasons that are not entirely clear, the p-value (p) has become the tool of choice, even in model selection. It represents the chance of seeing evidence of a difference, that is, against H_0, at least as strong as that seen in the experiment if H_0 were true. This will include for example hypotheses about model parameters. In other words, given the sampling distribution for a test statistic $U = U(Y)$ calculated from the random sample Y and its sampling distribution, when H_0 is true, compute

$$p = P[U(Y) > U(Y_{obs})].$$

Reject H_0 if $p < 0.05$, a widely accepted 'significance level'. This simple, seemingly natural, criterion came to be universally accepted as the perfect tool for implementing the scientific method as it was seen as representing evidence in support of H_0.

Fisher originally proposed the p-value and the method described above as a 'test of significance', although he did not intend it to be used in the way it is now for confirmatory analysis. Instead, he meant it to be a descriptive tool for exploratory analysis (Nuzzo, 2014). In particular, he did not see it controlling the probability of a false positive. That came with Neyman-Pearson theory, which formalized testing. If H_0 is true, the chances are no more than 5% of falsely rejecting H_0. While it seems plausible that the test criterion $p < 0.05$ will ensure the same result, it is not true. Notably, an alternative hypothesis does not need to be specified, unlike in Neyman-Pearson theory.

Berger (2012) finds this use of the p-value as one of the reasons published scientific studies are not reproducible. Citing Ioannidis (2005), Berger states that 'of the forty-nine most famous medical publications from 1990 – 2003 resulting from randomized trials; 45 claimed successful intervention'. Out of those 45 studies, 7 (16%) were contradicted by subsequent studies, 7 (16%) had found effects that were stronger than those of subsequent studies, 20 (44%) were replicated but with issues and 11 (24%) remained largely unchallenged. Of course, not all the replication failures were due to the use of the p-value, but their use was a factor in some cases and Berger elaborates on this point noting that few non-statisticians understand p-values.

Whether there is a sensible alternative to the p-value has been extensively explored (Bayarri and Berger, 2000; Sellke, Bayarri, and Berger, 1999). One approach, based on interpreting the p-value within a Bayesian testing framework, is to quote

$$B(p) = -eplog_e(p), \tag{7.19}$$

instead of the p-value as a measure of the evidence in the sample against the null hypothesis. This is a lower bound for the appropriate Bayes factor, giving the posterior odds in favor of H_0 over H_1 at least when a priori the two hypotheses are equally likely (the conservatively objective case) (Sellke et al., 1999). As we will see in more detail in Section 7.9.1, these factors are a ratio of the posterior probabilities of the models specified under H_0 over H_1, respectively, where for each model a prior has been put on the model parameters. The lower bound $B(p)$ is obtained by finding the minimum value over all reasonable choices of those priors. If $B(p)$ were substantially larger than p, then the evidence against H_0 would not be as strong as the p would suggest.

Example 7.7. *When a p-value might not be all it seems*

This is an example based on Bayarri and Berger (1999). Let $Y_i \sim_{iid} N(\mu, 1)$, $i = 1, \ldots, N$ be a random sample and $U(\mathbf{Y}) = \bar{Y}$ the test statistic you would use to test $H_0 : \mu = 0$ if the alternative hypothesis were $H_1 : \mu \neq 0$. If $U = u$ is observed then the p-value is

$$p = 2[1 - \Phi(\sqrt{N}u \mid)].$$

If the prior distribution were $p_1(\mu)$ under H_1, the Bayes factor would be

$$B = \frac{(2p/N)^{-1/2} \exp\{-Nu^2/2\}}{\int (2p/N)^{-1/2} \exp\{-N(u-\mu)^2/2\} p_1(\mu) d\mu}. \qquad (7.20)$$

Thus given any given p, we can find the observed value, u_p, of the test statistic that would yield that p. In turn, we can find the Bayes factor and $B(p)$; the minimum value over the priors, p_1. Table 7.2 shows the result, a B-value for any p-value. The table also contains the ratio for three specific priors under the alternative. For example, a value of $p = 0.01$, which would seemingly give strong evidence against H_0, yields a B-value of 0.13; which indicates much less evidence against it.

Table 7.2: A comparison of the p and B values for Example 7.7, the latter being a lower bound for the Bayes factor in favor of H_0 over H_1. Here, three different classes of priors under the alternative are considered. From the Bayesian perspective, the p-value substantially misrepresents the evidence in the data against H_0.

p	0.10	0.05	0.01	0.001
B	0.62	0.41	0.13	0.02
Normal	0.70	0.47	0.15	0.02
Unimodal – symmetric	0.64	0.41	0.12	0.02
Symmetric	0.52	0.29	0.07	0.01

In conclusion, although the p-value has been reported routinely by almost every statistical package for coefficients in a model for several decades and is routinely used by countless researchers to decide on the significance of model parameters, its value is the subject of controversy. In 2016 the American Statistical Association issued a statement on statistical significance and p-values (Wasserstein and Lazar, 2016) that provide six principles on the use of p-values. Following up this statement, in 2019 *The American Statistician* published a special issue titled 'Statistical Inference in the 21st Century: A World Beyond $p < 0.05$'. There is the real possibility that the use of p-values false rejection of null hypotheses in scientific inquiries and has contributed to the non-reproducibility of scientific findings.

7.9 Comparison of models

In this section, alternative model comparison criteria to AIC and BIC are discussed.

7.9.1 Bayes factors

In this section, an alternative to the likelihood ratio (LR) based methods of model comparison described in Chapter 2, Section (2.5.3) is introduced. In common with those methods, Bayes factors give an indication of how much more likely the data are to have arisen under one model than another, but unlike the LR tests, the models do not have to be nested. Further details on Bayes factors, their interpretation, and calculation can be found in Kass and Raftery (1995) and O'Hagan (1995).

For illustration, the simplest case is considered, where there are just two possible models, M_0 and M_1. If the two models are assigned prior probabilities $p(M_0)$ and $p(M_1)$ then these are compared with the probabilities of the data under each of the models, $P(y|M), i = 0, 1$, the *prior predictive*, to obtain *posterior model probabilities*, $p(M_0|y)$ and $p(M_1|y)$. Contained in each model is the uncertainly associated with its parameters. For each of the models, M_k,

$$p(y|M_k) = \int p(y|\theta_k, M_k) p(\theta_k|M_k) d\theta_k. \tag{7.21}$$

From Bayes' theorem, the probability that the data was generated under the first model can be obtained,

$$p(M_0|y) = \frac{p(y|M_0) p(M_0)}{p(y)} = \frac{p(y|M_0) p(M_0)}{p(y|M_0) p(M_0) + p(y|M_1) p(M_1)}. \tag{7.22}$$

As there are only two models under question, the posterior odds of model 1 in favor of model 2 can be expressed as

$$\frac{p(M_0|y)}{p(M_1|y)} = \frac{p(y|M_0)}{p(y|M_1)} \cdot \frac{p(M_0)}{p(M_1)}. \tag{7.23}$$

The term $p(y|M_0)/p(y|M_1)$ is known as the *Bayes' factor, B_{01}* in favor of model 0 over model 1. Therefore,

$$\text{Posterior Odds} = \text{Bayes factor} \times \text{Prior Odds}. \tag{7.24}$$

As described in Chapter 5, there are often difficulties associated with the often complex, integrals involved in obtaining the posteriors. One approach, suggested by E. Kass and Wasserman (1995), to approximating the posterior model probabilities is to restrict the choice of priors in such a way that approximations to the posterior model probabilities can be made that have no dependence on the prior distributions and don't involve performing integration. They suggest approximating the posterior model probabilities using the Bayesian Information Criteria, BIC, which was introduced in Section 7.7.2 under its more common use as a measure of model fit. When using the BIC approximation, the posterior probabilities are given by $\hat{P}(M_k|Y) = L_n(\hat{\theta})_k - \frac{r_k}{2}\log n$, where $L_n(\hat{\theta})_k$ is the log likelihood evaluated at the MLE under the model k and r_k is the number of parameters in the model. This is an approximation of order $O_P(1)$. For information, the notation, $O_P()$, known as 'big O_P' indicates that the error term series is *bounded in probability*, that is, for sufficiently large enough n, the sequence of error terms is bounded by some constant, K. The smaller order of the error term sequence (for example, $1/n, 1/n^2, ...$) the smaller the error terms become for large n, and thus the better the approximation. Further details on the subject of *stochastic order* are available in Bishop, Feinburg, and Holland (1975).

To calculate Bayes factors for generalized linear models, Raftery and Richardson (1996) suggest a Laplace approximation of the form seen in Chapter 6, Section 6.2. When this is used to approximate the Bayes factor (relative to the null model) the result is

$$\hat{m}_k = L(\hat{\theta}|Y)p(\hat{\theta})2p^{r_k/2}|H|^{1/2}, \tag{7.25}$$

where $\hat{\theta}$ is the mode of the posterior $P(\theta|Y)$ and H is the matrix of second derivatives of the log-posterior evaluated at θ. This approximation has an error of order $O_P(n^{-1})$. In order to use this, the posterior mode $\hat{\theta}$ and the inverse Hessian of the log-posterior evaluated at θ are required, which are not routinely available when using standard statistical software packages.

Raftery and Richardson (1996) suggest a way of using values of the MLE, Deviance and the Fisher information matrix, I_θ which are widely available when fitting generalized linear models (see Chapter 2, Section 2.5 and McCullagh and Nelder, 1989) to estimate Bayes factors for comparing two models, again using the Bayesian Information Criteria. This approximation is of the order, $O_P(n^{-1})$ when the expected Fisher information is used for F_k, but this can be improved to $O_P(n^{-1/2})$ if the observed information is used.

Gelman et al. (2013) points out that Bayes factor works well when the underlying model is truly discrete and the goal is to compare one or the other model. Gelman et al. (2013) discuss an example for continuous models where the Bayes factor can be sensitive to the prior specification of some parameters. In the following subsections, we discuss alternative model comparison criteria.

7.9.2   *Deviance information criterion – DIC*

The deviance information criterion (DIC) (Spiegelhalter, Best, Carlin, and Van Der Linde, 2002) can be seen as a Bayesian version of the AIC. It is based on the distribution of the deviance $D(\theta) = -2L_n(\theta)$ and is given by

$$DIC = \overline{D} + p_D = 2\overline{D} - D(\overline{\theta}), \tag{7.26}$$

where $\overline{D}$ is the posterior mean of the deviance, which measures the quality of the model fitting, and $p_D = \overline{D} - D(\overline{\theta})$ is the effective number of parameters, with $\overline{\theta}$ corresponding to the posterior mean of θ. Smaller values of DIC point to the best fitting models.

Although DIC is relatively easy to compute it has some limitations, for example, the component p_D is not invariant to reparametrization. See Spiegelhalter, Best, Carlin, and van der Linde (2014) for a discussion on the drawbacks of DIC and some proposed alternatives. Gelman et al. (2013) provides an alternative definition of the effective number of parameters which is more numerically stable.

7.9.3 Watanabe–Akaike information criterion – WAIC

Watanabe (2010) proposed the Watanabe–Akaike information criterion (WAIC) which is considered more fully Bayesian than the DIC. WAIC averages over the posterior distribution instead of conditioning on a point estimate (Gelman et al., 2013). Once a sample from the posterior distribution of the parameter vector θ based on sample $\mathbf{y} = (y_1, \cdots, y_n)'$ is available, it is computed as (Gelman et al., 2013)

$$WAIC = -2\left(\sum_{i=1}^{n} \log\left(\frac{1}{L} \sum_{l=1}^{L} p(y_i \mid \theta^{(l)}) \right) - \sum_{i=1}^{n} V_{l=1}^{L}(\log(p(y_i \mid \theta^{(l)}))) \right), \quad (7.27)$$

where $V_{l=1}^{L}(\log(p(y_i \mid \theta^{(l)})))$ is the posterior variance of the log predictive density for each observation y_i; this component represents the effective number of parameters to adjust for model overfitting (Gelman et al., 2013). Smaller values indicate the best fitting model. Both Nimble and Stan provide values of WAIC. In Stan, the user must compute the pointwise likelihood in the `Generated Quantities` block.

7.10 Bayesian model averaging

In Section 7.7.2, the traditional approach to model 'selection' was considered, that of choosing a single model which is then considered to be correct when drawing inference about the parameters of interest or performing prediction. This ignores the inherent uncertainty associated with the actual modeling process, and in particular the uncertainty which arises through selecting a subset of variables for inclusion, together with that due to distributional assumptions and/or transformations.

This section describes an alternative approach where, rather than choosing a single model, information from several models is combined to obtain averaged estimates and/or predicted values. To illustrate this concept, consider the notation for the regression example introduced in Section 7.7.1 with two potential covariates, X_1 and X_2, and $m = 4$ possible models, which are shown in Table 7.3.

Table 7.3: Possible models and posterior model probabilities using combinations of two covariates, with ε_i $(i = 1, 2, 3, 4) \sim$ i.i.d $N(0, \sigma_i^2)$.

Model	Formula	Posterior Probability
M_1	$Y = \beta_0^1 + \varepsilon_1$	$p(M_1\|y)$
M_2	$Y = \beta_0^2 + \beta_1^2 X_1 + \varepsilon_2$	$p(M_2\|y)$
M_3	$Y = \beta_0^3 + \beta_2^3 X_2 + \varepsilon_3$	$p(M_3\|y)$
M_4	$Y = \beta_0^4 + \beta_1^4 X_1 + \beta_2^4 X_2 + \varepsilon_4$	$p(M_4\|y)$

The choice is then to

1. choose the single model with the highest posterior probability, $p(M_i|Y)$, and use this to draw inference about the effects of the covariates (or to predict), ignoring the model uncertainty in the same way as would be done by picking a single model as the result of some likelihood comparison or stepwise procedure.

2. Examine the estimates from all four of the models separately, which introduces the problem of multiple comparisons and might not be very useful if a single estimate/predicted value is required.

3. Combine the information from the four models.

The last approach is the essence of the Bayesian modeling averaging approach, inference on the parameters of interest and/or prediction is performed using weighted averages of the values from the individual models. The process is carried out within a Bayesian framework; each of the candidate models is assigned a prior probability, which is updated using information from the data to obtain posterior model probabilities. Recently, Porwal and Raftery (2022) compared three adaptive Bayesian models averaging methods with the most popular Bayesian and penalized likelihood methods, resulting in 21 different approaches. For each of these approaches, the data generating model was based on 14 different datasets, from different fields. They found that Bayesian model average performed better than Bayesian model selection, when just one model is selected.

Consideration should be given to the fact that inference about an unknown parameter will be dependent on the structure of the model under examination, M_k, and the set of other variables included in that model. In order to calculate posterior probabilities for the parameters, one should condition not only on the observed data but also on the model in question. This is now incorporated into the model uncertainty framework. Given m candidate models, $M_1, ..., M_m$ ($m = 2^p$), each with prior probability, $p(M_i)$ (the simplest example being where all the models are considered equally likely before any data is observed, where $p(M_k) = 1/m$), then the posterior probability for the model, M_k can be found using Bayes' theorem in the following way:

$$p(M_k|y) = \frac{p(y|M_k)p(M_k)}{\sum_{l=1}^{m} p(y|M_l)p(M_l)}. \tag{7.28}$$

Contained in each model is the uncertainty associated with its parameters. For ease of illustration, the following description is given in terms of the regression parameters, β. For each of the models, M_k,

$$p(y|M_k) = \int p(y|\beta_k, M_k)p(\beta_k|M_k)d\beta_k. \tag{7.29}$$

Therefore, given prior probability distributions for the unknown parameters, $p(\beta|M_k)$, under a particular model, M_k, then, conditioning on the model, gives

$$p(\beta|Y, M_k) = \frac{p(y|\beta, M_k)p(\beta|M_k)}{p(y|M_k)},$$

with $p(y|M_k) = \int p(y|\beta, M_k)p(\beta|M_k)d\beta$.

In order to predict a future observation, $Z = \hat{Y}$, using the model in question, the predictive distribution is given by

$$p(Z|y, M_k) = \int p(Z|\theta, M_k)p(\theta|y, M_k)d\theta. \tag{7.30}$$

The Bayes factors comparing two models, M_k and M_l, is then defined as

$$B_{kl} = \frac{p(M_k|y)}{p(M_l|y)} = \frac{\int p(y|\beta_k)p_k(\beta_k)d\beta_k}{\int p(y|\beta_l)p_l(\beta_l)d\beta_l}. \tag{7.31}$$

When the posterior model probabilities have been obtained, the weighted posterior distributions of the individual parameters can be calculated, allowing the effect of individual covariates to be assessed. The weighted posterior density, mean and variance of the parameters of interest, β_j can be calculated as follows

$$
\begin{aligned}
p(\beta_j|y) &= \sum_{l=1}^{m} p(\beta_j^l|y, M_l)p(M_l|y) \\
E(\beta_j|y) &= \sum_{l=1}^{m} \overline{\beta}_j^l p(M_l|y) \\
\mathrm{VAR}(\beta_j|y) &= E_{M|y}[\mathrm{VAR}(\beta_j|y, M_l)] + \mathrm{VAR}_{M|y}[E(\beta_j|y, M_l)] \\
&= \sum_{l=1}^{m} (\sigma_j^l)^2 p(M_l|y) + \sum_{l=1}^{m} (\overline{\beta}_j^l - \overline{\beta}_j)^2 p(M_l|y) \\
&= \text{within model uncertainty} + \text{between model uncertainty},
\end{aligned}
$$

(7.32)

(7.33)

where $\overline{\beta}_j^l = E(\beta_j|y, M_l)$, is the posterior mean of value of the regression coefficient, β_j, under model M_l, and $\overline{\beta}_j = E(\beta_j|y)$.

When performing prediction of a new observation, $\hat{Y} = E(Z|y, X^*)$, using a particular model, the predictive distribution is given by

$$p(Z|y, M_k) = \int p(Z|\beta^k, X^*, M_k)p(\beta^k|y, M_k)d\beta^k. \tag{7.34}$$

When all models are considered, the resulting prediction will be a weighted average of the predicted values from all the possible models

$$p(Z|X^*) = \sum_{l=1}^{m} P_l(Z|M_l, y, X^*)p(M_l|y). \tag{7.35}$$

With expected value

$$
\begin{aligned}
E[Z|y, X^*] &= E_{M|y}[E[Z|y, X^*, M]] \\
&= \sum_{l=1}^{m} E[Z|y, X^*, M_l]p(M_l|y),
\end{aligned}
\tag{7.36}
$$

and variance

$$
\begin{aligned}
V[Z|y,X^*] &= E_{M|y}[VAR[Z|y,X^*,M]] + VAR_{M|y}[E[Z|y,X^*,M]] \\
&= \sum_{l=1}^{m} VAR[Z|y,X^*,M_l]p(M_l|Y) + \\
&\quad \sum_{l=1}^{m}(Z_l - \bar{Z})^2 p(M_l|y).
\end{aligned}
\tag{7.37}
$$

where Z_l is the predicted value using model M_l, and $\bar{Z} = E[Z|y,X^*]$.

7.10.1 Interpretation

It is natural to ask about the interpretation of a coefficient arising from a Bayesian model averaging procedure. For illustration, consider again the case of normal linear regression with just two covariates, X_1 and X_2 as described in Table 7.3. Considering Z, the predicted value given values of X_1 and X_2,

$$
E(Z|\beta_0,\beta_1,...,\beta_p,X_1,X_2,y) = \beta_0 + \beta_1 X_1 + \beta_2 X_2.
\tag{7.38}
$$

Expanding this expression over all the possible values of β gives,

$$
\begin{aligned}
E(Z|X,y) &= E_{\beta|y}(E(Z|X,\beta_0,\beta_1,\beta_2,y)) \\
&= E_{\beta|y}(\beta_0 + \beta_1 X_1 + \beta_2 X_2,y) \\
&= E(\beta_0|y) + E(\beta_1|y)X_1 + E(\beta_2|y)X_2.
\end{aligned}
\tag{7.39}
$$

Taking expectations over the set of possible models gives

$$
\begin{aligned}
E(Z|X) &= E_{M|y}(E(Z|X,M_k,y)) \\
&= E_{M|y}(E_{\beta|y}(E(Z|X,M_k,\beta,y))) \\
&= \sum_{l=1}^{4} E_{\beta|y}(E(Z|X,M_l,\beta,X,y))p(M_l|y),
\end{aligned}
\tag{7.40}
$$

where $X = (X_1,X_2)'$. Hence

$$
\begin{aligned}
E(Z|X) = {}& E(\beta_0|y,X,M_1)p(M_1|y) \\
+ {}& \{E(\beta_0|y,X,M_2) + E(\beta_1|y,X,M_2)\}\,p(M_2|y)) \\
+ {}& \{E(\beta_0|y,X,M_3) + E(\beta_2|y,X,M_3)\}\,p(M_3|y)) \\
+ {}& \{E(\beta_0|y,X,M_4) + E(\beta_1|y,X,M_4) + E(\beta_2|y,X,M_4)\}\,p(M_4|y)).
\end{aligned}
\tag{7.41}
$$

In the above, in model M_2 for example, $E(Z|X,\beta_0,\beta_1) = \beta_0 + \beta_1 X_1$, so that even if the value of X_2 were known, it wouldn't be used in that model. If $\beta^l = (\beta_0^l,\beta_1^l,\beta_2^l)$

is the set of parameter estimates found under model l then

$$
\begin{aligned}
E(Z|X_1,X_2,\beta^1,\beta^2,\beta^3,\beta^4,y) &= \beta_0^1 p(M_1|y) \\
&+ [\beta_0^2 + \beta_1^2 X_1]p(M_2|y) \\
&+ [\beta_0^3 + \beta_2^3 X_2]p(M_3|y) \qquad (7.42) \\
&+ [\beta_0^4 + \beta_1^4 X_1 + \beta_2^4 X_2]p(M_4|y).
\end{aligned}
$$

A unit increase in X_1 will therefore result in a predicted value of Z'

$$
\begin{aligned}
E(Z'|X_1+1,X_2,\beta^1,\beta^2,\beta^3,\beta^4,y) &= \beta_0^1 p(M_1|y) \\
&+ [\beta_0^2 + \beta_1^2 (X_1+1)]p(M_2|y) \\
&+ [\beta_0^3 + \beta_2^3 X_2]p(M_3|y) \qquad (7.43) \\
&+ [\beta_0^4 + \beta_1^4 (X_1+1) + \beta_2^4 X_2]p(M_4|y).
\end{aligned}
$$

The difference is

$$
\begin{aligned}
E(Z'|X_1+1,X_2,\beta^1,\beta^2,\beta^3,\beta^4,y) &- E(Z|X_1,X_2,\beta^1,\beta^2,\beta^3,\beta^4,y) \\
&= \beta_1^2 p(M_2|y) - \beta_1^4 p(M_4|y). \qquad (7.44)
\end{aligned}
$$

This weighted average (by the posterior model probabilities) of the effects from each of the models in which X_1 is included, gives a natural interpretation for a regression coefficient obtained using Bayesian model averaging.

Unlike the traditional approach of selecting just one model in which the estimate of a parameter of interest might be highly affected by the choice of which other variables to include/exclude in the model, this estimate allows for the fact that other variables may also be in the model. An estimate of the weight of support for including X_1 in the model can be found by summing the posterior probabilities for the models that include the variable

$$
p(X_1 \text{ should be included}) = \sum_{l=1}^{m} P(M_l|y, \text{ model } l \text{ contains } X_1). \qquad (7.45)
$$

Only models that contain the particular variable, X_1, and that have non-zero posterior probabilities will contribute to this sum, as is the case for the weighted averages in Equation 7.40.

Example 7.8. *Bayesian model averaging in studies of air pollution and health*

In studies of the effects of air pollution on mortality, it is often more appropriate to use Poisson regression, rather than simple linear regression. In this case, the expectation of the predicted value, Z, in the two covariate example is given by

$$E(Z|\beta_0,\beta_1,\beta_2,X_1,X_2,y) = \exp(\beta_0 + \beta_1 X_1 + \beta_2 X_2, y). \qquad (7.46)$$

When this expectation is expanded to condition on the possible models, as in Equation (7.40), it gives

$$
\begin{aligned}
E(Z|X) &= \sum_{l=1}^{4} E_\beta(E(Z|M_l,\beta,X,y))p(M_l|y) \\
&= \exp(\beta_0^1|y)p(M_1|y) \\
&+ \exp(\beta_0^2 + \beta_1^2 X_1|y)p(M_2|y) \\
&+ \exp(\beta_0^3 + \beta_2^3 X_2|y)p(M_3|y) \\
&+ \exp(\beta_0^4 + \beta_1^4 X_1 + \beta_2^4 X_2|y)p(M_4|y). \qquad (7.47)
\end{aligned}
$$

A unit change in X_1 (with X_2 remaining constant) again only results in changes in the predictions from the two models that contain X_1 (2 and 4), the difference between the two predicted values is now represented by

$$
\begin{aligned}
& p(M_2|y)[\exp(\beta_0^2 + \beta_1^2(X_1+1))/\exp(\beta_0^2 + \beta_1^2 X_1)] \\
+ & p(M_4|y)[\exp(\beta_0^4 + \beta_1^4(X_1+1) + \beta_2^4 X_2)/\exp(\beta_0^4 + \beta_1^4 X_1 + \beta_2^4 X_2)] \\
= & p(M_2|y)[\exp(\beta_1^2(X_1+1))/\exp(\beta_1^2 X_1)]) \qquad (7.48) \\
+ & p(M_4|y)[\exp(\beta_1^4(X_1+1) + \beta_2^4 X_2)/\exp(\beta_1^4 X_1 + \beta_2^4 X_2)].
\end{aligned}
$$

This non-linear expression of the regression coefficient for X_1 is not the same as would be obtained by simply calculating a weighted average of the coefficients from each model and taking the exponent, that is $\exp(p(M_2|y)\beta_1^1 + p(M_4|y)\beta_1^4)$. Despite this problem, the models can still be used for prediction, as the individual predictions are made under the conditions of the specific models and the resultant predicted values averaged to produce a single final predictive value. For prediction, the fact that the effects of the individual parameters have been lost is not important, as the interest is in the combined effect of all the covariates. In the case of pollution, for example, the ability to interpret the effect of a $25\mu\mathrm{gm}^{-3}$ increase of PM_{10} on the risk of respiratory deaths for all values of PM_{10} would be lost, but it could be found for categories of values, such as 0–25, 25–50, etc. and the ability to predict the additional number of respiratory deaths associated with an increase in PM_{10}, given values for other covariates, such as SO_2, CO, O_3 and temperature is retained.

7.11   Summary

This chapter considers both some wider issues related to modeling and the generalizability of results, together with more technical material on the effect of covariates and model selection. The reader will have gained an understanding of the following topics:

- Why having contrasts in the variables of interest is important in assessing the effects they have on the response variable.

- The biases that may arise in the presence of covariates and how covariates can affect variable selection and model choice.

- Hierarchical models and how that can be used to acknowledge dependence between observations.

- There are issues with using p-values as measures of evidence against a null hypothesis, and why basing scientific conclusions on it can lead to non-reproducible results.

- The use of predictions from exposure models, including acknowledging the additional uncertainty involved when using predictions as inputs to a health model.

- Methods for performing model selection, including the pros and cons of automatic selection procedures.

- Model selection within the Bayesian setting, and how the models themselves can be incorporated into the estimation process using Bayesian Model Averaging.

7.12   Exercises

Exercise 7.1. Elliott et al. (1996) performed a study to investigate the possible effects of municipal incinerators on health. Read this paper and consider the following issues:

(i) What was the population under study?

(ii) What factors might you want to know before generalizing the results, for example, to other countries?

(iii) What was the time period of the study? Are the results still valid today?

(iv) If an incinerator blew up, would you be happy applying the risk estimates obtained in this study to the surrounding population?

Exercise 7.2. In modeling the effects of land use covariates on NO_2 concentrations in Europe (Shaddick, Yan, et al., 2013), there were many possible explanatory variables. These variables are listed, together with their mean values, in Table 7.4. The models were fit on a training set, with predictions from the models used to predict concentrations at locations in a validation set. The concentrations were known at the validation locations, and so a comparison with the predictions could be made.

(i) Are there any substantial differences between the training and validation sets? What effect might such differences have on the assessment of the prediction model built using the training set?

(ii) Often, the sample size may not be large enough to split a dataset into a training and validation set in this way. What other methods can you think of to assess the predictive ability of the model?

Table 7.4: Summary (means) of covariates at locations of NO_2 monitoring sites in Europe; (1) variables constructed at 1 km and (21) at 21 km resolution.

Covariate	Training set	Validation set	EU
Altitude (m)	220	236	410
Distance to sea (m)	202	198	145
Climate factor 1 (1)	0.83	0.87	1.11
Climate factor 2 (1)	−0.42	−0.44	0.15
Climate factor 3 (1)	0.25	0.30	0.18
Climate factor 4 (1)	0.05	0.02	0.05
Climate factor 5 (1)	−0.03	−0.06	0.02
Non-Residential Built Up (21)	3.72	3.47	0.46
Forestry (1)	9.03	10.24	21.47
Agriculture (21)	45.95	46.97	52.08
Major roads (1)	0.65	0.62	0.10
Minor roads (1)	2.42	2.28	0.82
High density residential (1)	11.00	12.14	0.39
Low density residential (1)	38.83	35.9	2.47
Industry (1)	6.12	6.00	0.39
Transport (1)	0.93	0.87	0.04
Sea Ports (1)	0.30	0.44	0.03
Air Ports (1)	0.20	0.03	0.08
Construction (1)	0.56	0.35	0.20
Urban Greenery (1)	2.24	1.72	0.22
Forestry (1)	9.03	10.24	22.24

(iii) How would you choose the best set of variables from those in Table 7.4 to predict NO_2 concentrations?

(iv) Many of the variables seen in Table 7.4 are likely to be highly correlated. How might this affect your choice of which covariates should be included in the model?

(v) The data for this example are included in the online resources. Using this data, perform an appropriate statistical test, or tests, to quantify your answer to (i).

(vi) Perform an automatic stepwise procedure to choose a subset of the variables with which to predict NO_2 concentrations. Comment on whether you are happy with the choice of variables, considering your response to question (iv).

Exercise 7.3. Show that in the simplest case where the prior probabilities of two possible models, M_0 and M_1 are equal to 1/2 that posterior odds will equal the Bayes factor.

Exercise 7.4. In the case of the Poisson regression example shown in Example 7.8, consider the case where there are three covariates, X_1, X_2, X_3.

(i) Derive an equivalent expression to that seen in Equation 7.47 for the three covariate case.

(ii) Derive an expression for the relative risk when X_1 is increased by one unit.

(iii) Derive an expression for the relative risk when both X_1 and X_2 are simultaneously increased by one unit.

Chapter 8

The challenges of working with real-world data

8.1 Overview

Epidemiological studies require accurate measurements of both health outcomes, potential confounders and estimates of exposures that might drive associations with health (Finazzi, Scott, and Fassò, 2013). These may be measured with varying degrees of error. Considering measurements of air pollution, for example, there is a true underlying pollution surface which will form the basis of the exposures experienced by the population at risk. However, this surface is not directly observable and instead measurements are taken at locations over space and time. Differences between these exposure measurements and the unknown underlying field are often referred to as *measurement error*. Here the term measurement error is taken to refer to any difference between the underlying true values and what is measured. Traditionally measurement error has been based around the idea of repeated measurements of a value, for example, measuring blood pressure where repeated measurements will contain a component of error, often assumed to be random. In modeling exposures and in spatial epidemiology, error will possibly comprise several factors including monitor calibration error and random variation, but also variations in the underlying pollution field over time and space which aren't acknowledged in the analyzes. This may arise for example when modeling assumptions are too simplistic for the complex surface of the pollution field.

There are also likely to be periods of missing data in the exposure information. Simple methods for handling missing values are commonly used, including simply discarding them from the analysis or replacing them with a specific single value, for example, the overall mean. By discarding missing values, we may lose useful information and may introduce bias. When replacing missing values by a single value, for example, a sample mean of observations or the posterior mean from an exposure model, the intrinsic variability associated with the summary value may be ignored.

Where a health effects analysis uses predictions from an exposure model as substitutes for actual measures of exposures, as with regular measurement error, there is the possibility of bias in the estimation of risks. An additional issue termed the 'change of support' problem by Gelfand et al. (2001) occurs when the exposure and health outcome data are recorded at different levels of aggregation, for

DOI: 10.1201/9781003352655-8

example health counts for administrative areas and exposures from monitoring sites at point locations within, or outside, those areas.

It is also a common phenomenon that monitors in an environmental monitoring network are often located in a non-random fashion. For example, they are often located to check for adherence to statutory limits and if monitors are positioned close to known pollution sources, such as roads or industrial plants, then the estimated pollution surface is likely to be overestimated. This is known as *preferential sampling*. It is very important that the information coming from networks is accurate and reflects the levels of exposure that may be experienced by the populations at risk. This might be a problem if monitors are placed in locations where pollution might be expected to be high. Formally, preferential sampling occurs when the process that determines the locations of the monitoring sites and the process being modeled are in some ways dependent (Diggle, Menezes, and Su, 2010). For example, in the study of air pollution and health, Guttorp and Sampson (2010) state that the choice of locations for air pollution monitoring sites may be for several reasons, including measuring: (i) background levels outside urban areas; (ii) levels in residential areas and (iii) levels near pollutant sources. Geostatistical methods which assume sampling is non-preferential are often used despite preferential sampling (Diggle et al., 2010). Ignoring preferential sampling may lead to incorrect inferences and biased estimates of pollution concentrations and thus any subsequent estimation of health risks.

In this chapter, we review approaches to classifying missing values and consider measurement error and the effect that it may have on estimates obtained from regression models. We also provide a review of how preferential sampling can affect assessments of exposures that might be used within a health analysis and methods that might be used to adjust for its effects.

8.2   Missing values

In real-life applications, data are often incomplete and there are many reasons why observations may be missing. Here, we follow the notation proposed by Little and Rubin (2014) who classify the process which leads to missing data as either (i) completely random, (ii) random or (iii) informative. Let Y denote the complete set of data which would be available if there were no missing values. Since this situation is unlikely in practice we split the dataset into $Y = (Y_{obs}, Y_{mis})$ where Y_{obs} are the observed data and Y_{mis} the missing observations.

For the classification of the missing values, we denote R_i as a indicator which takes values 1 or 0 dependent on whether Y_i is a missing value or not. The missing data mechanism can therefore be classified in the following ways:

1. Completely random (MCAR): if R_i is independent of both Y_{obs} and Y_{mis}.

2. Random (MAR): if R_i is independent of Y_{mis}.

3. Informative: if R_i is dependent on Y_{mis}.

If the missing data mechanism can be assumed to be non-informative, that is MAR or MCAR and if $f(y_{obs}, y_{mis}, r)$ denotes the joint probability density function of

(Y_{obs}, Y_{mis}, R) then this can be factorized in

$$f(y_{obs}, y_{mis}, r) = f(y_{obs}, y_{mis}) f(r|y_{obs}, y_{mis}) \qquad (8.1)$$

Integrating out the missing values, the joint pdf of the observable random variables, (Y_{obs}, R), can be obtained

$$f(y_{obs}, r) = \int_{y_{mis}} f(y_{obs}, y_{mis}) f(r|y_{obs}, y_{mis}) dy_{mis} \qquad (8.2)$$

Under the assumption that the missing data mechanism is non-informative we conclude to the following equation

$$f(y_{obs}, r) \quad = f(r|y_{obs}) \int f(y_{obs}, y_{mis}) dy_{mis} \qquad (8.3)$$
$$= f(r|y_{obs}) f(y_{obs}) \qquad (8.4)$$

Taking logarithms gives

$$L = log(f(r|y_{obs}) + log(f(y_{obs})) \qquad (8.5)$$

Maximizing L here is achieved by maximizing the second part of the right-hand side, $log(f(y_{obs}))$, meaning that the estimation of the model parameters does not depend on the missing data mechanism.

8.2.1   Imputation

Trivial methods of handling missing values include simply discarding them from the analysis or replacing them with a specific single value, for example, the overall mean. By discarding missing values we may lose useful information, and by replacing a missing value with a single value we may ignore important features of the dataset and ignore intrinsic variability.

A more sophisticated method is multiple imputation (Little and Rubin, 2014). This replaces missing values with a set of plausible values that acknowledge the inherent uncertainty associated with the unobserved value. After the imputation of the missing values, multiple complete-value datasets are produced and a combined analysis of these datasets is performed. This results in valid statistical inferences that properly reflect the uncertainty due to missing values.

Two simple examples of imputation are presented here; the first is based in a regression method that assumes multivariate normality, and a description of how the imputed values are calculated and the complete-values datasets are obtained is given. The second method, set within a Bayesian framework, was proposed by J. Schafer (1997). Instead of producing multiple complete-value datasets, the missing values are drawn from a posterior distribution, given the observed data, in each iteration of an MCMC algorithm.

8.2.2   Regression method

The regression method requires that the missing values appear in a monotone pattern. The basic idea is that a regression model is fitted with the variable with missing values as the response, with previous values as covariates. For a variable Y_j, this can be represented with missing values as

$$Y_j = \beta_0 + \beta_1 Y_1 +, \ldots, + \beta_{j-1} Y_{j-1}$$

Since the data has missing values in monotone pattern, $Y_1, \ldots, Y_{j-1}$ do not have missing values. After estimation of the regression parameters $(\hat{\beta}_0, \hat{\beta}_1, \ldots, \hat{\beta}_{j-1})$ with corresponding covariance matrix $\sigma_j^2 V_j$, and after each imputation, new estimates of the parameters are drawn. The imputation is performed by replacing the missing values with

$$\hat{\beta}_0 + \hat{\beta}_1 y_1 +, \ldots, + \hat{\beta}_{j-1} y_{j-1} + z_i \sigma_j$$

where $(y_1, y_2, \ldots, y_{j-1})$ are the covariates and z_i follows a zero-mean normal distribution, $N(0, 1)$.

8.2.3   MCMC method

In Bayesian inference, a prior distribution is assigned to each parameter and after observing the data, information about these parameters is expressed in the form of a posterior distribution. Using imputation to treat the missing values in an MCMC algorithm is akin to treating missing values as unknown parameters. Once we obtain draws from the unknown parameters from their posterior distributions given the observed data, simulation-based estimates can be obtained for the missing values. This method is called Expectation – Maximization (EM). Basically, the EM algorithm is performed in two steps which are as follows:

i. In the Expectation or E-step, the unknown parameters of the model are assumed to have already been estimated. Estimates are drawn from the posterior distributions given Y_{obs}, $P(Y_{mis}|Y_{obs}, \theta^t)$ where t is the current number of iterations in the MCMC algorithm.

ii. In the maximization or M-step estimation, values of the unknown parameters, θ^{t+1} are drawn given the complete-value dataset and are used to perform the following E-step.

Further details of the EM algorithm and its properties can be found in J. Schafer (1997).

8.3   Measurement error

Measurement error is a general term used to encompass situations where the observed data do not represent the quantity of interest exactly. It can occur in both response variables and covariates. Epidemiological studies require accurate measurements of both health outcomes and exposures together with potential confounders. All of these data may be measured with varying degrees of error. Consider measurements of air pollution; there is a true underlying pollution surface that will drive the exposures experienced by the population at risk. However, this surface is not directly observable and instead measurements are taken at locations over space and time. Differences between these exposure measurements and the unknown underlying field is often referred to as measurement error. In this sense, the term measurement error is taken to refer to any difference between the underlying true values and what is measured.

Traditionally, measurement error has developed around the idea of repeated measurements of a value, for example measuring blood pressure, in which the repeated measurements will contain a component of error that is often assumed to be random. In spatio-temporal epidemiology, error may be comprised of several factors including monitor calibration error and random variation, but also variations in the underlying pollution field over time and space which aren't acknowledged in the model. This may arise for example when the modeling assumptions are too simplistic for the complex surface of the pollution field. Another issue that is often contained under the umbrella term of 'measurement error' is the misalignment of locations or times of exposure measurements and health outcomes. This arises because exposure and health data are often drawn from independent sources and not the result of a carefully designed study. In which case a straightforward comparison is not possible without a model to align these elements in the spatial and temporal domains (Gryparis et al., 2009; Peng and Bell, 2010). In such settings, health effects analysis may use predictions from an exposure model as substitutes for actual measures of exposures in the health model.

A brief review of measurement error models is given here while more comprehensive discussions can be found in Fuller (1987); Carroll, Ruppert, and Stefanski (1995). Measurement error models are based on four quantities:

- $Y^{(1)}$ – the response variable;

- Z – the true unobserved exposures;

- $Y^{(2)}$ – the observed exposures which are measurements of Z, potentially incorporating some measure of error;

- X – covariates, which are assumed to be measured exactly.

The joint likelihood of these quantities can be expressed as

$$f(Y^{(1)}, X, Y^{(2)} | Z) = f(Y^{(1)} | X, Y^{(2)}, Z) f(X, Y^{(2)} | Z) \tag{8.6}$$

where the covariates are conditioned on because they are fixed and known. The first element of Equation 8.6 is an exposure-response model, of the form described in Chapter 13, Section 13.5.1 and seen in Chapter 2. It is typically simplified to $f(Y^{(1)} | Z, X)$ by assuming the measurement error is non-differential, that is $Y^{(1)}$ and $Y^{(2)}$ are conditionally independent given Z. The second element in Equation 8.6 is a measurement error model, which represents the relationship between the unobserved exposure Z and the measured surrogate $Y^{(2)}$. There are two types of measurement error models; classical and Berkson, which are outlined below.

8.3.1   Classical measurement error

Classical measurement error models rely on the following factorization

$$f(Z, Y^{(2)} | X) = f(Y^{(2)} | Z, X) f(Z | X)$$

the first element of which is a conditional model for the measured surrogate $Y^{(2)}$ given the true (unobserved) exposure Z. Two common classical measurement error models are (i) additive and (ii) error calibration as follows.

(i) $Y_i^{(2)} \sim N(Z_i, \sigma^2)$ for $i = 1, ..., n$

(ii) $Y_i^{(2)} \sim N(\beta_0 + \beta_z Z_i + \sum_{j=1}^J \beta_j X_{ji}, \sigma^2)$ for $i = 1, ..., n$

In the simple additive formulation, the observed surrogate is assumed to be correct on average (i.e. $E[Y_i^{(2)}|Z_i] = Z_i$), while in model (ii) the surrogate is biased. Both models specify an additive relationship between $Y_i^{(2)}$ and Z_i, an alternative being a multiplicative error model $Y_i^{(2)} = Z_i v_i$, where v_i is a zero mean Gaussian error with variance σ^2. The remaining term $f(Z|X)$ can be based on knowledge of that true exposure or represent prior ignorance. In the latter case, a common choice is the production of normal distributions, each of which has a large variance, for example $\prod_{i=1}^n N(Z_i|\mu, \tau^2)$ where τ^2 is large. In a Bayesian setting $f(Z|X)$ acts as a prior for the unknown exposure Z.

8.3.2 Berkson measurement error

In contrast to the classical case, the Berkson measurement error model relies on the following factorization:

$$f(Z, Y^{(2)}|X) = f(Z|Y^{(2)}, X) f(Y^{(2)}|X)$$

where the first term is a conditional model for the true exposure Z given the measured surrogate $Y^{(2)}$. Again, there are two common approaches; (iii) additive and (iv) regression calibration. In common with the classical models $f(Z|Y^{(2)}, X)$ is a decomposition of independent distributions for each observation.

(iii) $Z_i \sim N(Y^{(2)}, \sigma^2)$ for $i = 1, ..., n$

(iv) $Z_i \sim N(\beta_0 Y_i^{(2)} + \beta_{Y(2)} Y_i^{(2)} + \sum_{j=1}^J \beta_p X_{ji}, \sigma^2)$ for $i = 1, ..., n$

In the simple additive model the true exposure is assumed to be equal to the surrogate on average (i.e. $E[Z_i|Y_i^{(2)}] = Y_i^{(2)}$), but this is not true for (iv). As with classical models, a multiplicative alternative can be used, which is implemented using an additive model on the log scale. In the Berkson model, as $Y^{(2)}$ are known measurements, the distribution $f(Y^{(2)}|X)$ can be ignored. The choice between classical and Berkson models will depend on the structure of the problem as well as the set of available data. Further details can be found in Carroll et al. (1995).

The measurement error models described above can only be used if additional data are available, because the information from $(Y^{(1)}, Y^{(2)}, X)$ is not sufficient to estimate the measurement error process. Examples of such additional data include repeated measurements of $Y^{(2)}$, which in a spatial setting may be measurements at each location over time. Alternatively, external data may be able to inform the process if observed values of Z and $Y^{(2)}$ were available at a subset of locations. The identifiability of a proposed model may also depend on the assumptions made about the measurement error process. There are two general classes of such assumptions;

functional and structural. Functional models are distribution invariant and specify minimal assumptions about the measurement error process. They do not specify a proper likelihood, and estimation is typically based on regression calibration and the SIMEX algorithm (Carroll et al., 1995). In contrast, structural models, such as those shown in (i) to (iv), are fully parametric and specify probability distributions for $f(Y^{(2)}|Z,X)$ or $f(Z|Y^{(2)},X)$. The choice between functional and structural models determines the method of estimation and inference that can be used, with structural models enabling likelihood and Bayesian methods to be applied. A brief outline of estimation techniques for measurement error models is given in the next section. For a more comprehensive treatment, the reader is referred to (Carroll et al., 1995).

8.3.3 Attenuation and bias

Covariate measurement error typically causes non-measurement error models to produce biased estimates of the regression parameters, and except for the simple linear model $Y_i^{(1)} \sim N(\beta_0 + \beta_Z X_i, \sigma_v^2)$, understanding the nature of this bias may not be straightforward. In this simple case replacing Z by $Y^{(2)}$ yields the model $Y_i^{(1)} \sim N(\beta_0 \times + \beta_{Y(2)} Y_i^{(2)}, \sigma_{v2}^2)$, which estimates $\beta_{Y(2)}$ instead of the relationship of interest, β_Z. As Z is unknown β_Z can only be estimated using measurement error methods, and a simple classical model is given by

$$
\begin{aligned}
Y_i^{(1)} &\sim N(\beta_0 + \beta_Z Z_i, \sigma_{v1}^2) \\
Y_i^{(2)} &\sim N(Z_i, \sigma_{v2}^2) \\
Z_i &\sim N(\mu, \sigma_z^2)
\end{aligned} \tag{8.7}
$$

For this model it can be shown that $\beta_{Y(2)} = \frac{\sigma_z^2}{\sigma_z^2 + \sigma_{v2}^2} \beta_z$ (Fuller, 1987) and so naively replacing Z with $Y^{(2)}$ and ignoring measurement error results in a biased estimate of β_Z. This bias is known as attenuation, with β_Z being shrunk towards zero by a factor of $\frac{\sigma_z^2}{\sigma_z^2 + \sigma_{v2}^2}$. In addition, allowing for measurement error inflates the variance from σ_{v1}^2 using the simple linear model to $\sigma_{v1}^2 + \frac{\beta_Z \sigma_{v2}^2 \sigma_z^2}{\sigma_z^2 + \sigma_{v2}^2}$ if Equation 8.7 is used.

In contrast with the Berkson error model,

$$
\begin{aligned}
Y_i^{(1)} &\sim N(\beta_0 + \beta_Z Z_i, \sigma_\varepsilon^2) \\
Z_i &\sim N(Y^{(2)}, \sigma_u^2)
\end{aligned} \tag{8.8}
$$

there is no attenuation, meaning that $\beta_{Y(2)} = \beta_Z$. However, in common with the classical model incorporating measurement error inflates the variance to $Var[Y_i^{(1)}|Y_i^{(2)}] = \sigma_\varepsilon^2 + \beta_Z^2 \sigma_u^2$.

Although the effects of measurement error are well known for the Gaussian linear model, the corresponding effects for more complex linear and non-linear models may be unknown.

8.3.4 Estimation

Here we concentrate on estimation for structural measurement error models. The parameters in the model are collectively denoted by Ω, which can be estimated by maximizing the joint likelihood of $(Y^{(1)}, Y^{(2)})$ given by

$$f(Y^{(1)}, Y^{(2)}|X, \Omega) = \int_Z f(Y^{(1)}, Z, Y^{(2)}|X, \Omega)dZ \qquad (8.9)$$

As previously described, $f(Y^{(1)}, Y^{(1)}|X, \Omega)$ can be factorized according to either classical or Berkson error models.

Classical:

$$f(Y^{(1)}, Z, Y^{(2)}|X, \Omega) = f(Y^{(1)}|Z, X, \omega_1)f(Y^{(2)}|Z, X, \omega_2)f(Z|X, \omega_3) \qquad (8.10)$$

or Berkson:

$$f(Y^{(1)}Z, Y^{(2)}|X, \Omega) = f(Y^{(1)}|Z, X, \omega_1)f(Z|Y^{(2)}, X, \omega_2)f(Y^{(2)}|X, \omega_3) \qquad (8.11)$$

where $\Omega = (\omega_1, \omega_2, \omega_3)$. However in the Berkson setting $Y^{(2)}$ is assumed to be a known measurement, meaning that Equation 8.9 is replaced by

$$f(Y^{(1)}, Y^{(2)}|X, \Omega) = \int_Z f(Y^{(1)}|Z, X, \omega_1)f(Z|Y^{(2)}, X, \omega_2)dx \qquad (8.12)$$

where $Y^{(2)}$ has been conditioned out of the joint likelihood. Likelihood methods estimate Ω by maximizing $f(Y^{(1)}, Y^{(2)}|Z, \Omega)$ or $f(Y^{(1)}|X, \Omega)$, where ω_1 is of primary interest because it describes the relationship between the response $Y^{(1)}$ and the true exposure Z. Neither Equation 8.9 nor 8.12 is typically available in closed form. In simple problems where the likelihood can be computed or well approximated analytically Ω can be estimated by iterative numerical methods, for example using the EM algorithm (D. W. Schafer, 2001). In more complex cases, Monte Carlo techniques can be used to approximate $f(Y^{(1)}, Y^{(2)}|X, \Omega)$ or $f(Y^{(1)}|X, \Omega)$, an example of which is given by Geyer and Thompson (1992). Alternatively, measurement error models can be viewed as missing data problems with Z being a missing covariate and estimation methods from the literature on missing data can be used. Further details of such methods can be found in Little and Rubin (2014).

Bayesian measurement error models comprise one of the likelihoods given by Equations 8.9 or 8.12 and a prior $f(\Omega)$, the latter of which is a product of marginal and conditional distributions. Bayesian inference is based on the posterior distribution of Ω, which for classical and Berkson models is proportional to

Classical $f(\Omega|Y^{(1)}, Y^{(2)}, X) \propto f(\Omega) \int_Z f(Y^{(1)}|Z, X, \omega_1)f(Y^{(2)}|Z, X, \omega_2) \times$

$$\ldots \times f(Z|X, \omega_3)dZ$$

Berkson $f(\Omega|Y^{(1)}, Y^{(2)}, X) \propto f(\Omega) \int_Z f(Y^{(1)}|Z, X, \omega_1)f(Z|Y^{(2)}, X, \omega_2)dZ$

The posterior distribution is typically calculated using MCMC simulation, where Z is treated as additional parameters to be estimated. Both Gibbs and Metropolis-Hastings algorithm have been used, and examples based on conditionally independent models (Richardson and Gilks, 1993), non-linear regression models (Dellaportas and Smith, 1993; S. M. Berry, Carroll, and Ruppert, 2002) and Gaussian mixture models (Richardson, Leblond, Jaussent, and Green, 2002).

8.4   Preferential sampling

Preferential sampling is a common phenomenon in environmental studies, as the monitoring locations in a spatial network are often chosen based on a subjective purpose, such as the change of government policies and the intention of monitoring high levels of pollution. For example, if monitors are positioned close to known pollution sources, such as at the roadside, near an industrial polluter, or within a city center, then the estimated pollution surface is likely to be overestimated. Both the number and locations of the pollution monitors will affect the accuracy with which pollution monitors will affect the accuracy with which non-preferential are often employed despite the presence of a preferential sampling scheme. It is often intrinsically assumed the true exposure surface is based on the random sampling of the complete spatio-temporal pollution field. However, this is extremely unlikely to be the case and the exposure measurements obtained from preferentially sampled networks may lead to an inaccurate estimation of exposure to air pollution and consequently to the estimation of relative risks in epidemiological studies.

Recently there have been a few papers published on the subject of preferential sampling in an environmental setting, which occurs when the process that determines the locations of the monitoring sites and the process being modeled is in some ways dependent (Diggle et al., 2010; Pati, Reich, and Dunson, 2011; Gelfand, Sahu, and Holland, 2012; Zidek, Shaddick, and Taylor, 2014). Diggle et al. (2010) extend the classical geostatistical model in two ways; (1) the monitoring locations are treated as random quantities of a log-Gaussian process rather than being fixed; (2) the exposures are modeled conditionally on the locations assuming a Gaussian spatial process. Through simulation examples, they show that ignoring preferential sampling can lead to misleading inferences, especially with spatial predictions. (Pati et al., 2011) adapt this approach within a Bayesian framework and demonstrate its use in a case study of ozone data over the eastern U.S. that shows significant evidence of preferential sampling. Other examples of the application of this approach include Lee, Ferguson, and Scott (2011) who implement it when constructing air quality indicators for a case study set in Greater London.

Gelfand et al. (2012) suggested another approach to deal with the effects of preferential sampling. Again, the locations are treated as a realization of a random process, but they use a deterministic model with informative covariates, such as population density, to indicate the underlying pollution surface. This approach is based on the assumption that if sampling locations are drawn as a reflection of covariate factors, then the covariates should be used in the exposure model to correct the preferential sampling bias. A simulation study shows the spatial predictions of exposures under preferential sampling are substantially biased when compared to those from random sampling. Lee and Shaddick (2010) investigated the influence of preferential sampling on the pollution concentration estimation on spatial prediction using a Bayesian spatio-temporal model, again showing significant biases in spatial predictions.

The majority of research in this area has focused on the predictions of exposure surface in a spatial network. The approach of Diggle et al. (2010) models the spatially continuous unobserved process to be used in the stochastic model of locations, but this process is unknown in practice, so it is difficult to specify its propriety. In addition, only a single realization of the underlying random field is used to generate the data for the locations in the study region. For the approach proposed by Gelfand, Banerjee, and Gamerman (2005), the difficulty is that it requires complete information on covariates used in the deterministic model, which is normally unavailable in practice.

An alternative approach to adjusting for preferential sampling from the spatial modeling approaches described above is that of response-biased regression modeling (Scott and Wild, 2001). Zidek, Shaddick, and Taylor (2014) proposed a method to model preferential sampling in environmental networks based on this approach. The idea is based on concepts from survey sampling in which sampling weights define the under- or oversampling of specific demographic groups. The resulting estimates can then be adjusted using the sampling weights to allow for the non-random design. They used the Horwitz-Thomson (HT) estimator to unbias estimates based on preferentially sampled data.

In short, the HT estimator weighs each observation against the probability that the particular observation is included in the sample. In the setting considered here, however, the sampling weights, which define the process of preferential sampling, are generally not known. The selection probabilities cannot, therefore, be characterized as they are in survey sampling. The idea of Zidek, Shaddick, and Taylor (2014) was to estimate these probabilities using logistic regression based on concentrations measured in previous years and locations.

A substantial extension of the approach outlined in the previous paragraph is seen in the recent work on preferential sampling of Watson, Zidek, and Shaddick (2019), hereafter denoted by WZS. That work was limited to the retrospective case where all the data are in hand. A latent spatio-temporal process with observable attributes has been monitored over time at a varying subset of spatial locations. The goal is an understanding of that natural process based on the data that has been collected. In particular, an understanding of what went on at the unmonitored sites through spatial mapping during the period of observation would be desirable.

Like WZS, we adopt the general framework described in Chapter 4. So we have a natural process of interest, a measurement process and a parameter process. The population consists of a set of space-time points $(s,t) \in \mathscr{S} \times \mathscr{T}$. The process model assumes the existence of a latent spatial field of attributes $Z_{\mathscr{S}t} = \{Z_{st} : s \in \mathscr{S}\}$ at each time point t. The measurement process will then yield a set of observations Y_{st} at points in a subset of the population $\mathbf{S}_t \subset \mathscr{S}$, for each $t \in T \subset \mathscr{T}$.

Often in practice, the process will not be observable at all sites in $\mathscr{S}$. Some will be remote or otherwise inaccessible. Some will not be in locations where monitoring stations are not allowed due to administrative restrictions, for example air pollution monitors are commonly found on public property such as a park or school grounds. Only a subset of locations, of size M, $\mathscr{P} \subset \mathscr{S}$, will be candidates for process monitoring stations. Thus, WZG consider two different populations, respectively $\mathscr{P}_1$ and $\mathscr{P}_2$, the actual population and the entire population of possibilities. Thus $\mathscr{P}_1 \subset \mathscr{P}_2 = \mathscr{S}$. At possible sites, the process is deemed to be assessable only at discrete times $t \in \{t_1, \ldots, t_N\} = \mathscr{T}$. And the latent process model has been characterized in various ways.

We may now set up the requisite model for modeling the spatio-temporal field. It needs to be flexible due to the large variety of spatio-temporal fields encountered in practice. To be practical, it must be able to handle the many monitoring sites now seen in the application. WZS achieves these objectives by adopting the framework provided by INLA (see Subsection 6.7). The requisite software is provided on the GitHub site associated with the book. A more detailed look at INLA is seen in Subsection 10.12. One by-product of WZS's use of INLA is a mesh that is grid that discretizes the continuum of points, the domain of interest. Thus, we may regard the full population of points $\mathscr{S}$ to be the grid points generated by this approximation.

The underlying process model has been represented in various ways, for example by Pati et al. (2011). The authors ignore time and according to WZS, model the process by $Z_s = \mu + \alpha^T \mathbf{X}_s + \beta \xi_s + \beta_1 \eta_s$. This reflects the important role that covariate vectors $\mathbf{X}$ may play in determining the level of the process. But as WZS points out, the second residual term is added to account for selection bias that may be due to such things as administrative considerations rather than the covariates X.

We now turn to the measurement process. To simplify notation, let Y_{ij} denote the assessed value of the latent process Z at time $t_j \in \mathscr{T}$ and site $s_i \in \mathscr{P}$, $i \in \{1, \ldots, M\}$ and $j \in \{1, \ldots, N\}$. Furthermore, let R_{ij} denote the binary random selection indicator for the site $s_i \in \mathscr{P}$ and time t_j. Covariates X_{st} play an important role as well, both in characterizing the latent process and the measurement process. Classical spatio-temporal modeling focused on the field where $R_{ij} = 1$. However, as noted by WZG, learning that $R_{ij} = 0$ is also informative. This knowledge helps provide the contrast needed when considering possible preferential sampling-induced bias.

In any case, WZG proposes for the site selection model:

$$(Y_{i,j} | R_{i,j} = 1) \quad \curvearrowleft \quad f_Y(g(\mu_{i,j}), \theta_Y), \quad f \curvearrowleft \text{Exponential family}$$

$$g(\mu_{i,j}) = \eta_{i,j} = \mathbf{x}_{i,j}^T \gamma + \sum_{k=1}^{q_1} u_{i,j,k} \beta_k(\mathbf{s}_i, t_j)$$

$$R_{i,j} \quad \curvearrowleft \quad \text{Bernoulli}(p_{i,j})$$

$$h(p_{i,j}) = v_{i,j} = \mathbf{v}_{i,j}^T \alpha + \sum_{l=1}^{q_2} d_l \sum_{m=1}^{q_1} w_{i,j,l,m} \beta_m(\mathbf{s}_i, \phi_{i,l,m}(t_j))$$

$$+ \sum_{n=1}^{q_3} w_{i,j,n}^\star \beta_n^\star(\mathbf{s}_i, t_j)$$

$$\beta_k(\mathbf{s}_i, t_j) \quad \backsim \quad \text{(possibly shared) latent effect with parameters } \theta_k,$$
$$k \in \{1, \ldots, q_1\}$$
$$\beta_l^\star(\mathbf{s}_i, t_j) \quad \backsim \quad \text{site} - \text{selection only latent effect with parameters } \theta_l^\star$$
$$l \in \{1, \ldots, q_3\}$$
$$\Theta \quad = \quad (\theta_Y, \alpha, \gamma, \mathbf{d}, \theta_1, \ldots, \theta_{q_1}, \theta_1^\star, \ldots, \theta_{q_3}^\star) \backsim \text{Priors}$$
$$\mathbf{x}_{i,j} \quad \in \quad R^{p_1}, \mathbf{u}_{i,j} \in R^{q_1}, \quad \mathbf{v}_{i,j} \in R^{p_2}, \quad \mathbf{W}_{i,j} \in R^{q_2 \times q_1}, \quad \mathbf{w}_{i,j}^{\star T} \in R^{q_3}$$

We will see in the sequel, an application in Example 8.1. A key feature of the model are the β_k terms. For it is these terms which link Y and R, thus yielding a bivariate distribution for these variables. However, the R package for implementing this model comes with the warning that it demands a lot of memory (about 64 GB. The simplified version called 'naive' in Example 8.1 is not so demanding.

Example 8.1. *Long-term monitoring of air pollution in the UK*

Black smoke (BS) has been routinely measured in the UK since the early 1960s as part of the UK Smoke and Sulfur Dioxide network and its predecessor the National Survey. In later years, the network was used to monitor compliance with the relevant EC Directives on sulfur dioxide and suspended particulate matter The monitoring network, which measures both SO_2 and BS, was established in the early 1960s and by 1971 included over 1200 sites. As levels of BS and SO_2 pollution has declined, the network has been progressively rationalized and reduced in size and by 2006 when the network ceased to be operational it comprised 65 sites. BS continues to be monitored, but on a much smaller scale (Fuller and Connolly, 2012), and as the network was reduced in size, there is the possibility of selection bias if there was a tendency for monitoring sites to be kept in the more polluted areas. This may occur for example, if the locations of sites remaining in the network were chosen to assess whether guidelines and policies were being adhered to. This will lead to preferential sampling.

Shaddick and Zidek (2014) consider the change in levels of pollution concentrations in relation to changes in the network from the 1960s until the 2000s; a period for which there were both reductions in the size of the network and in the concentrations being measured. Annual means fell from 237 μgm^{-3} in 1962 to 99 in 1966, 32 in 1976, 19 in 1986, 11 in 1996 and 5 μgm^{-3} in 2006. This period represents a unique period in history containing dramatic declines in the levels of air pollution together with the most marked reduction in the network providing the data on which these reported declines are based. During this period, there were a total of 1466 operational sites of which 35 consistent sites were operating throughout the entire period. Figure 8.1 shows the mean concentrations over all sites by year for four groups of sites; (i) the set of 35 consistent sites, (ii) 655 sites which were added (and remained) during the period of study, (iii) 133 sites which were dropped and (iv) 643 sites which were added then dropped. Concentrations are shown for all years

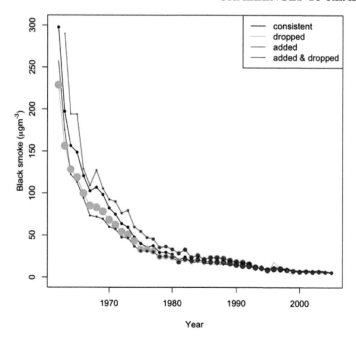

Figure 8.1: Annual means of BS concentrations by year (1962-2006). Dots denote the yearly mean value. The size of the dots is proportional to the number of sites which contributes to the calculation of the mean for each year. Values are given for: (i) sites for which measurements were consistently available throughout the period (black) together with those from sites which were (ii) dropped from (green) and (iii) added to (red) the network within the period of study. Values for (iv) the group of sites which were added and then dropped from the network are given in blue.

for which data were available, with the grouping derived using the main pe-riod of analysis. Very similar patterns are seen using different periods to define the groups, albeit with a smaller number of consistent sites when considering longer periods. There is a clear decline in the level of BS over this period with markedly higher concentrations in the consistent and added sites than those that were dropped, suggesting preferential sampling had taken place.

For simplicity in this part of our analysis, we now adapted the general model above for this example and in doing so, have split it into the site selection and mea-surement parts. First the site selection:

$$R_{i,j} \sim \text{Bernoulli}(p_{i,j})$$
$$\text{logit} p_{i,1} = \alpha_{0,0} + \alpha_1 t_1^\star + \alpha_2 (t_1^\star)^2 + \beta_1^\star(t_1)$$
$$+ \alpha_{rep} I_{i,1} + \beta_0^\star(\mathbf{s}_i)$$
$$+ d_b [b_{0,i} + b_{1,i}(t_1^\star)] +$$
$$d_\beta \left[\beta_0(\mathbf{s}_i) + \beta_1(\mathbf{s}_i)(t_1^\star) + \beta_2(\mathbf{s}_i)(t_1^\star)^2 \right]$$

$$\text{for } j \neq 1 \quad \text{logit} p_{i,j} \quad \alpha_{0,1} + \alpha_1 t_j^\star + \alpha_2 (t_j^\star)^2 + \beta_1^\star(t_j)$$
$$+ \alpha_{ret} r_{i,(j-1)} + \alpha_{rep} l_{i,j} + \beta_0^\star(\mathbf{s}_i)$$
$$+ d_b \left[b_{0,i} + b_{1,i}(t_{j-1}^\star) \right] +$$
$$d_\beta \left[\beta_0(\mathbf{s}_i) + \beta_1(\mathbf{s}_i)(t_{j-1}^\star) + \beta_2(\mathbf{s}_i)(t_{j-1}^\star)^2 \right]$$

$$l_{i,j} = \mathbb{I}\left[\sum_{l \neq i} r_{l,j-1} \mathbb{I}(\|s_i - s_l\| < c) \right]$$

$$[\beta_0^\star(\mathbf{s}_1), ..., \beta_0^\star(\mathbf{s}_m)]^T \quad \backsim \quad N(\mathbf{0}, \Sigma(\zeta_R))$$
$$[\beta_1^\star(t_1), ..., \beta_1^\star(t_T)]^T \quad \backsim \quad AR1(\rho_a, \sigma_a^2)$$
$$\theta_R = [\alpha, d_b, d_\beta, \rho_a, \sigma_a^2, \zeta_R] \quad \backsim \quad \text{Priors.}$$

Then the conditional measurement model:

$$(Y_{i,j} | R_{i,j} = 1) \quad \backsim \quad N\left(\mu_{i,j}, \sigma_\varepsilon^2\right)$$
$$\mu_{i,j} = (\gamma_0 + b_{0,i} + \beta_0(\mathbf{s}_i)) + (\gamma_1 + b_{1,i} + \beta_1(\mathbf{s}_i)) t_j^\star +$$
$$(\gamma_2 + \beta_2(\mathbf{s}_i))(t_j^\star)^2$$
$$[\beta_k(\mathbf{s}_1), \beta_k(\mathbf{s}_2), ..., \beta_k(\mathbf{s}_m)]^T \quad \backsim^{IID} \quad N(\mathbf{0}, \Sigma(\zeta_k)), \quad \text{for } k \in \{0,1,2\}$$
$$[b_{0,i}, b_{1,i}] \quad \backsim^{IID} \quad N(\mathbf{0}, \Sigma_b),$$
$$\Sigma_b = \begin{pmatrix} \sigma_{b,1}^2 & \rho_b \\ \rho_b & \sigma_{b,2}^2 \end{pmatrix}$$
$$\Sigma(\zeta_k) \quad \backsim \quad \text{Matern}(\zeta_k) = \text{Matern}(\tau_k, r_k, \nu_k)$$
$$\theta = (\sigma_\varepsilon^2, \gamma, \zeta_k, \sigma_{b,1}^2, \rho_b) \quad \backsim \quad \text{Priors.}$$

These models were implemented in three different ways that are now described along with the results seen in the figures that follow in this subsection.

Implementation 1-Independence between Y and R. Here the model parameters are constrained in such a way as to force on the model, a prior assumption of no stochastic dependence between the site-selection process and the observation process. This can be done by setting $d_b = 0$ and $d_\beta = 0$. In other words, no preferential sampling PS has occurred. That in turn, forces the same assumption on the posterior distribution of the measurement process. So in short we get the results that would obtain from the typical spatio-temporal analyzes conducted in practice. The result provides a baseline for comparison with results obtained when PS is incorporated into the model. Figure 8.2 shows the results.

The relative lack of sites in some regions of the UK might be expected to lead to them having relatively low levels of BS relative to $\mathscr{P}_1$. The latter includes many preferentially selected sites located in areas of heavy pollution. Thus, the model tends to predict unduly high levels in regions with low levels. This would be essentially the regression toward the mean effect seen in regression analysis. Overall, the results point to preferential sampling throughout the entire period over which the modeling was done, but the results are more nuanced than those seen in the empirical analysis of Shaddick and Zidek (shown in Figure 8.1). Further discussion of this can be found

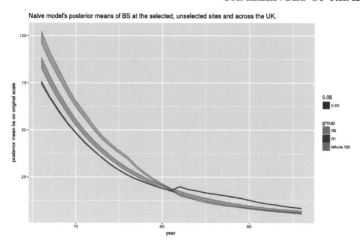

Naive model's posterior means of BS at the selected, unselected sites and across the UK.

Figure 8.2: Implementation 1. BS levels averaged over sites that were selected in $\mathscr{P}_1$ (i.e. operational) at time t are in green while those in red are the BS levels averaged over sites that were not selected in $\mathscr{P}_1$ (i.e. offline) at time t. Blue shows the BS levels averaged across Great Britain. With the posterior mean values are their 95% posterior credible intervals.

in WZS. The selection bias was reversed in about 1982 when the network in the UK underwent a major redesign.

Implementation 2-Dependence between Y and R but $\mathscr{P} = \mathscr{P}_1$ all ever-monitored sites. For Implementation 2, only the 1466 observed site-locations comprising the population of ever selected network sites and this population is assessed at time t. Thus $M = 1466$. This implementation of the model seeks to determine if the network evolved preferentially. In other words, were sites added and dropped from the network in a way that depended on the evolution of the concentrations of the black smoke concentrations?

Now the condition $d_b = 0$ and $d_\beta = 0$ is removed so that the relationship between Y and R may be more fully assessed. However, in their analysis WZS found only the former effect d_β significantly non-zero. It had a posterior estimated value of 0.66 and a 95% posterior credible interval of (0.34, 0.99). In contrast, the 95% posterior estimate for the short-range preferentiality contained 0, although just barely. Thus, WZS found positive preferentiality in both cases. Year-by-year, it would seem that site placements were positively associated with the relative levels of black smoke. At the same time, despite that finding, the posterior predictions of black smoke levels are similar to those of in Implementation 1, as can be seen in Figure 8.3. In particular, no obvious changes were seen in the predicted BS levels in the unsampled regions such as those in the Scottish Highlands.

These findings are 'in stark contrast with the observed debiasing of the regional mean witnessed ... under Implementation 3' according to WZS, all because we now move from populations $\mathscr{P}_1$ to $\mathscr{P}_2$.

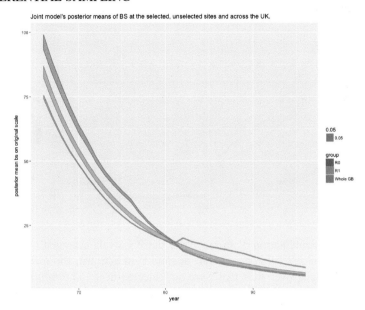

Figure 8.3: A plot of the year-by-year change in the logit of selection captured by the autoregressive $\beta_1^\star(t)$ process in the R process in Implementation 2. Note that the plot for Implementation 3 is very similar.

Implementation 3-Dependence between Y and R-but $\mathscr{P} = \mathscr{P}_2$ is all possible sites including $\mathscr{P}_1$. Thousands of pseudo-sites were now added to the list of sites considered for selection at each time, to those in $\mathscr{P}_1$. A massive number of sites in total and an analysis made possible only by using the INLA approximation. In effect, WZS were now exploring three different processes in Implementation 3: (i) the observation process; (ii) the initial site placement process; (iii) the site-retention process. The results are seen in Figure 8.4.

Overall, amongst other things, Implementations 2 and/or 3 sought to determine if sites were added or removed preferentially after accounting for the various covariates involved. The increasingly sharp contrast added by the new sites in $\mathscr{P}_3$ leads to a strong indication of significance in the credibility intervals for d_b and d_β. This might be considered a major product of using the more complex model and its INLA implementation. Thus, in both cases, the direction of preferentiality was significantly positive, suggesting that year-by-year, the site placements were positively associated with the relative levels of black smoke at the site location, both locally and regionally. Of particular note, we see in Figure 8.4 a striking difference in the appearance of the estimated black smoke field through time. According to WZS, '...this is a direct consequence of the strong preferential sampling detected is the dramatic drop in the posterior predictions of black smoke levels in under-sampled regions of GB relative to Implementation 1.' The paper contains much more detail.

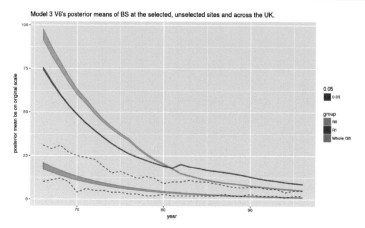

Figure 8.4: Implementation 3. In green are the BS levels averaged over sites that were selected in $\mathscr{P}_1$ (i.e. operational) at time t. In contrast, those in red are the BS levels averaged over sites that were not selected in $\mathscr{P}_1$ (i.e. offline) at time t. Finally, in blue are the BS levels averaged across Great Britain. Also included with the posterior mean values are their 95% posterior credible intervals. The black dashed lines denote the lower 10th percentile and lower quartile observed in the data. Note that the estimated black smoke trajectories from the pseudo-sites are not included in the mean calculations to form the red band.

8.4.1   Detecting and mitigating the effects of preferential sampling

The previous subsection describes a strategy for modeling spatio-temporal processes over space and time. But that model does not provide a test for detecting preferentiality in the selection of the sites at which the process will be monitored. Nor does it provide a way of mitigating the impact of the measurement bias generated by that bias. This section tackles both of these issues, beginning with testing.

Detection

The idea of detecting preferential sampling sounds like pulling yourself up by your bootstraps, as it is using potentially biased data to detect that bias. However, several techniques have been successfully proposed for doing just that.

An early paper on the topic of this subsection (Schlather, Ribeiro Jr, and Diggle, 2004), used two alternative MCMC tests and compared the observed value of various test statistics, using conventional methods, on the assumption that sampling was not preferential. A later approach (Guan and Afshartous, 2007) divided the observations into non-overlapping subregions, and assumed the results were approximately independent replicates of those test statistics. This method required a very large sample of $n = 4358$. Diggle et al. (2010) models the joint physical and sampling processes with shared spatio-temporal latent effects.

More recently, Watson (2021), hereafter denoted by 'WAT' for brevity, proposed a method based on a point process approach. The basic idea is that if the network were set up to detect high levels of the spatio-temporal field, you would expect site clustering to be induced with the result that overall intersite distances would be smaller than expected under a purely selection of the sites, say following a log Gaussian Cox point process model. Thus the concentration level and intersite distances would tend to be negatively correlated.

Based on this idea and to maximize the domain of applicability of the method, WAT proposed a test based on the non-parametric Spearman's Rho correlation between the ranked nearest neighbor distance and the ranked pollutant levels at the sites. If this score were unusually large, compared to a simulated metric-uncorrelated network, preferential sampling would be indicated.

The steps in the WAT test to detect preferential sampling are as follows:

- generate a point process for the observed locations under the null hypothesis of no preferential sampling;
- generate many sample networks of sites using that point process;
- compare the correlation of the observed point process to the distribution of the samples correlation.

The WAT algorithm compares the k nearest neighbors to each location, $k \geq 1$. The choice of k is a tuning parameter. Ideally, k tries to match the cluster size of the actual network to get the best power in the test. When the number of sites in a cluster is small (e.g. clusters cover smaller spatial scales) a smaller k is used and vice versa. As the number of nearest neighbors increases the power of the test increases. But it also becomes less precise, smoothed further out than the size of the clusters of high or low concentration (Watson, 2021).

Like any test, the WAT test has limitations. For example, WAT found that like all tests, his two-sided rank-based test has limitations, for example his test tends to be quite conservative. However, he sees its strengths, for example robustness and simplicity, outweighing its weaknesses.

The method has been published as the software package called PStestR. Its GitHub site describes it briefly as follows:

```
''PStestR is an R package for testing for preferential
    sampling in spatio-temporal data. This includes
    discrete (i.e. areal) and continuous (i.e. point-
    referenced) data. The package is compatible with many
    popular R packages for handling spatial data
    including the spatstat, sp, and sf packages. However,
    as always, the user will need to determine if the
    package will run on their current operating system.
```

```
PStestR uses two functions: PSTestInit and PSTestRun. The
    first is a helper function for creating an object in
    the necessary format for the test. The second function
    implements the test.

To install PStestR, make sure the devtools package is
    loaded in R and run $install_github('joenomiddlename/
    PStestR',
dependencies=T, build_vignettes=T)$

To use PStestR, read the tutorials found in the
    comprehensive vignette provided by typing vignette('
    PStestR') into R.''
\hfill\cite{watson2021perceptron}
```

The package may be downloaded from its GitHub site and installed as suggested in the following listing.

```
@ -3,6 +3,6 @@ PStestR is an R package for testing for
    preferential sampling in spatio-temporal processes

PStestR uses two functions: PSTestInit and PSTestRun. The
    first is a helper function for creating an object in
    the necessary format for the test. The second function
    implements the test.

To install PStestR, make sure the devtools package is
    loaded in R and run:
> install_github('joenomiddlename/PStestR', dependencies=T)

To install PStestR, make sure the devtools package is
    loaded in R and run

To use PStestR, read the tutorials found in the
    comprehensive vignette provided by typing vignette('
    PStestR') into R.
```

The user will be asked to make choices as the package is being installed. (You may need to install 'Rtools' for Windows before installing devtool. Mac users may need to install 'Xcode' or the command line tools.)

Assumptions underlying Watson's method:

- the preferential sampling is driven by some or all of the spatio-temporal latent effects $Y_{s,t}$;
- all latent effects $Y_{s,t}$ driving the preferential sampling are spatially smooth enough relative to both the size of the study region, $|S|$, and the number of locations chosen to sample the process;

- the density of points within S_t at space-time point $(s,t) \in (S \times T)$ depends monotonically on the values of the components of $Y_{s,t}$ driving the preferential sampling.

Watson (2021) explains that his test can be used under two different paradigms. In the first, the number of nearest neighbors to use is specified. Then a single test is performed. It compares the known sites to the distribution of the Monty Carlo samples. In the second, that number is uncertain. So an exploration of a range of options becomes part of the research inquiry. Multiple comparisons are made with varying values of k, the number of nearest neighbors used. PStestR then yields:

- A Test Rho: The calculated Spearman's Rho for the network during each year.
- An Empirical P-Value: It compares the Test Rho for the actual network to the distribution from the Monte Carlo simulation.

The test also has several tuning parameters that can be adjusted to optimize the test.

Example 8.2. *Preferential sampling: A Case Study*

Jones, Zidek, and Watson (2023) assesses the Watson test for preferential sampling detection. That study involved the sites that constituted the Southern California Air Quality Basin SOCAB network for monitoring particulate that is their air pollution, that is PM_{10}. Their identity may be found in the 2019 South Coast Air Quality Management District Report (Miyasato and Lowe, 2019). That case study is shown in its Figure 8.5, the sites that were selected and the period during which they actively monitored that pollutant.

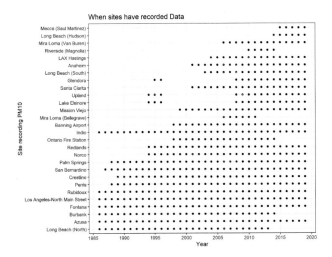

Figure 8.5: This figure shows how the network developed over time. We can see that sites are generally added to the network, that 5 sites have been removed, and that 5 sites started in 1986. A handful of sites have the unusual behavior of being taken offline and then removed. These are sites that only had Federal Reference Method monitoring, no Federal Equivalent Method.

As background, PM_{10} is one of the criteria pollutants for which Air Quality Standards AQS are mandatorily published by the Environmental Protection Agency EPA in the USA, as is required by the Clean Air Act of 1970. This air pollutant consists of airborne particulates with a diameter of less than 10 μgm^{-3} in diameter. They, like other pollutants, have negative impacts on human health and welfare, both short-term and long-term. For example in the short term, high concentrations of PM_{10} can result in acute respiratory problems while. Long-term exposure to even lower pollution concentrations can result in a chronic reduction in functionality of the lungs and cardiovascular system (EPA, 2002) and, on the welfare side, PM_{10} also damages property, crops, and reduces visibility (EPA, 2002).

At the Federal level, the EPA defines standards for air quality levels, monitoring and reporting. These standards define:

1. the levels of pollution that must not be exceeded;
2. how they should be monitored;
3. policies regarding the reporting requirements imposed by the EPA.

In return, the EPA regularly revises and publishes AQS for its criteria pollutants, for example PM_{10}.

Turning to the analysis, after a logarithmic transformation of the recorded PM_{10} concentrations, the PSTestR was applied to determine if there was evidence of preferential selection of the SOCAB sites. The analysis proceeded as follows. Having obtained a predicted pollutant surface and knowing the location of sites, the package calculated the mean of the k nearest neighbors at each site. It then calculated the correlation metric with the estimated concentration of the pollutant. The same result is then produced for many Monte Carlo samples of possible sites over the whole network area.

Turning to the analysis of these data, briefly here is what JZW chose to use to implement that WAT test described above:

- Number of Nearest neighbors, k: After examining a map of the largest cluster seems to be about 3 and $k = 3$ was chosen.
- Number of Monte Carlo Samples: The number of Monte Carlo samples M to use needed to be specified and in this case, $M = 1000$ seemed a good compromise between accuracy and processor time.
- Year: The annual concentration levels are autocorrelated to some degree, making a multiple comparison procedure complex, in deciding if there were evidence of preferential selection. So instead, for the purpose of this case study the year 2019 was chosen.

The results: It was found, for the SOCAB network in 2019, a correlation of -0.822 (p-Value $= 0.00300$. This correlation, being very close to -1, makes it seem very unlikely that this subset of sites could have been chosen at random. In other words, that selection was stochastically dependent upon the PM_{10} field.

Mitigation

Zidek, Shaddick, and Taylor (2014) propose a general framework for dealing with the effects of preferential sampling in environmental monitoring. Strategies for implementation are proposed, leading to a method for improving the accuracy of official statistics used to report trends and inform regulatory policy. An essential feature of the method is its capacity to learn the preferential selection process over time and hence to reduce bias in these statistics, such as annual means and exceedances.

As noted in the discussion preceding this example, an alternative method can be found from principles underlying survey sampling, in which sampling weights, which are part of the sampling design and may for example over-sample certain age groups, are used to correct the results of the survey (Scott and Wild, 2011). However, in this setting, the location of sites in monitoring networks is not often the result of a carefully designed study design, but instead site selection is complex involving committees, guidelines and negotiations, and political considerations. In practice then the process that selects the monitoring sites is non-random and generally not known. Thus, the selection probabilities cannot be characterized as they are in multi-stage survey sampling, for example. However, having a time series of samples of sites from the finite the population of N possible sites enables the selection process to be modeled and those probabilities estimated and (Zidek, Shaddick, and Taylor, 2014) describe a logistic regression approach that may be used when such information is available.

It is assumed that at time t, the sample of S_t among the population of N sites is selected by a PPS (probability proportional to size) sample survey design, $u \in S_t$ being included with probability π_{tu}. That probability is assumed to depend on all responses, both on observed data but also the unmeasured responses at the unsampled sites over the period $1 : (t-1)$, the latter of which is treated as latent variables. Thus, in terms of the measured and unmeasured responses, Y and vector of binary indicators of selected/rejected sites R, the conditional distribution of the probability of selection is

$$
\begin{aligned}
logit[\pi_{tu}] &= logit[P(R_{tu} = 1 \mid \mathbf{y}^{(1)}{}_{1:(t-1)}, \mathbf{r}_{1:(t-1)})] \\
&= G(\mathbf{y}^{(1)}{}_{1:(t-1)}, \mathbf{r}_{1:(t-1)})
\end{aligned}
\tag{8.13}
$$

for some function $0 \leq G \leq 1$. That function is analogous to the preferential sampling intensity seen in (Diggle et al., 2010).

Under the assumption of a superpopulation model (see Zidek, Shaddick, Taylor (2014) for details) there will be a predictive probability distribution for the unmeasured responses. Values for these might be obtained using for example geostatistical methods as described in Chapter 10, which under repeated imputation will allow $k = 1, \ldots, K$ replicate datasets. Each replicate enables G to be fitted $\hat{\pi}_{tu}^k$, $k = 1, \ldots, K$.

From these replicates, multiple values of the Horvitz – Thompson estimator can be obtained. In a spatial setting R is defined to be a sampled site indicator so that R_u

is 1 or 0 according as site u is selected into the sample or not. Let

$$\pi_u = \pi(y_u, x_u) = P\{R_u = 1 | y_u, x_u\}$$

be the selection probability for site u. The HT approach estimates the first-order parameter β above by solving the estimating equations

$$\sum_u \frac{R_u}{\pi_u} \frac{\partial \log[y_u | x_u, \beta]}{\partial \beta} = 0 \tag{8.14}$$

assuming $\pi_u > 0, u \in \mathscr{S}$ are known at the sampled sites.

In the simplified case of a strictly decreasing network, at each time point the logistic regression model described in Equation 8.13 is used to predict the inclusion probabilities at each time point, t,

$$logit(\hat{\pi}_{tu}) = \beta_0 + \beta_1 [y_{tu}^{(1)} - \bar{y}_{t.}^{(1)}] \tag{8.15}$$

for the N binary select – reject indicators for all sites u where $y^{(1)}$ are the observed values at time t which have mean $\bar{y}_{t.}^{(1)}$

The unconditional site selection probabilities are then calculated, $\hat{\pi}_{tu}^*$. Note that $u \in S_t$ implies $u \in S_{t'}$, $t' \leq t$ so under the assumption of no autocorrelation

$$\hat{\pi}_{tu}^* = \Pi_{t=1}^t \hat{\pi}_{tu}$$

Horvitz – Thompson adjusted summaries can then be calculated for each time point. The estimate of the annual mean will be

$$\hat{\mu}_t = \sum_{u \in S_t} \frac{y_{tu}^{(1)}}{N \hat{\pi}_{tu}^*}$$

Example 8.3. *Adjusting annual means and exceedances of black smoke*

As seen above, in Example 8.1, there is evidence of preferential sampling in the long-term network of black smoke in the UK. Here we present adjustments for two characteristics associated with the responses which are of interest. The first is the set of annual averages as this information could be published to show the effect of regulatory policy over time. The left-hand panel of Figure 8.6 shows the estimated geometric annual mean levels over time (blue line) together with the Horvitz–Thompson adjusted ones (red line). It clearly shows the adjustment reduces the estimates of the average levels. Since the standard unit for calculating relative risks of particulates in health effects analysis is 10 μgm^{-3} the difference seems important, being more than one of these standard units over much of the period.

The second characteristic may potentially be of even greater operational importance; the number of sites in non-attainment, that do not comply with air quality standards in any year. This number is a surrogate for the cost of

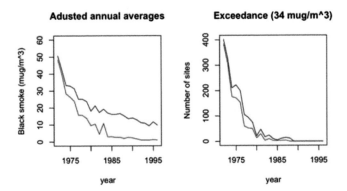

Figure 8.6: Changes in the levels of black smoke within the UK from 1970-1996 and the effects of adjusting estimates of annual indices. The left-hand panel shows the annual means over all sites (blue line) together with adjusted values (red line). The right-hand panel shows the number of sites exceeding the EU guide value of 34 μgm^{-3} (blue line) together with the corrected values (red line).

mitigation for putting the BS concentrations into compliance. The right-hand panel of Figure 8.6 shows the number of sites each year that exceed the 1980 EU guide value of 34 μgm^{-3} (European Commision, 1980). The blue line is the number of exceeding sites based on the recorded data with the red line the numbers after adjustment for the preferential sampling. The unadjusted numbers are the fraction of the monitoring network out-of-compliance multiplied by the finite population total of $N = 624$. Their adjusted counterparts are found by using the Horvitz–Thompson weights in the summation used to calculate that fraction. For example, in 1974, the crude estimate gives 211 of the 624 sites out of compliance with the 34 μgm^{-3} criterion, while its adjusted counterpart is just 189. This is a substantial difference, especially considering the large costs that can be involved in achieving compliance.

8.5   Summary

This chapter considers some of the issues that will arise when dealing with 'real data'. Data will commonly have missing values and may be measured with error. This error might be random or may be due to systematic patterns arising from the data collection mechanism. The reader will have gained an understanding of the following topics:

- Classification of missing values into missing at random or not at random.
- Methods for imputing missing values.
- Different measurement error models, including classical and Berkson.
- The attenuation of regression coefficients under measurement error.

- Preferential sampling, where there are dependencies between processes that determines the locations of monitoring sites and the process being modeled;
- How preferential sampling can bias the measurements that arise from environmental monitoring networks.

8.6 Exercises

Exercise 8.1. The `Amelia` R package provides several methods for estimating missing values using multiple imputations.

(i) Investigate the use of multiple imputation by analyzing the `freetrade` dataset supplied with the package. Produce ten simulated datasets with missing values imputed.

(ii) Perform an analysis of the variation between the simulated datasets and show your results graphically.

(iii) Show how you might use these multiple datasets in a regression analysis where `tariff` is the response variable. How will you ensure that the variability between the datasets is reflected in the standard errors associated with the regression
coefficients?

Exercise 8.2. Show that the attenuation factor for the measurement error model shown in Equation (8.7) is $\beta_{Y^{(2)}} = \frac{\sigma_z^2}{\sigma_z^2 + \sigma_{v2}^2} \beta_z$

Exercise 8.3. (i) Simulate a set of true exposures Z based on the model shown in Equation 8.7 using a fixed variance, σ_Z^2.

(ii) For a value of $\beta_Z = 2$ generate a set of $Y^{(1)}$'s (using a fixed σ_{v1}^2) and perform a linear regression. Note your estimate of β_Z.

(iii) Generate a set of data measured with error, $Y^{(2)}$, for a fixed σ_{v2}^2 and perform a linear regression of $Y^{(1)}$ on $Y^{(1)}$.

(iv) Compare the two values of β you get from the two models. Does the difference between them correspond to the attenuation factor you would obtain if you used the equation in part (i)?

(v) Show the effect of the attenuation graphically.

Exercise 8.4. Repeat the simulation exercise in Exercise 8.3 using different values for the variances, σ_{v1}^2 and σ_{v2}^2. What do you conclude about the relative importance of these two variances?

Exercise 8.5. Repeat the simulation exercise in Exercise 8.3 but now generate the set of responses, $Y^{(1)}$, using a Poisson distribution. Note, the linear part of the model will now be on the log scale, and so care should be taken in regard to the magnitude of the values that will be exponentiated. What do you conclude about the effects of measurement error in this case? For further reading on the subject of measurement error in non-linear models, see Carroll et al. (1995).

Exercise 8.6. Return to Example 8.1 and model a different air pollution field using the Watson method (Watson et al., 2019). It could for example be a different air pollutant field over the UK.

Exercise 8.7. The data and code to perform the preferential sampling approach given in Diggle et al. (2010) is available on the R-INLA website. Use this to perform an analysis of the data from Galicia shown in the paper, with and without adjustment for preferential sampling.

Exercise 8.8. The data and code to perform the preferential sampling approach given in the GitHub site for this book. Use it to reproduce Figure 8.2.

Exercise 8.9. Repeat the case study in Example 8.2 for the SOCAB region for PM_{10} and a different year after downloading the data from sources described in that Example. Note that the sites ultimately chosen from the SOCAB region were:

SOCAB Site				
Anaheim	Azusa	Banning Airport	Burbank	Crestline
Fontana	Glendora	Indio	Lake Elsinore	LAX Hastings
Long Beach & Long Beach	Long Beach	Los Angeles	Mecca	
(Hudson)	(North)	(South)	(N Main Str)	(Saul Martinez)
Mira Loma	Mira Loma	Mission Viejo	Norco	Ontario Fire
(Bellegrave)	(Van Buren)			(Station)
Palm Springs	Perris	Redlands	Riverside	Rubidoux
			(Magnola)	
San Bernardino	Santa Clarita	Upland		

Chapter 9

Spatial modeling: areal data

9.1 Overview

Disease mapping has a long history in epidemiology, starting with John Snow's map of cholera cases in London in 1854 (Hempel, 2014). The aims of disease mapping range from simple spatial description of health data and hypothesis generation to the estimation of risks over space. In the latter, allowance should be made for differing sized populations, which may provide varying levels of uncertainty in the estimation of risks. Area-based mapping has also been used for the assessment of inequalities and the allocation of health care resources.

In terms of the areas used for disease mapping, there will be a trade-off in relation to the geographical scale that is used: rates calculated using larger geographical areas will be more stable but summaries of risk, such as relative risks, may be affected by the aggregation of large numbers of individuals. If there is substantial variation between risks within a particular area, this information will be lost. An effect of a high risk in a subregion will be diluted under aggregation. Detecting elevated risks in such subregions will not be possible unless data are available at a lower level of aggregation.

For small areas, and in particular rare diseases, estimates of risk may be dominated by sampling variability. This issue has led to methods being developed to produce 'smoothed' estimates of risk using hierarchical/random effects models. These use data from the individual areas together with global measures of risk estimated using data from all the areas to provide more reliable estimates in each of the constituent areas.

There are three main types of spatial data that are commonly encountered in environmental epidemiology. They are (i) lattice, (ii) point-referenced and (iii) point-process data.

(i) Lattices refer to situations in which the spatial domain consists of a discrete set of 'lattice points'. These points may index the corners of cells in a regular or irregular grid. Alternatively, they may index geographical regions such as administrative units or health districts (see for example Figure 1.2), This is an important topic in spatio-temporal epidemiology and detailed discussions can be found in Gotway and Young (2002); Cressie and Wikle (2011) and Banerjee et al. (2015). We denote the set of all lattice points by $\mathscr{L}$ with data available at a set of N_L points, $l \in L$ where $L = l_1, ..., l_{N_L}$. In many applications, such

DOI: 10.1201/9781003352655-9

as disease mapping, L is commonly equal to $\mathscr{L}$. A key feature of this class is its neighborhood structure; a process that generates the data at a location has a distribution that can be characterized in terms of its neighbors.

(ii) Point-referenced data are measured at a fixed, and often sparse, set of 'spatial points' in a spatial domain or region $\mathscr{S}$. $\mathscr{S}$ may be a continuum. But in the applications considered in this book the domain will be treated as a finite set of points both to reduce technical complexity and to reflect the practicalities of siting monitors of environmental processes (e.g. on land that is accessible). For example, when monitoring air pollution, the number of monitors may be limited by financial considerations, and they may have to be sited on public land. Measurements are available at a selection of N_S sites, $s \in S$ where $S = s_1, ..., s_{N_S}$. Sites would usually be defined in terms of their geographical coordinates such as longitude and latitude, that is $s_l = (a_l, b_l)$.

(iii) Point-process data consists of a set of points, S, that are randomly chosen by a spatial point process (Diggle, 2013). These points could mark, for example, the incidence of a disease such as childhood leukemia (Gatrell, Bailey, Diggle, and Rowlingson, 1996). Despite the importance of spatial point process modeling, we do not cover this topic and its range of applications in this book. The reader is directed to P. J. Diggle (1993) and Diggle (2013) for further reading on this subject.

9.1.1 Smoothing models

In disease mapping we assume that the spatial data is in the lattice domain $L = \mathscr{L} = \{1, ..., N_L\}$ and assume that disease counts, Y_l, in an area l are Poisson distributed with the rate being a combination of the overall relative risk, μ, multiplied by the expected number of health outcomes, E_l (as seen in Chapter 2, Section 2.7) and the risk in that particular area, θ_l. For simplicity, here we assume there are no covariates. The model for the health counts in each area is given by

$$Y_l | \theta_l, \mu, E_l \sim_{ind} \text{Poisson}(\mu E_l \theta_l), \tag{9.1}$$

for all $l \in L$ where *ind* means 'independently distributed' and μ is the overall relative risk that reflects differences between the reference rates and the rates in the study region as a whole.

At the second stage, the random effects θ_l are assigned a distribution which will reflect the deviations of the relative risks from the overall mean, μ. A common choice of distribution is the Gamma distribution which is conjugate to the Poisson as seen in Chapter 6, Example 6.2. They are modeled by

$$\theta_l | \alpha \sim_{iid} \text{Gam}(\alpha, \alpha), \ l = 1, ..., N_L. \tag{9.2}$$

Here, the marginal prior relative risks for each individual area follow a gamma distribution with mean 1, and variance $1/\alpha$.

In this case, it can be shown that the marginal distribution of $Y_l|\mu,\alpha$ with respect to θ_l is negative binomial. This is obtained by integrating out the random effects θ_l, that is, $p(Y_l|\mu,\alpha,E_l) = \int_\theta p(Y|\mu,\theta_l)p(\theta_l\mid\alpha)d\theta_l$.

Marginally, the mean and variance are given, respectively, by

$$
\begin{aligned}
E[Y_l|\mu,E_l] &= E_l\mu \\
\text{Var}(Y_l|\mu,\alpha,E_l) &= E[Y_l|\mu,\alpha,E_l](1+E[Y_l|\mu,\alpha,E_l]/\alpha).
\end{aligned}
\tag{9.3}
$$

Therefore the variance increases as a quadratic function of the mean, and the scale parameter α can accommodate different levels of 'over-dispersion' (see Chapter 2, Section 2.7.2).

9.1.2 Empirical Bayes smoothing

In empirical Bayes, the prior distribution is estimated from the data (Carlin and Louis, 2000). This is in contrast to fully Bayesian analyzes, in which the prior distribution is chosen before any data are observed. If we have estimates $\hat\mu,\hat a$ then the posterior distribution would be

$$
\theta_l|\mathbf{y},\hat\mu,\hat\alpha \sim \text{Ga}(\hat\alpha+y_l,\hat\alpha+E_l\hat\mu).
$$

The relative risk that would be applied to the expected numbers of health outcomes, E_l, is given by $\text{RR}_l = \mu\theta_l$, and has mean

$$
\begin{aligned}
\widehat{RR}_l &= \hat\mu\times E[\theta_l|\mathbf{y},\hat\mu,\hat\alpha] = \hat\mu\left(\frac{\hat\alpha+Y_l}{\hat\alpha+\hat\mu E_l}\right) \\
&= E[\text{RR}_l]\times(1-w_l)+\text{SMR}_l\times w_l.
\end{aligned}
\tag{9.4}
$$

This is a weighted combination of the prior estimate $E[\text{RR}_l]=\mu$, which will be the global RR over the entire set of areas, $l\in L$, and the SMR (Y_l/E_l) in area l.

The *weight*,

$$
w_l = \frac{E_l\hat\mu}{\hat\alpha+E_l\hat\mu},
$$

given the observed SMR using the data increases as E_l, which represents the size of the population, increases. Therefore, for areas with large populations, the estimate is dominated by the data in that area rather than the overall RR. If α is large then there will be less variability in the random effects than with small α and so there will be more shrinkage towards the overall RR.

It can be seen that the estimates will be less variable than the original SMRs. However, this does mean that a very high SMR, which might be important in detecting potential risk factors, may be shrunk if it is based on a small population and so may be overlooked.

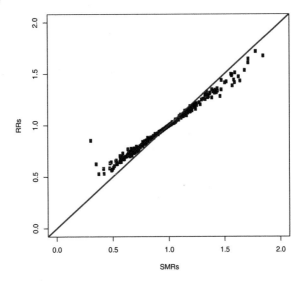

Figure 9.1: The effect of smoothing SMRs using an empirical Bayes approach. The red line has a slope of one and helps show the shrinkage effect with estimates being brought towards the overall mean relative risk.

Example 9.1. *Empirical Bayes and Bayes smoothing of COPD mortality for 2010*

Here we consider hospitalization for a respiratory condition, chronic obstructive pulmonary disease (COPD), in England in 2010. There are $N_l = 324$ local authority administrative areas each with an observed, Y_l and expected, E_l, number of cases, $l = 1, ..., 324$. As described in Section 2.4 the expected numbers were calculated using indirect standardization by applying the age–sex specific rates for the whole of England to the age–sex population profile of each of the areas. In order to perform empirical Bayes smoothing, we will use the eBayes function in the SpatialEpi package.

```
# requires SpatialEpi package
library(SpatialEpi)
RRs = eBayes(Y,E)
plot(RRs$SMR, RRs$RR, xlim=c(0,2),ylim=c(0,2), xlab="
    SMRs",ylab="RRs")
abline(a=0,b=1, col="red", lwd=3)
```

The result can be seen in Figure 9.1 in which the smoothing can be seen with lower and higher SMRs being brought close to the overall average, μ which in this case is $\exp(-0.0309) = 0.9696$. Note that in this example, the areas are relatively large and would be expected to have substantial populations, so the effect of the smoothing is limited. In this example, α was estimated to be 14.6. For a fully Bayesian, rather than empirical Bayes, analysis we can use NIMBLE using the following code:

```
model{
  for (i in 1 : N) {
      Y[i]    ~ dpois(mu[i])
      mu[i]  <- E[i]*exp(beta0)*theta[i]
      RR[i]  <- exp(beta0)*theta[i]
      theta[i] ~ dgamma(alpha,alpha)
  }
```

```
# Priors
  alpha  ~ dgamma(1,1)
  beta0  ~ dnorm(0,10)
  overall.risk <- exp(beta0)
}
```

The results of this analysis are available on the book's GitHub site.

9.2   The Markov random field (MRF)

We now introduce some basic theory that underlies the processes used in disease mapping. The starting point is the seminal paper of Besag (1974) which introduced what has proven to be a very important idea for modeling areal data, the Markov random field. For a fixed time point a lattice process, Z_l, over domain $L = \{1, \ldots, N_L\}$, $Z_l, l \in L$ has a distribution determined by its conditional distribution given its values at the neighboring points. Thus, if for example Z_l were observed with error, yielding, Y_l then the conditional distribution could be used for inference about Z_l by borrowing strength from data collected at the neighboring lattice points.

In his celebrated paper, Besag builds on earlier work, including one of the most famous unpublished papers in the history of statistical science, the 1971 paper of Hammersley and Clifford. In personal communications with the second author, Peter Clifford said he was a postdoctoral summer visitor at the University of California, Berkeley, when by then the distinguished Hammersley delivered a series of lectures, one of which contained a false claim that sparked the collaboration that led to the famous result. As we understand it, the authors were not satisfied with the progress they made that summer and did not feel the result worthy of submission for publication!

As with Hammersley and Clifford, Besag makes an important assumption of positivity throughout his paper. More precisely, after ordering the lattice points in an arbitrary order (which will not matter as far as the results are concerned) let $\mathbf{Z} = (Z_1, \ldots, Z_{N_L})$, and f denote its joint PDF, that is, $f_{\mathbf{Z}}(\mathbf{z}) = f(\mathbf{z})$ while $f(z_l)$ denotes that of Z_l for lattice point l. Then positivity means that $f(z_l) > 0$ for all l implies $f(z_1, \ldots, z_{N_L}) > 0$ over the range of Z that is $\mathscr{Z} = \{\mathbf{z} : f(z_1, \ldots, z_{N_L}) > 0\}$.

Under the positivity assumption, Besag presents the surprising result now referred to as Brook's lemma (Brook, 1964), that for any two points $\mathbf{z}, \mathbf{z}^0 \in \mathcal{Z}$, we have

$$f(\mathbf{z}) = f(\mathbf{z}^0) \Pi_{j=1}^{N_L} \frac{f(z_j \mid z_1, \ldots, z_{j-1}, z_{j+1}^0 \ldots, z_{N_L}^0)}{f(z_j^0 \mid z_1, \ldots, z_{j-1}, z_{j+1}^0 \ldots, z_{N_L}^0)}. \qquad (9.5)$$

As observed in Banerjee et al. (2015), this means that the joint distribution is determined by the full set of conditional densities for $\mathbf{Z}$, with each coordinate conditional on all the others. Knowing these conditionals, fixing $\mathbf{z}^0$, then determining the second factor in Equation (9.5) as a function of $\mathbf{z}$ and finally integrating the right-hand side over $\mathbf{z}$ would determine $f(\mathbf{z}^0)$. That is because the latter does not depend on $\mathbf{z}$ while the left-hand side of the equation would become 1. That discovery is important for Gibbs sampling, as it means sampling from those conditionals sequentially would yield samples from the joint distribution, which is at the heart of Gibbs sampling.

Besag recognizes some important implications of Brook's lemma in modeling lattice random fields. He states that the lemma highlights a fundamental difficulty:

> '...concerning the specification of a system through its conditional probability structure. ... the labelling of individual sites in the system being arbitrary implies that many factorizations of $P(\mathbf{x})/P(\mathbf{y})$ are possible. All ... must be equivalent, and this ... implies the existence of severe restrictions on the available functional forms ... to achieve a mathematically consistent joint probability structure'.

In other words, the form of the distribution must not depend on the way in which we happened to label the lattice points from 1 to N_L.

The Brook's lemma would not be very useful for modeling the joint distribution of a random field when N_L is large, as specifying all these conditionals would not be easy. More preferable would be a simplified model where the conditional distribution of a site depends on just a small subset of them. Besag approaches this using a neighborhood structure. Using the notation in Banerjee et al. (2015), the set $\partial_l \subset L$ is a neighborhood of l if it satisfies

$$[Z_l \mid \{Z_{l'} : l' \in L\}] = [Z_l \mid \{Z_{l'} : l' \in \partial_l\}]. \qquad (9.6)$$

Here we are using the general bracket notion $[U]$, $[U \mid V = v]$ and $[U \mid A]$ for arbitrary random variables U and V, where an event A means respectively the distribution of U, the conditional distribution of U given $V = v$ and the conditional distribution of U given that the event A occurs.

It would simplify things if the joint distribution were determined by just the conditional distributions given just the responses for the neighborhoods. For example, suppose the random responses were independent. Then the neighborhood of each response would be a null set. Moreover, the analysis could be carried out for each response separately. In other words, the joint distribution would be completely specified just by its marginals.

The problem of finding a set of such neighborhoods proves challenging. Yet in practice that neighborhood structure would need to be specified by the modeller for all $l \in L$, as in Equation (9.6), along with the conditional distributions. In a regular lattice, for example, these may be the nearest four points to the north, south, east and west of l in the lattice. Then again, there are cases where this is not appropriate, for example, for widely separated lattice points on high peaks that have similar temperatures on opposite sides of a valley. (see Example 14.14 for further discussion on this point).

Even at the theoretical level, finding admissible neighborhood structures is difficult. Initially, based on Besag's quotation above, we anticipate a strong restriction that these neighbors must be invariant in some sense under permutations of the site labels. However, given such a set of invariant neighborhoods, what kind of joint distributions would be consistent with them? Does such a joint distribution even exist? There is certainly no reason to be optimistic, after all, specifying just local dependence properties of the process is far from specifying a *bona fide* joint distribution over the whole lattice domain. That is the central issue Besag addressed in his paper, and his representation of joint lattice process probabilities is a central result.

That result is given first in the discrete case, albeit by a somewhat heuristic argument. A rigorous, constructive proof of that representation is given in a general theorem of Hosseini, Le, and Zidek (2011) where like Besag they have to exclude 0 from the list of possible values.

Theorem 1. Suppose, $h : \prod_{i=1}^{p} M_l \to R$, M_l being finite with $|M_l| = c_l$ and $0 \in M_l$, $\forall l$, $1 \le l \le p$. Let $M_l^* = M_l - \{0\}$. Then there exists a unique family of functions

$$\{G_{i_1,\cdots,i_k} : M_{i_1}^* \times M_{i_2}^* \times \cdots \times M_{i_k}^* \to R, \ 1 \le k \le r, \ 1 \le i_1 < i_2 < \cdots < i_k \le p\},$$

such that,

$$
\begin{aligned}
h(z_1,\cdots,z_p) \ = \ & h(0,\cdots,0) + \sum_{i=1}^{p} z_l G_l(z_l) + \cdots + \\
& \sum_{1 \le i_1 < i_2 < \ldots < i_k \le r} (z_{i_1} \cdots z_{i_k}) G_{i_1,\cdots,i_k}(z_{i_1},\cdots,z_{i_k}) \qquad (9.7) \\
& + \cdots + (z_1 z_2 \cdots z_{N_L}) G_{12\cdots p}(z_1,\cdots,z_{N_L}).
\end{aligned}
$$

In an extension of this theorem, Hosseini et al. (2011) replace 0 by an arbitrary point to get a more general representation. They apply their result to derive a class of Markov chain models in a temporal context. There, since time is ordered and invariance under permutations would not make sense, the issues around invariant neighborhood structures do not arise.

Leaving the general result above and returning to the case of lattice processes, we note that Besag applies his result to the function

$$h = \log\{f(\mathbf{z})/f(\mathbf{0})\}, \qquad (9.8)$$

assuming $f(\mathbf{0}) > 0$ and embraces the need expressed in his quotation above by incorporating, in his expansion, the idea of a 'clique'. This is a set, C, of location indices with the property that every one of its points is in the neighborhood of every other point in C thus ensuring its invariance under a permutation of their site labels. In the context of his application, the functions G in the expansion above are non-null only if the subscripts correspond to the members of a clique, for otherwise the required invariance will be lost.

We now turn to the Hammersley-Clifford theorem and the work of Geman and Geman (1984), which gives its inverse. Banerjee et al. (2015) give a very clear account of that work. We start with the set of all cliques of size $l = 1, \ldots, N_L$ in the expansion shown in Equation (9.7). Any clique $c_j \subset L$ of size j corresponds to a vector $\mathbf{z}_{c_j}$ of values. By inverting Besag's function h in the form given by Geman and Geman (and presented by Banerjee et al., 2015) we get the density function of the so-called Gibbs distribution named after Josiah Willard Gibbs (1803–1903) from his original work in statistical mechanics:

$$f(\mathbf{z}) = \exp\left\{ \tau \left(\sum_{c_1 \subset L} H_1(\mathbf{z}_{c_1}) + \sum_{c_2 \subset L} H_2(\mathbf{z}_{c_2}) + \ldots + c_{N_L} H_{N_L}(\mathbf{z}) \right) \right\}. \qquad (9.9)$$

The H's, which are required to be invariant under permutations of their arguments, are called potentials, τ the 'temperature', and the expression in brackets in Equation (9.9), the energy function. The Hammersley-Clifford theorem says a valid MRF model must yield a Gibbs distribution, while Geman's paper proves the inverse. An update to this theory can be found in Kaiser and Cressie (2000).

Example 9.2. *The Ising model*

One well known Gibbs distribution comes from the Ising model, where the process is binary and each $z \in \{-1, 1\}$. The distribution models pairwise interactions between the sites through

$$f(\mathbf{z}) = \exp(\tau \sum_{(l,l') \in L_2} z_l z_{l'}),$$

where L_2 defines pairs of neighboring sites, which are neighbors of each other. In other words, $c_2 = \{l, l'\}$, $\mathbf{z}_{c_2} = (z_l, z_{l'})$ and $H_2(\mathbf{z}_{c_2}) = z_l z_{l'}$. When the temperature is high, the probability tends to be higher than when the values at different sites are alike.

An assessment of the MRF approach

The MRF approach would be considered in situations where processes of interest manifest themselves through observable responses that generate the data. It is assumed that such data are available for all indices $\{l\}$ and it provides a natural way of building up a Bayesian hierarchical model in such situations.

However, identifying appropriate neighborhoods may be difficult. (See Section 9.4.1 for discussion of this issue). Unlike classical geostatistical methods, which allow extrapolation as well as smoothing, the MRF will only be of value when there are neighbors. Finally, the change of support problem can make this approach difficult to use, in other words Z may be measured at point-referenced points s while Y is for lattice points l.

9.3   The conditional autoregressive (CAR) model

Since space, unlike time, is not ordered, we cannot use the classes of models such as the AR(1) that depend on that ordering. However, Besag proposes a spatial autoregressive model that resembles its temporal counterpart that is known as the conditional autoregressive (CAR) model.

Assume that a region, L, is sub-divided into areas that are denoted by $l \in L$ where $L = l_1, ..., l_{N_L}$ with Y_l the variable of interest in area l, $\mathbf{Y}_{-l}$ the set observables after removing Y_l and ∂_l denoting the neighbors of l. The CAR model is defined as follows for all l:

$$[Y_l \mid \mathbf{Y}_{-l} = \mathbf{y}_{-l}] \quad \sim \quad N\left(\mu_l, \sigma_l^2\right), \tag{9.10}$$

where $\mu_l = E(Y_l | \mathbf{Y}_{-l} = \mathbf{y}_{-l})$ and $\sigma_l^2 = Var(Y_l | \mathbf{Y}_{-l} = \mathbf{y}_{-l})$. The mean term can be expressed in terms of covariates, $\mathbf{x}$, and associated (regression) parameters, β: $\mu_l = \mathbf{x}_l^T \beta + \sum_{l'} c_{ll'}(y_{l'} - \mathbf{x}_{l'}^T \beta)$, with $c_{ll'} > 0$, $l \neq l'$ and $c_{ll} = 0$ (De Oliveira, 2012).

It now follows that

$$f(\mathbf{y}) \propto \exp\left[-\frac{1}{2}(\mathbf{y} - \mathbf{X}\beta)^T L^{-1}(I - C)(\mathbf{y} - \mathbf{X}\beta)\right], \tag{9.11}$$

where $D = diag\{\sigma_1^2, ..., \sigma_{N_L}^2\}$, $C = (c_{ll'})$ with $c_{ll} = 0$, and $c_{ll'}\sigma_{l'}^2 = c_{l'l}\sigma_l^2$, the last condition being to ensure that $L^{-1}(I - C)$ is a positive definite symmetric matrix (Gelfand et al., 2005).

In the CAR model, the advantage of the neighborhood structure has the disadvantage that the coefficients $c_{ll'}$ now need to be specified. An obvious and intuitively appealing solution to this problem is based on the idea the conditional mean in Equation (9.10) should be a weighted average of means in the neighboring points. For this purpose, we need the idea of adjacency weights $w_{ll'}$ that are non-negative only if l and l' are adjoining points while $w_{ll} = 0$. We now take, $c_{ll'} = w_{ll'}/w_{l+}, l \neq l'$ and $\sigma_l^2 = \tau/w_{l+}$, where $w_{l+} = \sum_{l'} w_{ll'}$. This way we can take account of the degree to which l' is seen as like l when it comes to borrowing strength. We now find that $D^{-1}(I - C) = \tau^{-2}(C_w - W)$ in Equation (9.11) where $C_w = diag\{w_{1+}, ..., w_{N_L+}\}$.

If we don't have the mean term in Equation (9.10) then this distribution would be singular. That is because the sum of the columns of $(C_w - W)$ is a vector of zeros (Banerjee et al., 2015),

$$\mathbf{y}^T D^{-1}(I - C)\mathbf{y} = \sum_{l \neq l'} w_{ll'}(y_l - y_l')^2. \tag{9.12}$$

This singularity makes this joint distribution unsuitable to describe the behavior of observed quantities, since the joint distribution of $\mathbf{Y}$ does not result in a proper (that integrates to 1) density. This distribution is called an intrinsically autoregressive (IAR) process. One way around the impropriety of the IAR distribution is to introduce an additional parameter and replace W with ϕW in this case with a suitable ϕ so that the covariance matrix has full rank, that is the columns of the $(C_w - \phi W)$ no longer sum to one (De Oliveira, 2012). Other reparametrizations of the IAR model have been proposed, and these will be discussed in Section 9.4.

Other versions of the CAR model have been developed, notably a multivariate extension called the MCAR model (Gelfand et al., 2005).

9.3.1   The intrinsic conditional autoregressive (ICAR) model

A common approach is to assign the spatial random effects an intrinsic conditional autoregressive (ICAR) prior. Under this specification, the neighborhood structure is such that $w_{ll'} = 1$ if l and l' are neighbors, and 0 otherwise. This results in the following conditional distributions

$$Y_l | Y_{l'}, l' \in \partial_l \sim N\left(\overline{Y}_l, \frac{\tau^2}{m_l}\right),$$

where ∂l is the set of neighbors of the lattice point l, m_l is the number of neighbors and $\overline{Y}_l$ is the mean of the spatial random effects of these neighbors. τ^2 is a conditional variance, and its magnitude determines the amount of spatial variation. Notice that if τ^2 is 'small' then, although the residual is strongly dependent on the neighboring value, the overall contribution to the residual relative risk is small. This is a little counterintuitive but stems from spatial models having two aspects, strength of dependence and total amount of spatial dependence, and in the ICAR model there is only a single parameter which controls both aspects.

9.3.2   The simultaneous autoregressive (SAR) model

The simultaneous autoregressive (SAR) model, a very natural choice, resembles the CAR (Whittle, 1954) but is specified through a regression model resembling the AR(1) model. Thus, it is defined this way when we ignore measurement error:

$$Y_l - \mu_l = \sum_{l'} c_{ll'}(Y_{l'} - \mu_{l'}) + v_l, \tag{9.13}$$

where $v_l \sim_{iid} N(0, \sigma_l^2)$ and $c_{ll} = 0$ is designed to capture spatial structure. Thus Y_l is regressed on all the remaining responses. In vector-matrix form:

$$\mathbf{Y} - \mu = \mathbf{C}(\mathbf{Y} - \mu) + \mathbf{v}, \tag{9.14}$$

where $\mathbf{C}$ is chosen to be invertible and $\mathbf{v}$ represents a combination of process and data model error. It follows that

$$(\mathbf{I} - \mathbf{C})(\mathbf{Y} - \mu) = \mathbf{v},$$

from which, it follows that

$$\mathbf{Y} = \mu + \mathbf{v}^*$$

where $\mathbf{v}^* \sim N_{N_L}(0, (\mathbf{I}-\mathbf{C})^{-1}\Sigma(\mathbf{I}-\mathbf{C}^T)^{-1})$ with $\Sigma = diag\{\sigma_1^2, \ldots, \sigma_{N_L}^2\}$. This model captures spatial independence through the mean structure – a moving average of the $\{v_l\}$.

Banerjee et al. (2015) note that the SAR is commonly used to model regression residuals where $\mu = \mathbf{X}\beta$ incorporates, through the design matrix $\mathbf{X}$, the covariates that might explain the spatial variation in the process. Then we have for the residuals $\mathbf{U} = \mathbf{Y} - \mathbf{X}\beta$ the equation, $\mathbf{U} = \mathbf{C}\mathbf{U} + \mathbf{v}[$ or equivalently $\mathbf{Y} = \mathbf{C}\mathbf{Y} + (\mathbf{I}-\mathbf{C}^T)\mathbf{X}\beta + \mathbf{v}$. In this form, we see $\mathbf{Y}$ as a weighted mixture of $\mathbf{Y}$, recalling that the diagonal elements of $\mathbf{C}$ are equal to zero, that is $c_{ll} = 0$, and a regression model for the spatial mean is based on covariates. Thus, we are borrowing strength from the neighbors as well as the covariates.

9.4   Spatial models for disease mapping

In general, we might expect to observe similar residual relative risks in areas that are 'close' to one another or at least more alike in some sense, than they would be for areas that are further apart. Ideally, we would exploit this information and provide more reliable estimates of relative risk in each area. This is analogous to the use of a covariate; if we knew that a covariate, X, had an effect on risk, then we might expect areas with similar X values to have similar relative risks. The idea here is that spatial location is acting as a surrogate for unobserved covariates that will induce a spatial pattern.

9.4.1   Poisson-lognormal models

The Poisson-gamma model is analytically tractable, but does not easily allow the incorporation of spatial random effects. Spatial random effects can be incorporated in a Poisson log-normal model in a straightforward and interpretable fashion. Whereas in the Poisson–Gamma model we have $\theta \sim Ga(\alpha, \alpha)$, here we have $\theta = e^{V_l} \sim LogNormal(0, \sigma^2)$. A Poisson-lognormal non-spatial random effect model is given by

$$Y_l | \beta, V_l \sim_{ind} \text{Poisson}(E_l \mu_l e^{V_l}), \quad V_l \sim_{iid} N(0, \sigma_v^2), \tag{9.15}$$

where V_l are area-specific random effects that capture the unexplained (log) relative risk of disease in area $l \in L, L = l_1, \ldots, l_{N_L}$.

However, the model shown in Equation (9.15) does not give a marginal distribution of known form. The marginal variance is of the same quadratic form as that seen in Equation (9.3) and Chapter 2, Section 2.7.2. In order to implement this model, it is easier to consider a fully Bayesian analysis rather than an empirical Bayes approach. This is because the marginal distribution of Y_l when integrated out with respect to V_l

does not have a closed form. Therefore, a prior distribution to the vector containing the unknowns of the model needs to be specified; then, a fully Bayesian approach is followed when estimating the parameters of the model.

The prior specification follows by assuming prior independence among the parameters of the model. We need to specify priors for the regression coefficients, β, and the variance of the random effects σ_v^2. For a rare disease, a log-linear link is a natural choice for the link function (between the response and the linear predictor):

$$\log \mu(\mathbf{x}_l, \beta) = \beta_0 + \sum_{j=1}^{J} \beta_j' x_{lj},$$

where x_{lj} is the value of the j-th covariate in area l. For regression parameters $\beta = (\beta_0, \beta_1, ..., \beta_J)$, vague, for example $N(0, 1000)$ or improper priors $p(\beta) \propto 1$ are often used. However, in some circumstances that latter choice may lead to an improper posterior. If there are numerous covariates, or high dependence amongst them, more informative priors may be required; or regularization methods (see Section 7.7.3) can also be used.

If one aims at accounting for a spatial structure that is left after adjusting for the covariates x_{lj}, one can assume a CAR prior distribution as discussed in Section 9.3, that is, assume

$$Y_l | \beta, \gamma, U_l \sim_{ind} \text{Poisson} \left(E_l \mu_l e^{U_l} \right)$$
$$U_l \mid U_{l'}, l' \in \partial_l \sim N \left(\frac{\sum_{l'} w_{ll'} u_{l'}}{w_{l+}}, \frac{\tau^2}{w_{l+}} \right), \tag{9.16}$$

such that $\mathbf{U} = (U_1, ..., U_{N_L})$ follows a CAR prior distribution as discussed in Section 9.3.

Here we consider *conditional* models that are amenable to area level (lattice) data as discussed in Section 9.3. As discussed there, in this approach we specify the distribution of each U_l as if we knew the values of the spatial random effects $U_{l'}$ in 'neighboring areas'. In order to do this, we need to be able to specify the 'neighbors' of each area. A simple approach is to define areas l' and l as neighbors if they share a *common boundary*. Other neighborhood structures can be explored, for example, one based on the Euclidean distance among centroids of the areas. Ferreira and Schmidt (2006) investigate the use of different neighborhood structures that take into account the particular landscape of the region under study. They noticed that the importance of some covariates in the mean structure changed when different neighborhoods structures were assumed.

Besag, York, and Mollié (1991) propose a convolution prior model (also known as BYM), wherein an independent (across areas) random effect, V_l, is added to Equation (9.16), such that

$$Y_l | \beta, \gamma, U_l, V_l \sim_{ind} \text{Poisson}(E_l \mu_l e^{U_l + V_l}), \tag{9.17}$$

where U_l and V_l are assumed independent, *a priori*. Note that if $\tau^2 \to 0$ then the U_l's are constants, whereas large values of τ^2 imply large but spatially structured variation. On the other hand, if $\sigma_v^2 \to 0$ then $V_l = 0$, whereas large σ_v^2 implies large unstructured variability (Besag et al., 1991). More importantly, the likelihood involves the sum $U_l + V_l$, so it is challenging to identify each of these components from a single realization of the process under study. Also, note that the variances τ^2 and σ_v^2 are in different scales; the former is the variance of the *conditional* distribution of U_l given its neighbors, whereas the latter is the *marginal* variance of the independent random effect V_l.

Because of the identifiability issue present in the BYM model, reparametrizations of the CAR model have been proposed. Leroux, Lei, and Breslow (1999) propose to remove V_l from Equation (9.17) and include a component λ in the CAR prior specification, such that

$$E(U_l \mid \mathbf{u}_{-l}) = \left(\frac{\lambda}{1 - \lambda q_{ii}} \right) \sum_{j \in \partial_i} u_j, \ \text{and} \ V(U_i \mid \mathbf{u}_{-i}) = \frac{\tau^2}{1 - \lambda + \lambda q_{ii}}, \qquad (9.18)$$

where $0 \leq \lambda \leq 1$ denotes a spatial dependence parameter, such that $\lambda = 0$ defines a non-spatial model, and the level of spatial dependence increases with λ. In this case, the joint prior distribution of the vector $\mathbf{U}$ is a zero mean normal distribution, with covariance matrix $\Sigma_u = \tau^2 \left[\lambda Q + (1 - \lambda) I_n \right]^{-1}$, where the diagonal elements of Q, q_{ii}, contain the number of neighbors of region l, and $q_{ll'} = -1$ if $l \sim l'$, and 0 otherwise. When $\lambda = 1$ the distribution of $\mathbf{U}$ is improper, as it results in the ICAR specification.

More recently, D. Simpson, Rue, Riebler, Martins, Sørbye, et al. (2017) claim that the components U_l and V_l in Equation (9.17) should not be assumed to be independent $\forall l$, suggesting that the priors on τ^2 and σ_v^2 should be dependent. Simpson, Rue, Riebler, Martins, Sørbye, et al. (2017) propose a parametrization of the model in Equation (9.17), wherein the component $U_l + V_l$ is substituted by $\frac{1}{\tau} \left(\sqrt{1 - \phi} V_l + \sqrt{\phi} U_l^* \right)$, with $0 \leq \phi \leq 1$ being a mixing parameter. The component U_l^* is a scaled spatially structured component where the generalized variance, computed as the geometric mean of the marginal variances, is equal to one. In this case, $1/\tau$ represents the marginal precision contribution from U_l^* and V_l, with ϕ representing the fraction of this variance explained by U_l^*, and $(1 - \phi)$ the fraction explained by V_l. See Riebler, Sørbye, Simpson, and Rue (2016) on how to obtain the scaled neighborhood matrix of $\mathbf{U}^*$ using R-INLA.

The inference procedure of the models previously described can be performed via MCMC or INLA. As the CAR prior distribution is improper, one needs to guarantee that the posterior distribution is proper. One possible approach is to impose a linear constraint such that $\sum_l u_l = 0$. In a MCMC algorithm this is done by centering the random effects, that is, by replacing u_l by $u_l - \overline{u}$, for all l at each MCMC iteration (Gelfand and Sahu, 1999; Banerjee et al., 2015).

There are different pieces of software and packages in R that can be used to fit models with CAR components. If the approximation to the posterior distribution is to be performed via MCMC, we suggest using NIMBLE, STAN or CARBayes (D. Lee, 2013).

Example 9.3. *Fitting a conditional spatial model in NIMBLE*

In this example, we see how to fit the Poisson log-normal model seen in Section 9.4 with spatial random effects coming from the ICAR model described in Section 9.3.1.

The ICAR model can be specified via the function dcar_normal:

```
U[1:N] ~ dcar_normal(adj[1:L], weights[1:L], num[1:N],
                     tau, zero_mean=1)
```

where:

- adj[1:L] : A vector listing the ID numbers of the adjacent areas for each area.
- weights[1:L] : A vector the same length as adj[] giving unnormalized weights associated with each pair of areas.
- num[1:N]: A vector of length N (the total number of areas) giving the number of neighbors m_l for each area.
- The dcar_normal distribution is parameterized to include a sum-to-zero constraint on the random effects. In this case, a separate intercept must be used, and the option zero_mean should be set to 1 in the specification of dcar_normal.

We now use the Poisson log-normal model with the data for respiratory admissions seen in Example 9.4.

The NIMBLE code is as follows:

```
CAR_Code <- nimbleCode({
  # Likelihood
  for(i in 1:N){
    y[i] ~ dpois(lambda[i])
    log(lambda[i]) <- log(E[i])+ u[i] + inprod(X[i,1:p
      ],beta[1:p])
  }
  # Priors
  beta0 ~ dnorm(0, sd=0.98)
  for(k in 1:p){
    beta[k] ~ dnorm(0, sd=0.98)
  }
  u[1:N] ~ dcar_normal(adj[1:L], weights[1:L], num[1:N
    ], tau, zero_mean=1)
  tau <- 1/(sigma_u^2)
  #half-Cauchy prior for sigma_u
  sigma_u ~ T(dnorm(0,sd=1),0,)
  # Fitted values and likelihood for WAIC
  for(i in 1:N){
    fitted[i] ~ dpois(lambda[i])
  }
})
```

Example 9.4. *Fitting a conditional spatial model in CARBayes*

Here we consider fitting the Poisson log-normal with spatial effects to the data for respiratory admissions seen in Example 9.4 using the R package CARBayes. Again, the spatial effects come from the ICAR model described in Section 9.3.1 and this requires a set of observed and expected values together with an adjacency matrix. In this example, we created the required adjacency matrix from a shapefile using the spdep and shapefiles packages (although the maptools package could also be used). CARBayes performs MCMC simulation similarly to using NIMBLE but has the distinct advantage that the simulations are performed within R. NIMBLE is of course a much more general platform for fitting a wide variety of complex models using MCMC, as described in Section 6.5.

```
# requires CARBAyes, spdep and shapefiles libraries
library(CARBAyes)
library(spdep)
library(shapefiles)

# read in the shape file
shp <- read.shp(shp.name="england local authority.shp"
    )
```

```
# read in the details of the areas
dbf <- read.dbf(dbf.name="england local authority.dbf"
    )

# calculate the SMRs and combine with the spatial
    information
SMR <- Y/E
SMRspatial <- combine.data.shapefile(SMR, shp, dbf)

# Create the neighborhood matrix
W.nb <- poly2nb(SMRspatial, row.names = rownames(SMR))
W.list <- nb2listw(W.nb, style="B")
W.mat <- nb2mat(W.nb, style="B")

# Fit a  CAR smoothing model
formula <- observed~offset(log(expected))

model <- iarCAR.re(formula=formula, family="poisson",
    W=W.mat,
      burnin=20000, n.sample=100000, thin=10)
risk <- model$fitted.values[ ,1] / expected
```

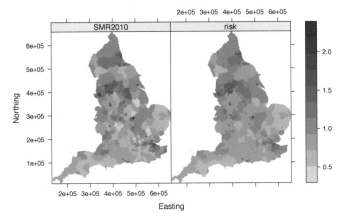

Figure 9.2: Maps of the spatial distribution of risks of hospital admission for a respiratory condition, chronic obstructive pulmonary disease (COPD), in the UK for 2001. The left-hand side map shows the SMR estimates. The right-hand map shows the smoothed risks which were estimated using the BYM Bayesian model. Darker shades indicate higher rates of hospitalization, allowing for the underlying age–sex profile of the population within the area.

The CARBayes package allows a number of CAR models to be used including non-intrinsic models. For further details see D. Lee (2013).

Again, Figure 9.2 is used to show the resulting map of the estimates of relative risks from applying the intrinsic CAR model as the results are the same as those using NIMBLE.

Example 9.5. *Fitting a conditional spatial model using R–INLA*

In this final example of implementing the Poisson log-normal with spatial effects, we use R-INLA. Again, the spatial effects come from the ICAR model described in Section 9.3.1. This form of spatial data, for example areas, is already in the form that can be used by R-INLA. Chapter 10, Section 10.12 considers the case when spatial data takes the form of points rather than areas and details are given of the methods that need to be employed to transform point referenced data into a form that INLA can use.

The intrinsic, and non-intrinsic, CAR models are two of a set of defined latent models in R-INLA. As such the syntax is very simple with the random effects being defined following the form f(ID, model="besag", graph="UK.adj") where UK.adj is an adjacency matrix that is suitable for use with R-INLA. The code to perform the model is as follows and follows on from the component of the code seen in Example 9.4 which sets up the data and adjacency matrix.

```
# requires INLA
library(INLA)

### Create the neighborhood matrix
W.nb  <- poly2nb(SMRspatial, row.names = rownames(SMR))
W.list <- nb2listw(W.nb, style="B")
W.mat <- nb2mat(W.nb, style="B")

#Convert the adjacency matrix
  into a file in the INLA format
nb2INLA("UK.adj", W.nb)
```

```
#Create areas IDs to match the values in UK.adj
data=as.data.frame(cbind(Y, E))
data$ID<-1:324

# run the INLA model
m1<-inla(Y~f(ID, model="besag", graph="UK.adj"),
    family="poisson", E=E,data = data,
    control.predictor=list(compute=TRUE))
```

As mentioned in the previous two examples, Figure 9.2. shows the result-ing map of the estimates of relative risks from applying the intrinsic CAR model.

The online resources provide the analysis of the COPD example comparing the CAR prior specification with the Leroux and BYM2 alternative prior distributions. It also includes the code for these models in Stan.

9.5 Summary

This chapter contains an introduction to different types of spatial data, the theory of spatial lattice processes and introduces disease mapping and models for performing smoothing of risks over space. The reader will have gained an understanding of the following topics:

- Disease mapping and how to improve estimates of risk by borrowing strength from adjacent regions which can reduce the instability inherent in risk estimates based on small (expected) numbers;

- How smoothing can be performed using either the empirical Bayes or fully Bayesian approaches;

- Computational methods for handling areal data;

- Besag's seminal contributions to the field of spatial statistics including the very important concept of a Markov random field;

- Approaches to modeling areal data including conditional autoregressive models;

- How Bayesian spatial models for lattice data can be fit using NIMBLE, RStan and R-INLA.

9.6 Exercises

Exercise 9.1. Find a Gibbs distribution when all cliques are of size 1. Repeat when all cliques are of size 2 that tends to put high probability on sites in cliques of size 2 where the two values tend to be different.

Exercise 9.2. Show that a random walk process of order 1 can be expressed in terms of an intrinsic CAR model, that is, if $p(\theta_t|\theta_{t-1}) \sim N(\theta_{t-1}, \sigma_w^2)$ then

$$p(\theta_t|\theta_{-t}, \sigma_w^2) \sim \begin{cases} N(\theta_{t+1}, \sigma_w^2) & \text{for } t = 1 \\ N\left(\frac{\theta_{t-1}+\theta_{t+1}}{2}, \frac{\sigma_w^2}{2}\right) & \text{for } t = 2, ..., T-1 \\ N(\theta_{t-1}, \sigma_w^2) & \text{for } t = T \end{cases}$$

where θ_{-t} represents the vector of θ's with θ_t removed. Pay particular attention to any assumptions that need to be made when $t = 1$ and $t = T$.

Exercise 9.3. Using Brook's lemma, prove the assertion in and Equation (9.11).

Exercise 9.4. Prove the assertion in and Equation (9.12).

Exercise 9.5. The data used to produce the map for hospital admissions for COPD in 2001 are included in the online resources. Using that data, reproduce the map of smoothed risks shown in Figure 9.2.

(i) Perform the analysis using NIMBLE, the CARBayes package in R and R-INLA. Compare the results from the three approaches.

(ii) Investigate the sensitivity of the results to the choice of priors for the variance terms. For example, in NIMBLE change,

```
alpha1 ~ dnorm(0.0, sd=100)
tau   ~ dgamma(0.5, 0.0005)
```

(iii) Make the same changes using CARBayes and R-INLA. Compare the results obtained using the different packages.

Exercise 9.6. The online resources also have data for COPD admissions for other years.

(i) Choose two other years of data and reproduce your analysis from Exercise 9.5. Is there any evidence of any changes in the patterns of risk over time?

(ii) After covering the material in Chapter 12, construct a spatio-temporal model for this data and fit it in NIMBLE and/or R-INLA.

(iii) Do the results from your model in part (ii) agree with your initial findings from considering the years separately?

Chapter 10

Spatial modeling: point-referenced data

10.1 Overview

The study of exposures to environmental hazards and their potential effects on health outcomes begins with understanding the underlying structure of, and variation in, the hazard over space and time. Changes in exposures to the hazard will be used to estimate the associated health effects, together with associated measures of uncertainty. An important aspect of this is to provide the contrasts in exposures over space and time that will drive the health outcome. In addition, being able to model the underlying structure of the exposure field will enable predictions to be made at locations where data are not available due to the absence of monitoring. Often there will be locations and periods of time in which exposure data will not be available. This may be due to a fault in monitoring equipment or may be due to design.

In many epidemiological studies the locations and times of exposure measurements and health assessments do not match, in part, because the health and exposure data will have arisen from different data sources. The ability to predict levels of exposures at all locations for which health data is available can therefore maximize the use of the available health data. In this chapter we concentrate on spatial models for exposures, and in the next two chapters we will encounter exposure models that produce similar contrasts over time (Chapter 11) and both space and time (Chapter 12).

This chapter focuses on processes for point referenced spatial data, that is, observations are obtained across fixed locations over a region of interest rather than area-level data on a lattice as seen in Chapter 9. Methods for characterizing underlying spatial processes and for modeling exposures over space are described.

10.2 A brief history of spatial modeling

Techniques for modeling random spatial fields began in earnest in the 1950s, when the foundation of the subject of geostatistics was laid by Krige and Matheron (Cressie, 1990). Its origins lay in the mining industry and the need to predict ore deposits beneath the surface of the earth. The approach was to use a few core samples taken at a few selected locations to map ore deposits by predicting deposits at locations which were unsampled. The method has come to be known as kriging,

DOI: 10.1201/9781003352655-10

after Krige, a South African mining engineer. His method relied on estimating spatial correlation between observed concentrations at the sampling sites (Krige, 1951).

The concept of spatial variation goes back a long way, at least to Kolmogorov (1941) although it was Matheron (1963) in the 1960s who first published a detailed account of geostatistics. He called the optimal linear unbiased prediction of responses at unsampled locations 'Kriging' to honor Krige's contributions. Kriging expanded to include the environmental sciences, with Eynon and Switzer (1983) amongst the first statisticians to see its potential in that area. Spatial statistics has since become an extremely important topic within statistical science (Cressie, 1993).

10.3   Exploring spatial data

A number of exploratory methods have been developed for the analysis of spatial data, and in this section we introduce a selection of them through a series of examples. A number of R packages have been designed specifically to display and model spatial data, including gstat and geoR. Where such packages are used, they are indicated within the given R code. The first stage of a spatial analysis is to investigate the distribution of the exposure of interest, for example concentrations of lead, in order to assess whether the assumptions necessary for applying subsequent methods are tenable.

Example 10.1. *Spatial patterns in lead concentrations in the soil of the Meuse River flood plain*

The Meuse River is one of the largest in Europe, and a great deal of research has been performed in relation to potential environmental hazards within its flood plain (Ashagrie, De Laat, De Wit, Tu, and Uhlenbrook, 2006). A comprehensive survey of concentrations of a variety of elements in the river was collected at 155 sampling sites in 1990. We now consider how the measurements at these locations can be visualized using R.

Figure 10.1 shows the locations of the 155 sampling locations and indicates the lead concentrations measured at those sites. The plot suggests the possibility of spatial patterns in the concentrations. Figure 10.2 shows a set of four plots of the Meuse valley lead concentrations using geoR. The four plots show: (i) the locations of the sampling sites (as seen in Figure 10.1); the concentrations in relation to (ii) x and (iii) y coordinates and (iv) a histogram of the concentrations indicating the distribution of concentrations together with an estimate of the density. The latter of these shows that the distribution is very skewed to the right.

The online resources provide an analysis of the levels of benzene (Zapata-Marin et al., 2022) observed at monitoring sites located in Montreal and provide the code to produce similar plots.

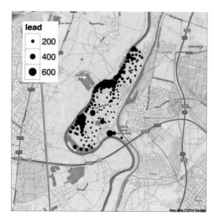

Figure 10.1: Bubble plot showing the size of lead concentrations measured in samples taken at 155 locations in the Meuse River flood plain.

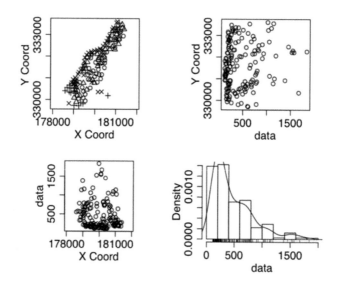

Figure 10.2: Summaries of the concentrations of lead measured at 155 sampling sites within the Meuse River plain. The top left panel shows the location of the sampling sites, the off-diagonal panels show scatter plots of concentrations against x and y coordinates and the fourth panel shows the distribution of lead concentration levels. The plots were produced by the R package geoR.

10.3.1 *Transformations and units of measurement*

Based on the distribution of the concentrations shown in Figure 10.2 (bottom right panel), before embarking on the analysis, we will log-transform the lead concentration due to the strong right skew in the data.

Before performing such a transformation, we need to consider the effects on the units of measurement. The logarithm is defined as the reciprocal operation of exponentiation, that is

$$x = \log_b(y) \text{ if } y = x^b$$

where b, x, and y are real numbers, b being the base of the logarithm. This definition precludes the association of any physical dimension to any of the three variables, b, x or y. Therefore, the data, y, needs to be 'normalized' before transforming it. Failure to do so can lead to results that can be difficult, or even impossible, to interpret. For example, consider a weight of 10.2 kg. Applied directly, its log would be $\log(10.2 \text{ kg})$ which could be expressed as $\log(2) + \log(5.1 \text{kg})$ which has a less obvious interpretation! Similarly, if the mean, μ and standard deviation, σ, of a log-Normally distributed variable, $Y \sim LN(\mu, \sigma^2)$, had units of measurement then the expectation $E(Y) = E(e^{\log(Y)}) = e^{(\mu + \frac{1}{2}\sigma^2)}$ would have units which were a mixture of two different scales.

Example 10.2. *Examining the log concentrations of lead in the Meuse River flood plain*

In Figure 10.3 we see a histogram and a qq-plot for the log values of the concentrations of lead. Even after taking logs, the data still does not follow a Gaussian distribution exactly, but the assumption (of normality) doesn't seem entirely unreasonable.

Investigating further the possible relationship between concentrations and spatial location, Figure 10.4 shows the result of using the coplot function in the graphics package in R. This fixes the x coordinate at six levels and, for each, shows how the concentrations change as y increases. The code for this plot is included in the online resources. The top panel shows the six x coordinates on which we are conditioning, and for each of these we see the scatter plots of lead concentrations against y coordinates. We see intriguing

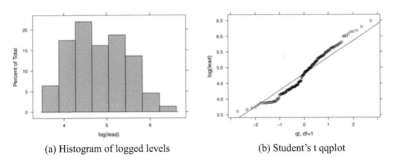

(a) Histogram of logged levels   (b) Student's t qqplot

Figure 10.3: Assessment of the assumption of normality for logged concentrations of lead in the Meuse River plain. Plot (a) shows a histogram of the logged concentrations and plot (b) a qq-plot using a t-distribution with 10 degrees of freedom.

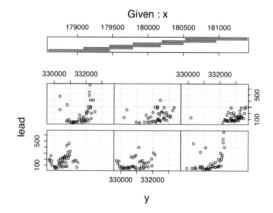

Figure 10.4: Trends in the level of lead concentrations in the soil of the Meuse River flood plain in relation to location. The top panel shows the distribution of x coordinates for a set of selected y coordinates. The corresponding scatter plots of lead concentrations against y coordinates is given for a set of six fixed x coordinates. The plots were produced by the R package gstat and show distinct spatial patterns in lead concentrations.

patterns in these scatter plots, suggesting a need for a spatial mean function when modeling the lead concentrations, that is, one that includes x and y coordinates.

10.4   Modeling spatial data

When modeling spatial data, we distinguish between the underlying spatial process and the process in which measurements are made. A spatial random field is a stochastic process over a region, $Z_s : s \in \mathcal{S} \subset \mathcal{R}^d$, $d = 1, 2$, or 3. This underlying process is not directly measurable, but realizations of it can be obtained by taking measurements, possibly with error, at a set of N_S known locations, $S \in \mathcal{S}$ where the points in S are labelled $s_1, ..., s_{N_S}$ and commonly $s_l = (a_l, b_l)$. One way of representing a random field is as a combination of an overall spatial trend together with a process that has spatial structure. In this case, we have,

$$
\begin{aligned}
Y_s &= Z_s + v_s \\
Z_s &= \mu_s + m_s \\
\mu_s &= \sum_{j=1}^{J} \beta_j f_j(X_s),
\end{aligned}
\tag{10.1}
$$

where v_s is measurement error. The first component of the second line, μ_s, is the mean of the underlying process. The latter is modeled as a function of the location, information about which is contained in X_s, with associated coefficients, β. The second term in the middle line, m_s, is a process with spatial structure. Commonly, it follows a zero mean Gaussian process with a valid covariance function.

The observable data, Y_s, at the first level of the model are considered conditionally independent given the value of the underlying process, Z_s. In this case, spatial structure is incorporated through the spatial component of the underlying process, m_s, which will have spatial structure in its covariance, $Cov(m_s, m_{s'})$. In a fully Bayesian analysis, a third level of the model would assign prior distributions to the hyperparameters from the first two levels. An alternative approach is to estimate them from the data (Diggle, Tawn, and Moyeed, 1998; Le and Zidek, 2006).

In a purely spatial analysis, repeated observations at a specific location over time are treated as independent realizations of the underlying process. The mean and covariance function are then estimated from the data and used to describe the spatial trend and association and for prediction at unsampled locations.

10.5   Spatial trend

A *spatial trend* refers to the case where the mean term (in Equation 10.1) is allowed to vary over space. The mean, μ_s, may be modeled directly as a function of s (Diggle and Ribeiro, 2007) which is often done by using a polynomial regression model with the coordinates of s used as explanatory variables. When replicates are available over time these can be used, after incorporating appropriate temporal structure in the model, to improve the modeling of the spatial trend (Guttorp, Meiring, and Sampson, 1994; Sahu and Mardia, 2005; Sahu, Gelfand, and Holland, 2006, 2007; Giannitrapani, Bowman, Scott, and Smith, 2007; Fanshawe et al., 2008; Bowman, Giannitrapani, and Scott, 2009; Paciorek, Yanosky, Puett, Laden, and Suh, 2009). Varying coefficient models have also been used in order to allow the mean to vary over space by assuming that the model parameters vary over the study region (Gelfand, Kim, Sirmans, and Banerjee, 2003).

When values of potential explanatory variables are available, these may be used to model the spatial trend. This method offers an appealing approach that allows the mean trend to vary over the study region and to be modeled as a function of explanatory variables, the effect of which can be scientifically interpreted. When the same set of explanatory variables is also available at locations for which predictions might be required, then we can use values of the explanatory variable at the new location(s) to produce the mean at that location. One drawback of this method is that it relies highly on data availability. It is often the case that such explanatory variables are only available at the locations where measurements are made, so prediction will have to rely solely on spatial prediction methods as described in the following sections.

10.6   Spatial prediction

Typically, fields of environmental hazards are sampled at a sparse set of spatial sites over an area of interest. For example, the US Environmental Protection Agency is charged with setting air quality standards that must be met. Ozone is strongly associated with adverse health outcomes and therefore must be regulated according to the US Clean Air Act of 1970 with concentrations monitored, in part, to ensure adherence with the act. Figure 10.5 shows an example of an ozone monitoring network, showing the locations of ozone monitoring sites within New York State. Note the relatively small number of monitors for such a large area. In many areas, especially rural ones, monitoring may be sparse despite the need for accurate information related to exposure levels given the potentially negative impacts of air pollution on human health and welfare.

Example 10.3. *Mapping the locations of ozone monitoring sites in New York State*

In this example, we show how the locations of monitoring sites can be superimposed onto a background map. The R code to produce the map shown in Figure 10.5 is given together with commented details of how the background map is defined in Google Maps and then downloaded into R.

This sparsity of such sites has led to the need to interpolate or extrapolate measured values using spatial prediction. For pollutants such as ozone, a photooxidant produced by atmospheric chemistry, pollution fields are relatively flat meaning that measurements at any one site are highly correlated with those at other nearby sites meaning that interpolating such fields between sites is feasible.

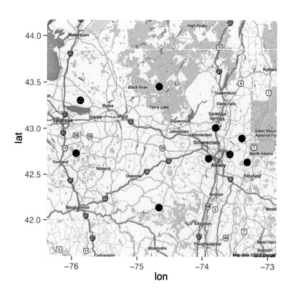

Figure 10.5: Locations of ozone (O_3) monitoring sites in New York State.

```
library(sp)
library(ggmap)

## Load the metadata giving the site coordinates
ny_data <- read.csv("NY.metadata.txt", sep="")

## Now copy ny_data into ny_data_sp and convert data
 to "sp" format
ny_data_sp <- ny_data
coordinates(ny_data_sp) <- ~Longitude+Latitude

## assign a reference system to ny_data_sp
proj4string(ny_data_sp) <-
        CRS("+proj=longlat +ellps=WGS84")

### We next specify a bounding box - a 2 x 2 matrix of
### corners of the geographic area. Then specify the
###   range of locations within the box.
###   Note: location must be in left-bottom-right-top
### bounding box format
latLongBox = bbox(ny_data_sp)
location = c(latLongBox[1, 1]-0.2, latLongBox[2, 1]-0,
             latLongBox[1, 2]+0.2, latLongBox[2,
               2]+0.2)

######## Now create the map with location dots
NYmap <- get_map(location = location, source = "google
    ",
 color="bw", maptype="roadmap")
NYmap <- ggmap(NYmap)
NYmap <- NYmap + geom_point(data=ny_data,
  aes(x=Longitude, y=Latitude), size=4)
```

Here the ggmap library, which is a geographical mapping tool for the ggplot2 package, is used. It allows maps such as the one shown to be obtained from a variety of sources, and in this example the map is obtained from Google Maps.

A simple approach for spatial prediction would be to calculate a weighted average of all points within a certain neighborhood of a chosen point, s_0. The weights may be chosen to reflect the distance between the point in question and a set of monitored locations, S containing points labelled $s_1, ..., s_{N_S}$. There are many possible ways of weighting the samples, all leading to different estimators. For example, the inverse of the squared distance between the points may be used, $\sum_{i=1}^{N_S} (||s_i - s_0||)^{-2}$.

Kriging is one of the most popular methods used for spatial prediction. It is a method of interpolation in which interpolated values are modeled by a Gaussian process. Under suitable assumptions, it gives the best linear unbiased prediction of the intermediate values (Cressie, 1985). The class of kriging models includes *simple kriging, ordinary kriging, universal kriging, indicator kriging, probability kriging, disjunctive kriging* and *cokriging* amongst others (Cressie, 1993). Further details on kriging can be found in Section 10.10.

10.7 Stationary and isotropic spatial processes

A stationary random field is a stochastic process over a region, $Z_s, s \in \mathcal{S}$ where s is a location in Euclidean space, $\mathcal{R}^d$, $d = 1, 2$ or 3. Commonly in spatial analysis, d will be equal to two and represent x, y coordinates, for example longitude and latitude, UTM or some other coordinate system.

The joint cumulative distribution function of a realization of the spatial process $\mathbf{Z} = (Z_{s_1}, \ldots, Z_{s_{N_S}})$ for any integer N_S is given by

$$F_{1,\ldots,N_S}(\mathbf{z}) = F_{1,\ldots,N_S}(z_{s_1}, \ldots, z_{s_{N_S}}) \equiv P\{Z_1 \leq z_1, \ldots, Z_{N_S} \leq z_{N_S}\},$$

for all $\mathbf{z} \in R^{N_S}$.

Definition 1. Strict stationarity.

A spatial process, Z, is strictly stationarity if

$$F_{1,\ldots,N_S}(\mathbf{z}) = F_{1+h,\ldots,N_S+h}(\mathbf{z}),$$

for any vector h and arbitrary N_S when $\mathcal{S} \subset \mathcal{R}$ is a continuum.

Definition 2. Second-order stationarity.

A weaker assumption is one of *weak* or *second-order* stationarity. Here, the mean is constant over space and the covariance depends only on the distance between locations and not their actual locations in space. This, on its own, would not imply strict stationarity.

A spatial process, Z, is second-order stationary if for all $s \in \mathcal{S}$ and arbitrary h,

$$
\begin{aligned}
\mu_s &= E[Z_s] \equiv \mu \text{ and} \\
Cov(Z_s, Z_{s'}) &= C(s + h, s' + h) \equiv C(h).
\end{aligned}
$$

Note that when we have $h = 0$, we have $Cov(Z_s, Z_s) = C(s, s) = C(0) = Var[Z(s)]$. The covariance kernel $C(h)$ here has a number of important properties. First, observe that for any pair of points s and s', $Cov(Z_s, Z_{s'}) = C(||s - s'||) = C(h_{ss'})$ so that all inter-site correlations can be obtained from the kernel. The kernel must be positive definite, meaning that if $\Sigma = C(h_{ss'})$ is the $N_S \times N_S$ dimensional covariance matrix for, $(Z(s_1), \ldots, Z(s_{N_S}))$ then it must be positive definite. This means that for any vector a

$$\sum_i \sum_j a_i a_j C(h_{ij}) > 0. \tag{10.2}$$

Definition 3. Isotropic stationary processes.

An *isotropic* stationary process is one where the covariance kernel depends only on the Euclidean distance between two points s and s' irrespective of the direction of one from the other. Any process that is not isotropic is called *anisotropic*.

A process, Z, is an isotropic second-order stationary if it is second-order stationary and in addition

$$C(h) \;\; = \;\; C(||h||),$$

where $||h||$ denotes the length of the vector h.

Example 10.4. *Gaussian random fields (GRFs)*

A special case of a stationary process is the *Gaussian random field (GRF)* in which the realizations come from the multivariate normal distribution with mean zero, $E(Z_s) = 0$, and covariance, $Cov(Z_s, Z_{s'}) = \sigma_s^2 \rho(||s - s'||)$. It has strong stationarity, where the joint distribution between locations is constant over the entire region, which implies second-order stationarity. Using Gaussian assumptions makes the theory for estimation and prediction considerably more straightforward than might otherwise be the case. This is because once the mean and covariance functions are defined, the spatial process is fully specified. Moreover, spatial interpolation is easily obtained using properties of the multivariate normal distribution.

Definition 4. A relaxed form of stationarity is *intrinsic stationarity* which is based on the difference in the process between locations. For a choice of two locations, the difference in means will be zero and the difference in variances is defined through the *semi-variogram*.

A process Z is intrinsically stationary if

$$\frac{1}{2} Var(Z_s - Z_{s'}) = \gamma(||s - s'||) = \gamma(h), \tag{10.3}$$

where $h = ||s - s'||$ and $E[Z_s - Z_{s'}] = 0$.

If two locations are close together, their difference would typically be small, and hence so would the variance of their differences. As the locations get farther apart, their differences get larger, and usually the variance of the difference will increase. This is similar to the definition of second-order stationarity although here stationarity is defined in terms of the variance of the difference between the process at different locations and not the covariance.

Here $\gamma(h)$ is the semi-variogram which plays a major role in modeling spatial processes through classical kriging.

10.8 Variograms

The covariance function and the semi-variogram are both functions that summarize the strength of association as a function of distance and, in the case of anisotropy, direction. When dealing with a purely spatial process where there are no independent realizations, patterns in correlation and variances from different parts of the overall region of study are used as if they were replications of the underlying process.

Under the assumption of stationarity, a common covariance function for all parts of the regions can then be estimated.

The semi-variogram will be zero at a distance of zero, as the value at a single spot is constant and has no variance. It may then rise and reach a plateau, indicating that past a certain distance, the correlation between two units is zero. This plateau will occur when the semi-variogram reaches the variance of Z. Assuming second-order stationarity, the relationship between the covariance and the semi-variogram is as follows:

$$
\begin{aligned}
\gamma(d) &= \frac{1}{2}Var(Z_s - Z_{s'}) \\
&= \frac{1}{2}\{Var(Z_s) + Var(Z_{s'}) - 2Cov(Z_s, Z_{s'})\}.
\end{aligned}
\tag{10.4}
$$

If $Var(Z_s) = Var(Z_{s'}) = \sigma_s^2$ and $C(Z_s, Z_{s'}) = C(h)$ for all s, s', then

$$
\begin{aligned}
\gamma(h) &= \frac{1}{2}(2\sigma_s^2 - 2C(h)) \\
&= \sigma_s^2 - C(h).
\end{aligned}
$$

Therefore, at $h = 0$, the semi-variogram is $\gamma(0) = \sigma_s^2 - C(0) = \sigma_s^2 - \sigma_s^2 = 0$, where $C(0) = Cov(Z_s, Z_s) = Var(Z_s)$ when d is large, that is, when $C(d) = 0, \gamma(d) = \sigma_s^2 - C(d) = \sigma_s^2$. Valid variograms must be *conditional negative definite* (Cressie, 1993), namely $\sum_{i=1}^{m}\sum_{j=1}^{m} a_i a_j 2\gamma(Z_s, Z_{s'}) \leq 0$, for any $\sum_{i=1}^{m} a_i = 0$. Given an intrinsically stationary process, they must satisfy the condition,

$$
2\gamma(d)/d^2 \to 0, \quad \text{as} \quad d \to \infty.
\tag{10.5}
$$

For many years, the semi-variogram was often preferred to the covariance function because of the relaxed rules of stationarity and also because it only uses pairs of locations d units apart, and does not involve the overall mean; so if there is a shift in the mean (trend) that is not explicitly modeled, the semi-variogram is likely to be less affected than the covariance function. However, in the last 20 years, when following a model based approach, like the one discussed in Section 10.11, it has become common practice to model the covariance structure as the product between a common variance and a valid correlation function.

The variogram is a realization of the covariance function and under second-order stationarity the functions are related as follows,

$$
\begin{aligned}
2\gamma(h) &= Var(Z_{s+h} - Z_s) \\
&= Var(Z_{s+h}) + Var(Z_s) - 2Cov(Z_{s+h}, Z_s) \\
&= C(0) + C(0) - 2C(h) \\
&= 2[C(0) - C(h)].
\end{aligned}
\tag{10.6}
$$

Thus $\gamma(h) = C(0) - C(h)$ and from this relationship it can be seen that from the covariance $C(\cdot)$ we can easily determine the semi-variogram $\gamma(\cdot)$. In general, obtaining

$C(\cdot)$ from $\gamma()$ is not as straightforward. If $C(h) \to 0$ as, $|h| \to \infty$ then the covariance goes to zero as distance goes to infinity. If we take the limit on both sides of Equation (10.6) then we get $\lim_{h \to \infty} \gamma(h) = C(0)$. However, the limit may not exist, an example of this being the case of a linear variogram. In such cases, additional assumptions about the spatial process, such as ergodicity, will be required (Cressie, 1993; Banerjee et al., 2015).

10.8.1 The nugget effect

The semi-variogram of two observations taken at the same place is zero by definition since $Var(Z_s - Z_s) = 0$. However, there may be 'microscale variations' and measurement error, so that two measurements taken at the same location are not exactly the same. This *nugget effect*, or nugget variance, is a discontinuity in the semi-variogram at the origin, the difference between zero and at a lag distance just greater than zero. This is represented by the component v_s in Equation (10.1) and it is assumed to be independent of z_s.

10.8.2 Variogram models

Although it is possible to create empirical estimates of the semi-variogram, these are often less than ideal for modeling spatial data as there may only be a few points at particular lag distances and so estimates of the covariance may not be stable. In addition, the matrix of sample covariances, $\hat{C}$, may not be positive definite and thus may not be a valid covariance matrix $(Var(q'\hat{C}q) \geq 0)$. Often it will be better to pool the data at different lags and fit a smooth curve through the resulting estimate of the semi-variogram using an appropriate model. Such semi-variogram models do not always produce well-defined covariance matrices for the underlying processes, as often the exact variance function is not specified.

Figure 10.6 shows variograms for NO_2 concentrations throughout Europe in 2001 and for the residuals after fitting a set of land-use covariates (Shaddick, Yan, et al., 2013). It illustrates three important features of a variogram:

(i) The *nugget* – when, $\gamma(0) = 0$ by definition, $\gamma(0^+) \equiv lim_{h \to 0+} \gamma(h) = \tau^2$, this quantity is the nugget, the variation of the difference of observations at the same sites.

(ii) The *sill* – the asymptotic value of the semi-variogram $lim_{h \to \infty} \gamma(h) = \tau^2 + \sigma_s^2$. The the difference between the sill and τ^2, and called the *partial sill*.

(iii) The *range* – the distance at which the plateau starts and after which there is little association between correlation and distance.

Here, we provide a brief discussion of a subset of possible variogram models. Details of a number of other models for this purpose can be found in N. A. C. Cressie (1993) and Le and Zidek (2006). The linear semi-variogram has the simplest functional form, but the sill and range are both infinite. The spherical variogram yields a stationary process, and the corresponding covariance function is easily computed. However, it fails to correspond to a valid spatial covariance matrix when the dimension is $d \geq 4$.

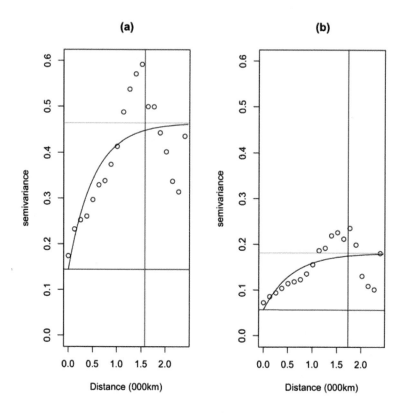

Figure 10.6: Variograms for (a) log values of Nitrogen Dioxide (NO_2) measured at monitoring sites throughout Europe in 2001; (b) residuals after fitting a model with land-use covariates. Lines show fitted exponential curve (black), nugget (blue), partial sill (green) and effective range at which correlation falls to 0.05 (red). Note the apparent lack of intrinsic stationarity suggested by the points on the right-hand side of the plots where the variogram appears to decline as the distance between locations increases.

A common class of models used for variogram models is the Matérn class (Matérn, 1986).

Matérn class of models

$$\gamma(h|\theta) = \begin{cases} 0 & h = 0, \\ \sigma^2 \left[1 - \frac{(\theta_1 h)^{\theta_2}}{2^{\theta_2 - 1}\Gamma(\theta_2)} K_{\theta_2}(\theta_1 h) \right] & h > 0, \end{cases} \quad (10.7)$$

where σ^2 is the variance of the process, $\theta_1 > 0$ is a scalable parameter controlling the range of the spatial correlation and $\theta_2 > 0$ is the smoothness parameter. K_{θ_2} is the modified Bessel function of order θ_2. The associated Matérn covariance function is $C(h) = \sigma^2 \frac{(\theta_1 h)^{\theta_2}}{2^{\theta_2-1}\Gamma(\theta_2)} K_{\theta_2}(\theta_1 h)$ for $h > 0$.

Exponential model

$$\gamma(h|\theta) = \begin{cases} 0 & h = 0, \\ \sigma^2 [1 - \exp(-h\,\theta_1)] & h > 0, \end{cases}$$

where σ^2 is the variance of the process and $\theta_1 > 0$ is the range of the spatial correlation. The associated exponential covariance function is $C(h) = \sigma^2 \exp(-\theta_1 h)$. The exponential model is a special case of the Matérn, with $\theta_2 = 1/2$. The limiting case of the Matérn class of models, when $\theta_2 \to \infty$, is the squared exponential model, $C(h) = \sigma^2 \exp\{-(\theta_1 h)^2\}$. This covariance function is rarely used in the modeling of environmental processes because it leads to spatial surfaces that are too smooth.

The variogram models discussed above do not include a nugget effect, that is the variance of the measurement error, say τ^2. This is because they represent the variogram of the process Z. If a nugget effect is included, as described in equation (10.1) for Y, then the variogram (or covariance) function should be added τ^2 times an indicator variable which is equal to 1 if $h = 0$ and 0 otherwise.

10.9 Fitting variogram models

The simplest method of fitting a variogram model is by least squares, although this assumes linearity and that the observations are uncorrelated with each other and have the same variance. That is unlikely to be the case, as estimates for different distances may be based on different numbers of pairs and will be correlated with each other. Simple weighted least squares can be used under certain stationarity and sampling conditions (Cressie, 1993), or the observations can be transformed to ensure that they are not correlated, that is, $Y^* = (V')^{-1/2}Y$, where $V = Var(Y)$, which results in performing generalized least squares regression.

It is often not easy to judge which variogram model is the most appropriate for a set of data. The 'goodness' of fit (based on nugget, sill, and range) can be judged visually or by using criterion such as least squares. More formal approaches to this problem are detailed in Cressie (1993); Cressie and Hawkins (1980); Omre (1984).

Matheron (1963) proposed a simple non-parametric estimate of the semi-variogram:

$$\hat{\gamma}(h) = \frac{1}{2N(h)} \sum_{(s,s') \in N(h)} [Z_s - Z_{s'}]^2, \tag{10.8}$$

where $N(h)$ is the set of pairs of points such that $||s - s'|| = h$, and $|N(h)|$ is the number of pairs in this set. Notice that the difference between the sites will all be different unless the observations fall on a regular grid and therefore a modification is used,

$$N(h_k) = (s,s') : ||s - s'|| \in I_k, \text{for}, k = 1, ..., K,$$

where $I_1 = (0, h_1)$, $I_2 = (h_1, h_2)$ and so on, up to $I_k = (h_{k-1}, h_K)$, see Banerjee et al. (2015) for further details. For each interval, it has been suggested at least 30 pairs of data should be included (Journel and Huijbregts, 1978).

It is noted that when fitting a variogram model a good characterization of spatial trend, that is, spatial mean function, is vital. Otherwise, the semi-variogram may include the square of a large bias (spatial mean estimation error) and hence give a misleading characterization of inter-site correlation.

10.10   Kriging

Kriging has been used extensively as a method for spatial prediction. As originally conceived, it was a distribution free method for developing predictive distributions. In what follows, for reasons of simplicity and clarity, we describe the methods for prediction as though we are working with the underlying 'true' process, Z. In practice, there will be microscale variations (represented by the nugget; see Section 10.8.1) and measurement error which give rise to the measurement level of the heirarchical model presented in Chapter 7, Section 7.5. If we assume the process is measured without error, that is $Y = Z$, then kriging produces the best linear unbiased predictor, $\hat{Z}_{s_0} = \sum_{s=1}^{N_S} \alpha_s z_s$ of Z_{s_0}, that is, the one that minimizes $E[(Z_{s_0} - \hat{Z}_{s_0})^2]$ under certain conditions (Cressie, 1993). No distributional assumptions are explicitly made, so this is a robust method in that sense.

The choice of a linear predictor is largely made for simplicity, but this may not necessarily be a sensible assumption unless Z has a multivariate normal distribution. In general, therefore, modeling a geostatistical analysis should begin with an exploration of the distribution of Z, based on available data and a decision on how best to proceed based on that analysis. If the assumption of a Gaussian random field is not justified, another approach will be required. A number of these are described in Sections 10.10.1 and 10.11.3.

If the use of linear prediction is deemed appropriate, then the two-step approach suggested by Webster and Oliver (2007) can be used.

Step 1. Model the spatial variation: Determine if the assumption of a stationary random field is valid and if it is, then model its correlation structure.

Step 2. Develop the spatial predictor: The classical technique is kriging, which incorporates spatial correlation and yield the best linear unbiased predictor (BLUP) for unsampled sites.

Although on the face of it, Step 1 is based on variances and correlations, these second-order properties are not really separable from the first-order properties. The spatial trend must therefore also be characterized as part of this step. To clarify this point, suppose the spatial trend given by $E(Z_s) = \mu_s$, $s \in \mathscr{S}$ is mis-specified as μ_s^*. In this case, the assumed variance would be $E(Z_s - \mu_s^*)^2 = Var(Z_s) + b_s^2$ where b_s denotes the bias $b_s = (\mu_s - \mu_s^*)$. A badly misspecified trend surface can greatly distort the apparent variance (and covariance) structure of the random field, and hence the accuracy of the BLUP.

As described in Section 10.6 spatial prediction can be performed by using a weighted average of measurements from all the points within a certain range. In ordinary kriging, the estimator incorporates correlations among the Z_s into the weights for predicting Z_{s_0}. The weights are based on the covariances among points in the sample and the covariances between sample points and the point to be predicted. To compute kriging estimates the covariances among all points, $\tilde{C}_{ss'} = Cov(Z_s, Z_{s'})$, and between each of the observed points and the point to be predicted, $C_{s0} = Cov(Z_s, Z_{s_0})$, need to be estimated using a covariance function or semi-variogram. The kriging estimator is the optimal estimator in that it minimizes the prediction variance or mean squared prediction error, $E(Z_s - \hat{Z}_s)^2$. Ordinary kriging gives optimal predictions under the assumption that the mean is constant (but unknown), with the weights obtained by solving the system of *kriging equations*,

$$
w = \begin{bmatrix} w_1 \\ w_2 \\ \vdots \\ w_{N_s} \\ \lambda \end{bmatrix} = \begin{bmatrix} C_{11} & \cdots & C_{1p} & 1 \\ \vdots & & \vdots & \vdots \\ C_{p1} & \cdots & C_{pp} & 1 \\ 1 & \cdots & 0 & 0 \end{bmatrix}^{-1} \times \begin{bmatrix} C_{11} \\ \vdots \\ C_{p1} \\ 1 \end{bmatrix}, \tag{10.9}
$$

where λ is a Lagrange multiplier that imposes the constraint $\sum w_s = 1$. Only intrinsic stationarity is required to obtain the ordinary kriging estimator, and so the results can thus be derived using semi-variograms instead of covariances.

Using kriging, the prediction variances $Var[Z_{s_0}|z]$ are generally small at locations close to the sampling locations because the location close to observation sites obtains greater influence through the weights w_s.

Example 10.5. *Spatial prediction of temperatures in California*

In this example we use measurements from seventeen temperature monitors in California to predict temperatures across the rest of the state. Note that this example is meant to be illustrative; a fully fledged analysis would look at all sites in the state and not just this subset. We now describe how to map the maximum daily temperatures. First we load the appropriate R libraries for the spatial analyzes: sp, gstat, together with some others for data manipulation and plotting. We then read in the measurement data and information on the locations of the monitoring sites. Both are stored in .csv files and here we load them using the read.csv function, although we could have used RStudio's 'Import Dataset' feature (as described in Chapter 4, Section 4.2.1).

```
library(sp)
library(utils)
library(gstat)
library(tidyverse)
library(readr)
library(cowplot)
```

```
###   load the data
CAmetadata<- read.csv("metadataCA.csv",header=TRUE)
CATemp<-read.csv("MaxCaliforniaTemp.csv",header=TRUE)
```

Next we load the data, changing the names of the latitude and longitude in the data file to *x* and *y* respectively, and augment it with the spatial locations of the sites. We also extract the temperatures for a single day (4th November 2011).

```
### Change names of lat, long
CAmetadata <- dplyr::rename(CAmetadata, x = Long , y =
    Lat)

## Temp data contains site Bakersfield, not present in
    Meta data
CATemp <- CATemp[, -grep("Bakersfield", names(CATemp))
    ]
choose_date <- 20121104
CATemp_date <- subset(CATemp,  Date==choose_date)[,-1]

### Augment data file with coordinates
CATemp_combined <- cbind(CAmetadata, t(CATemp_date))
names(CATemp_combined)[7] <- "Temp"
CATemp_combined <- CATemp_combined[,-1]
```

We need to define a grid on which the predictions will be made, and identify which of the data are the co-ordinates in both the measurement data and the prediction grid.

```
coordinates(CATemp_combined_geo) = ~x+y

### Create the grid on which to make the spatial
    predictions
CAPred.loci<-expand.grid(seq(-125,-115,.1),seq
    (32,42,.1))
names(CAPred.loci)[names(CAPred.loci)=="Var1"]<-"x"
names(CAPred.loci)[names(CAPred.loci)=="Var2"]<-"y"
coordinates(CAPred.loci) = ~ x + y
gridded(CAPred.loci) = TRUE
```

The final step is to produce the spatial predictions. We have to define a model structure, in this case an exponential model (for the relationship between correlation and diatance) and then use the krige function to fit the variogram.

```
mod <- vgm(5000, "Exp", 2.9, .04)
TheVariogram=variogram(Temp~x+y, data=CATemp_combined_
    geo)
FittedModel <- fit.variogram(TheVariogram, model=mod)
# ordinary kriging:
o_k1 <- krige(formula = Temp ~ 1, CATemp_combined_geo,
     CAPred.loci, model = mod)
o_krig_pred_1 <- spplot(o_k1["var1.pred"], main = "
   Predictions",
                      col.regions = viridis::plasma(60),
                      sp.layout = list(monitor_loc),
)
o_krig_var_2 <- spplot(o_k1["var1.var"],  main = "
   Variance",
                      col.regions = viridis::plasma(60),
                      sp.layout = list(monitor_loc),
)

# with x and y in the mean term:
m_k1 <- krige(formula = Temp_resid ~ x + y, CATemp_
    combined_geo,  CAPred.loci, model = FittedModel)

m_krig_pred_1 <- spplot(m_k1["var1.pred"], main = "
   Predictions",
                       col.regions = viridis::plasma
                          (60),
                       sp.layout = list(monitor_loc),
)

m_krig_var_2 <- spplot(m_k1["var1.var"],  main = "
   Variance",
                       col.regions = viridis::plasma(60)
                          ,
                       sp.layout = list(monitor_loc),
)

# monitor locations to be plotted
monitor_loc <- list('sp.points', CATemp_combined_geo,
    pch=19, cex=.8, col='cornsilk4')

# plot ordinary kriging
plot_grid(o_krig_pred_1, o_krig_var_2, labels = "")
# plot model with mean term (x and y)
plot_grid(m_krig_pred_1,m_krig_var_2, labels = "")
```

Predictions   **Variance**

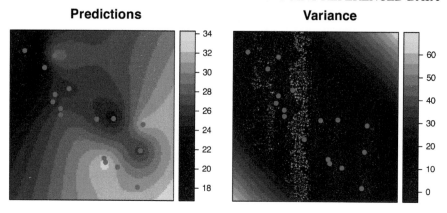

Figure 10.7: Predictions of the maximum daily temperature field in California on 14th November 2012 using kriging based on observed temperatures at seventeen monitoring sites. The left hand panel shows predicted temperatures using kriging and the left hand panel shows the prediction variances.

The result of mapping the California maximum daily temperature field using a model with a mean term that includes the x and y coordinates can be seen in Figure 10.7. The yellow subregions are where the daily maximum tempereratures are relatively high. The purple subregions are where they are relatively low. In the right hand panel we see the prediction variances that are smaller at points near the monitoring sites as might be expected. In Chapter 14 we will see how the locations of sites being added to a monitoring network can be determined in order to minimise prediction variances.

10.10.1 Extensions of simple kriging

We now describe some of the enhancements of the basic kriging principle that have been made for spatial prediction.

10.10.2 Co-kriging

If one or more covariates are measured along with the response variable, and if the cross correlation functions are known or can be estimated, then the covariates can be used to improve prediction, even when they are not measured at the same locations as the response variable. This is especially useful when there are few observations of the variable to be predicted, but many observations of some other variable which is highly correlated with the first. The co-kriging prediction is then a weighted average of nearby values of all the variables.

A function for multivariate or co-kriging is included in the gstat package for the case where a multiplicity of responses are present at each spatial site. This topic has not received nearly the attention it deserves in the spatial statistical literature, since even when interest lies in only one of the random responses, strength can be borrowed from the other responses in making spatial predictions.

10.10.3   Trans-Gaussian kriging

Transformed-Gaussian kriging is based on the assumption that if the random field is not Gaussian then it can be transformed to a Gaussian one by a suitable transformation function. It applies the kriging method on Box-Cox transformed data where y_s is transformed by the Box-Cox transformation into

$$\begin{cases} (y_s^\lambda - 1)/\lambda, \text{ or} \\ \log(y_s), \text{ if } \lambda = 0. \end{cases} \tag{10.10}$$

The latter option obtains by letting $\lambda \to 0$.

At the root of the problem is the requirement $y_s > 0$ for the Box-Cox transformation to be applicable, putting it on a ratio scale rather than an interval one. A positive scale σ has to be assigned and the size of the measurement measured against it by taking y_s/σ. The user has to choose the scale in order to make the results of the analysis interpretable in the context of the specific application. With this understanding a positive field of measurements can be transformed to an interval scale by the Box-Cox transformation or logarithm for application of a Gaussian distribution and kriging.

10.10.4   Non-linear kriging

Long ago geostatisticians recognised the need to spatially predict the presence or absence of material and developed a method called indicator or probability kriging. And non-linear kriging or disjunctive kriging was introduced where the predictor was $\hat{Z}_0 = \sum_{s=1}^{N_s} f_s(Z_s)$ where the fs are selected to minimise $E[\hat{Z}_0 - Z_0]^2$. The resulting solutions are more difficult to find than those for trans-Gaussian kriging, but less restrictive (Cressie, 1993; Wackernagel, 2003).

10.11   Bayesian kriging

From a Bayesian point of view, the model described in Equation (10.1) can be seen as a hierarchical model. We give details of a hierarchical model described by Shaddick and Wakefield (2002).

Stage 1 – Observational model
Assume that, for any $s \in \mathscr{S}$

$$y_s = z_s + v_s, \tag{10.11}$$

where y_s denotes the observed level of the exposure at a spatial location s. Assume $\mathbf{y} = (y_{s_1}, \cdots, y_{s_{N_S}})'$ is the vector containing the observed values at N_S locations,

$s_1, \ldots, s_{N_S}$. The component v_s represents measurement error and is assumed to be independent and identically distributed, $N(0, \sigma_v^2)$, or equivalently, $\mathbf{v} = (v_{s_1}, \cdots, v_{s_{N_S}})' \sim MVN_{N_S}(0_{N_S}, \sigma_v^2 I_{N_S})$ follows a zero mean multivariate normal distribution, with I_{N_S} the N_S-dimensional identity matrix.

Stage 2 – Process Model

In this stage the underlying levels of the exposure are modeled as a stationary spatial process, that is,

$$z_s = \mu_s + m_s,$$

where μ_s is a spatial mean term, for example, $\mu_s = \sum_{j=1}^{J} \beta_j X_{js}$ and m_s follows a Gaussian process. Therefore, the spatial random effects $\mathbf{m} = (m_{s_1}, \ldots, m_{s_{N_S}})'$ at locations s arise from the multivariate normal distribution

$$\mathbf{m} \sim MVN_{N_S}(0_{N_S}, \sigma_m^2 \Sigma_m),$$

where 0_{N_S} is an N_S-dimensional vector of 0s, σ_m^2 is the between location variance and Σ_m is the N_S x N_S correlation matrix, in which element (s, s') represents the correlation between sites s and s'. The covariance between the sites s and s' is assumed to be a function of the distance, $h = ||s - s'||$, between them. Often a member of the Matérn class is used, the most common choice being the exponential covariance function

$$f(h, \phi) = \exp(-\phi h),$$

where $\phi > 0$ describes the strength of the correlation.

Stage 3 – Hyperpriors

Let $\theta = (\beta, \sigma_m^2, \phi, \sigma_v^2)$ be the parameter vector to be estimated. Commonly, θ also includes predictions of the process at unobserved locations. It is common to assume prior independence among the components of θ, such that β_i follows a zero mean normal prior distribution with some reasonably large variance. The vector ϕ involves the parameters in the correlation function. Say that an exponential correlation function is used (i.e. $\exp(-\phi h)$) then it is common to assign a gamma prior distribution to ϕ with some reasonably large variance. Mean prior specification usually follows the idea of practical range: the prior mean of ϕ is such that when the correlation is 0.05 the range is reached at half of the observed maximum distance, that is, $E(\phi^*) = \frac{6}{dmax}$, a priori.

The prior for β_i can be flat but one must be careful about the prior specification of σ_m^2, σ_v^2 and ϕ. If the model does not have a nugget effect, σ_v^2, then it is not possible to identify both σ_m^2 and ϕ (Zhang, 2004). If a nugget effect is included, then ϕ and at least one of σ_m^2 and σ_v^2 require informative priors. If one uses a Matérn covariance function, and if the prior on β, σ_m^2, ϕ is of the form $\frac{\pi(\phi)}{(\sigma_m^2)^\alpha}$ with $\pi(\cdot)$ uniform, then the resultant posterior is improper if $\alpha < 2$. For σ_m^2 and σ_v^2 it is safer to assign inverse gamma priors $IG(a, b)$ with $a \geq 1$.

10.11.1 MCMC implementation

The MCMC implementation can follow two possible avenues. Note that at each iteration of the algorithm, the determinant and inverse of a n-dimensional covariance matrix needs to be computed.

One possible implementation is to write the likelihood function conditional on m_s as described in Equation (10.11). The advantage of doing so is that if a multivariate normal prior distribution is assigned to β and independent inverse gamma priors are assigned to σ_m^2 and σ_v^2, then their posterior full conditional distributions will have closed form and can be sampled through a Gibbs step. The posterior full conditional distribution of $\mathbf{m}$ follows a multivariate normal distribution and is easy to sample from. Assuming the above prior specification, the range parameter, ϕ, is the only one that results in an unknown posterior full conditional distribution. It is commonly sampled through a Metropolis-Hastings step.

The algorithm above requires, at each iteration of the MCMC, the sampling from a n-dimensional multivariate normal distribution. An alternative is to marginalize the distribution of $\mathbf{y}$ with respect to $\mathbf{m}$. This results in a multivariate normal distribution with mean $\mu = \mathbf{X}'\beta$ with $\mathbf{X}$ a $n \times p$ matrix of covariates, and covariance matrix $\Sigma_y = \sigma_m^2 \mathbf{R} + \sigma_v^2 \mathbf{I}_n$, where $\mathbf{R}_{ij} = \rho(||s_i - s_j||; \phi)$. The advantage of this integration is that, at each iteration of the MCMC, there is no need to sample from the posterior full conditional distribution of $\mathbf{m}$. However, as σ_m^2 and σ_v^2 are involved in Σ through a sum, their posterior full conditional does not have a closed form any longer. This is not an issue; usually, a Metropolis-Hastings step with a random walk on the log scale tends to work well when sampling from their resultant posterior full conditional distributions. Once a sample from the posterior distribution of β, σ_m^2, σ_v^2 and ϕ are available, a sample from the posterior distribution of $\mathbf{z}$ can be obtained using composition sampling, as

$$p(\mathbf{m} \mid \mathbf{y}) = \int_\theta p(\mathbf{m} \mid \theta, \mathbf{y}) p(\theta \mid \mathbf{y}) d\theta = E_{\theta \mid \mathbf{y}}[\mathbf{m} \mid \theta, \mathbf{y}],$$

where $p(m \mid \theta, \mathbf{y}) \propto l(\mathbf{y}; \mathbf{z}, \theta, \sigma_v^2) p(\mathbf{z} \mid \sigma_m^2, \phi)$ is a multivariate normal distribution.

10.11.2 Spatial interpolation

If the goal is to predict the process at r unobserved locations, $\mathbf{Y}_u = (Y_{s_{u_1}}, \cdots, Y_{s_{u_r}})'$, because of the GP assumption, the joint distribution of $\mathbf{Y}$ and $\mathbf{Y}_u$, conditional on θ, is given by

$$\begin{pmatrix} \mathbf{Y}_u \\ \mathbf{Y} \end{pmatrix} \mid \theta \sim N_{n+r}\left(\begin{pmatrix} \mu_u \\ \mu \end{pmatrix}; \begin{pmatrix} \Sigma_u & \Psi' \\ \Psi & \Sigma \end{pmatrix} \right), \tag{10.12}$$

where $N_k(\mathbf{a}, \mathbf{A})$ stands for the k-th multivariate normal distribution with mean vector $\mathbf{a}$ and covariance matrix $\mathbf{A}$; μ is a n-dimension vector representing the mean at the observed sites; μ_u is a r-dimensional vector representing the mean at the unobserved sites; Σ_u is a r-dimensional covariance matrix, containing the covariances of the process among unobserved sites; Ψ, is a $n \times r$ matrix, representing the covariance between i-th observed site and j-th unobserved site, $i = 1, \cdots, n$ and $j = 1, \cdots, r$.

From a Bayesian point of view, spatial interpolation proceeds through the posterior predictive distribution at new sites $s_{u1}, \cdots, s_{ur}$ that is, by obtaining samples from

$$p(\mathbf{Y}_u \mid \mathbf{y}) \;=\; \int_\theta p(\mathbf{Y}_u \mid \mathbf{y}, \theta) \pi(\theta \mid \mathbf{y}) d\theta = E_{\pi(\theta|Y)} \left[p(\mathbf{Y}_u \mid \mathbf{y}, \theta) \right]. \quad (10.13)$$

If a sample of size L is available from the posterior distribution of θ, the integral in (10.13) can be approximated through Monte Carlo integration, that is, $p(\mathbf{Y}_u \mid \mathbf{Y}) \approx \frac{1}{L} \sum_{l=1}^{L} p(\mathbf{Y}_u \mid \theta^l)$. From the properties of the partition of the multivariate normal distribution, it follows that

$$\left(\mathbf{Y}_u \middle| \mathbf{Y}, \theta \right) \sim N_r \left(\mu_u + \Psi' \Sigma^{-1} \left(\mathbf{Y} - \mu \right) ; \Sigma_u - \Psi' \Sigma^{-1} \Psi \right). \quad (10.14)$$

Assume that a sample of size L from the posterior distribution of θ is available, $\theta^{(1)}, \cdots, \theta^{(L)}$; one can use composition sampling to obtain samples from (10.13): for each $\theta^{(l)}$ drawn from $\pi(\theta \mid Y)$, draw $\mathbf{Y}_u$ from the normal distribution in Equation (10.14).

Example 10.6. *Fitting a Bayesian exponential spatial model using NIMBLE*

Here we discuss how to obtain samples from the posterior distribution of the model discussed above using MCMC using NIMBLE. In particular, the code in NIMBLE is written considering the likelihood marginalized with respect to **m** as discussed above. We consider the case of a collection of N_S monitoring sites measuring an environmental hazard and use the structure just shown in this section to represent the link between the measured data and the underlying spatial field.

In order to fit an exponential model in NIMBLE we define a covariance matrix with the elements as a function of the exponential correlation function. In NIMBLE, prediction of the process at r unobserved locations is performed by defining the matrices Ψ and Σ_u and the vector μ_u as described in equation (10.14).

```
Example10_6Code <-   nimbleCode ({
  # covariance among observed locations  - Sigma
  Sigma_obs [1:n, 1:n] <-
    sigma_sq * exp(-distMatrix [1:n, 1:n] / phi) + tau_
      sq * identityMatrix (d = n)

# covariance among unobserved locations  - Sigma_u
  Sigma_pred [1:nu, 1:nu] <-
    sigma_sq * exp(-distMatrixUnobs [1:nu, 1:nu] / phi)
      + tau_sq * identityMatrix (d = nu)

# covariance among observed and unobserved locations  -
    Psi
  Sigma_obs_pred [1:n, 1:nu] <-
    sigma_sq * exp(-distMatrixObsUnobs [1:n, 1:nu] /
      phi)
```

```
# mean structure for observed sites
  for (site in 1:n) {
    mean.site[site] <-
        beta0 + beta1 * X1[site] + beta2 * X2[site]
  }
  #likelihood function
  y[1:n]    ~   dmnorm(mean.site[1:n], cov = Sigma_obs[1:
      n, 1:n])

#mean structure at unobserved sites
  for (usite in 1:nu) {
    mean.pred.site[usite] <-
        beta0 + beta1 * X1[usite] + beta2 * X2[usite]
  }
#computing the elements of the conditional normal
    distribution
  mean_sigma[1:nu] <- t(Sigma_obs_pred[1:n, 1:nu])%*%
    inverse(Sigma_obs[1:n, 1:n])%*%(y[1:n] - mean.site
      [1:n])

  mu_pred[1:nu] <-
    mean.pred.site[1:nu] + mean_sigma[1:nu]
    cov_pred[1:nu, 1:nu] <-
    Sigma_pred[1:nu, 1:nu] - t(Sigma_obs_pred[1:n, 1:
        nu]) %*% inverse(Sigma_obs[1:n, 1:n]) %*%
        Sigma_obs_pred[1:n, 1:nu]

  #sampling from the distribution in equation (10.14)
  y_pred[1:nu]    ~   dmnorm(mu_pred[1:nu], cov = cov_
      pred[1:nu, 1:nu])
```

In the above, y_pred contains a sample from the posterior predictive distribution at the nu locations provided by the user.

```
# Prior specification
#half-Cauchy priors for variances
sigma ~ T(dt(mu = 0, sigma = 1, df = 1), 0, Inf)
sigma_sq <- sigma ^ 2
tau ~ T(dt(mu = 0, sigma = 1, df = 1), 0, Inf)
tau_sq <- tau ^ 2
phi_inv ~ dgamma(shape =  5, rate = 5)
phi <- 1 / phi_inv
# prior specification for coefficients
beta0 ~ dnorm (0, 10)
beta1 ~ dnorm (0, 10)
beta2 ~ dnorm (0, 10)
})
```

Example 10.7. *Spatial prediction of PM$_{2.5}$ in Europe*

In this example, we use the model and code introduced in Example 10.6 to produce a map of fine particulate matter air pollution. Measurements of PM$_{2.5}$ from monitors in selected countries in Western Europe were extracted from the WHO ambient air pollution database introduced in Chapter 4, Section 4.2.1. These data were used to fit an exponential model for the relationship between distance (between monitoring locations) and correlation (between the measurements at those sites). In addition to the spatial component, a (non-zero) mean term was used that included the effect of (log) population and altitude, $X1$ and $X2$ respectively in the NIMBLE code shown in Example 10.6.

Predictions from the model were made at points on a 10 km × 10 km grid defined over the entire study region. To produce predictions from the model, values of any covariates used in the model ((log) population and altitude in this example) need to be available at each location in order to calculate the value of the mean term. Each each prediction location, there will be not just a single prediction, but samples from the posterior distribution (or predicted values). Summaries from the posterior distributions can be taken, for example the medians, and used to produce maps of concentrations using R. An example can be seen in Figure 10.8, which shows the medians of the (predicted) concentrations for 2016. Using the samples from the posterior predictive distributions, it is also straightforward to obtain not just a single measure of the prediction at each point but also measures of uncertainty (e.g. width of credible intervals) and functions of the predictions (e.g. probabilities of exceeding a threshold).

In cases where there are a large numbers of prediction locations, as here, where there are ca. 50,000 grid points, producing predictions within MCMC can be computationally prohibitive. Here, single site predictions were used with calculations being performed off-line or out-of-simulation using posterior medians of the required parameters in Equation 10.14. Although computationally efficient, this approach does ignore the inherent uncertainty in the parameter estimates and the uncertainty associated with the predictions will therefore be underestimated. In Example 12.6 (in Chapter 12) we show how a method for performing Bayesian inference using integrated nested Laplace approximations can be used to fit spatial, and spatio-temporal, models with large datasets (i.e. monitoring data and covariates) along with a large number of prediction locations.

10.11.3 *Modeling spatial processes in the exponential family*

Bayesian kriging can be considered as part of a more general framework denoted model-based kriging (Diggle and Ribeiro, 2007). The normal case can be seen as a particular case of a broader class of models where observations are conditionally

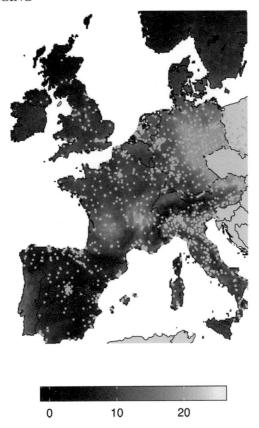

Figure 10.8: Predictions of fine particulate matter air pollution (PM$_{2.5}$) concentrations in Europe for 2016. Predictions are from a Bayesian spatial model fit using NIMBLE and represent the posterior medians from predictions on a 10 km × 10 km grid covering Western Europe. The locations of ground monitors in the WHO ambient air quality database are shown in pink.

independent given the spatial process $Z(\cdot)$. The broader class extends the response distribution to the exponential family (Diggle et al., 1998) and the kriging predictor is obtained as a non-linear function of a latent spatial process. Next we discuss an example based on binary responses.

Example 10.8. *Model-based kriging with binary responses*

Suppose Y_s, $s \in \mathscr{S}$ is a measurable binary response representing presence or absence of an outcome, for example disease, at a location s and Z_s is a realization from a latent Gaussian spatial process (at s). A predictive model for unmeasured binary responses may be constructed by assuming that for any two sites s, s', these responses are conditionally independent as follows:

$$[Y_s = y_s, Y_{s'} = y_{s'} \mid Z_s = z_s, Z_{s'} = z_{s'}, \theta]$$

$$= [Y_s = y_s \mid Z_s = z_s, \theta][Y_{s'} = y_{s'} \mid Z_{s'} = z_{s'}, \theta],$$

where the notation $[w \mid u]$ denotes the distribution of the random variable w conditioned on u, θ denotes the vector of model parameters. More specifically we may assume that given $Z_s = z_s$,

$$Y_s \mid Z_s \;\sim\; Bernoulli(p_s)$$

$$\log \frac{p_s}{1 - p_s} \;=\; X_s'\beta + Z_s,$$

where $p_s = P[Y_s = y_s \mid Z_s = z_s, \beta]$. Embedding this model in a hierarchical Bayesian model with a prior distribution for β and the parameters involved in the Gaussian process $Z(\cdot)$ provides a very flexible model for the binary field.

Inference procedure can be performed using MCMC. As the likelihood function does not follow a normal distribution, it is not possible to marginalize the distribution of y with respect to z. Regardless of the prior specification all posterior full conditional distributions do not have closed forms. Commonly, Metropolis-Hastings steps are used to sample from the resultant full conditionals. Once a sample from the posterior distribution of the parameters is available, predictions to unobserved locations of interest follow a similar partition of the multivariate normal distribution as in Equation (10.14) but changing $Y(\cdot)$ for $Z(\cdot)$. Sometimes, to improve the convergence of some of the coefficients β, hierarchical centering is used, such that $X_s'\beta$ is moved into the mean of the multivariate normal distribution of Z.

The online resources include the analysis of the malaria data in Gambia analyzed in Diggle, Moyeed, Rowlingson, and Thomson (2002).

10.12   INLA and spatial modeling in a continuous domain

The methods presented in this chapter are for use with point-referenced data and particularly cases where there is a Gaussian field (GF) with responses measured with error. A GF itself has no natural Markov structure and so INLA, as originally developed and described in Chapter 6, does not apply directly as it does with Gaussian Markov random fields (GMRFs) as would be the case when using areal data as in Chapter 9.

It is possible to use a bridge between a GF and a GMRF to which INLA can be applied. This is done using the stochastic partial differential equation (SPDE) approach presented by Lindgren, Rue, and Lindström (2011). This starts with a GF over a continuous domain of arbitrary dimension and from it induces a GMRF. Key elements of this method are the use of GFs, that are characterised by their second order properties, and the restriction that the field must have a Matérn covariance structure. Lindgren, Rue, and Lindström (2011) show that such a field can be expressed as the solution of an SPDE that can be approximated using a finite element method whose elements are triangles over the field's domain. The induced Gaussian random weights attached to its vertices then determine the joint distribution of the induced GMRF representation of the original GF. The precision matrix for this GMRF is approximated by a sparse precision matrix, $\mathbf{Q}$, that represents the covariance Σ of the GF well, i.e with $\mathbf{Q}^{-1}$ close to Σ, in order to achieve computational simplicity.

The result is a GF model for the process but with an associated GMRF that can be used (by INLA) for performing the computations that would be computationally prohibitive using the GF directly. The resulting algorithm is implemented in R-INLA.

10.12.1 Implementing the SPDE approach

We now describe the SPDE-GRMF approximation following Lindgren, Rue, and Lindström (2011). INLA assumes the GF $Z_s, s \in \mathscr{S}$ has a Matérn spatial covariance as given by (10.7) that is the solution of the SPDE

$$(\kappa^2 - \Delta)^{\alpha/2} Z_s = v_s, \alpha = v + d/2, \kappa > 0, v > 0, \qquad (10.15)$$

where $(\kappa^2 - \Delta)^{\alpha/2}$ is a pseudo-difference operator, Δ is the Laplacian and v is spatial white noise with unit variance. The marginal variance of the process is given by

$$\sigma^2 = \frac{\Gamma(v)}{\Gamma(v+d/2)(4\pi)^{d/2}\kappa^{2v}}. \qquad (10.16)$$

Representing the process in this way is key to the developments that follow; it provides the bridge over which we can cross from the GF to the GMRF via an approximate solution to the SPDE.

An infinite dimensional solution, Z_s, of the SPDE over its domain, $\mathscr{S}$, is characterised by the requirement that for all members of an appropriate class of test functions, ϕ,

$$\int \phi_{js}(\kappa^2 - \Delta)^{\alpha/2} Z_s dZ. = \int \phi_{js} v_s ds. \qquad (10.17)$$

However in practice, only approximate solutions are available and Lindgren, Rue, and Lindström (2011) use the conventional finite element approach, which uses a Delauney triangulation (DT) over $\mathscr{S}$. Initially the triangles are formed with vertices at the points of the sparse network where observations are available with additional triangles added until $\mathscr{S}$ is covered, leading to an irregular array of locations (vertices).

Example 10.9. *Creating a mesh: black smoke monitoring locations in the UK*

Figure 10.9 shows the mesh that was constructed using Delauney triangulation for the locations of black smoke monitors in the UK. The R code for producing the mesh is as follows.

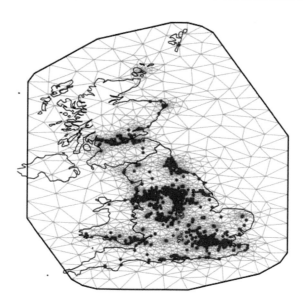

Figure 10.9: Triangulation for the black smoke network in the UK. The red dots show the locations of black smoke monitoring sites.

```
mesh = inla.mesh.create(locations[,1:2],
extend=list( offset=-0.1), cutoff=1,
# Refined triangulation,
# minimal angles >=26 degrees,
# interior maximal edge lengths 0.08,
# exterior maximal edge lengths 0.2:
refine=(list(min.angle=26,
max.edge.data = 100,
max.edge.extra=200))
)
```

where locations is a matrix with two columns, containing the x and y coordinates of the monitoring sites. With the plot created as follows:

```
ukmap <- readShapeLines("uk_BNG.shp")
plot(mesh, col="gray", main="")
lines(ukmap)
points(locations, col="red", pch=20,bg="red")
```

Here the file uk_BNG.shp is the shapefile for the UK using the British National Grid projection that provides the outline of the UK coastline and is included in the online resources. In this case, the distance between the points is expressed in metres and so the distances used in creating the mesh to ensure the plots will overlay should also be in metres.

In this case, there are 3799 edges and the mesh was constructed using triangles that have minimum angles of 26 and a maximum edge length of 100 km. There are 1466 monitoring locations being considered over the period of study and these are highlighted in red. This lattice underlies the GRMF and gives a finite element representation of the solution of that shown in Equation (10.15),

$$Z_s = \sum_{k=1}^{n} \psi_{ks} w_k, \qquad (10.18)$$

where n is the number of vertices of the DT, $\{w_k\}$ are Gaussian weights and ψ_{ks} are piecewise linear in each triangle (1 at vertex k and 0 at all other vertices). The ψ_{ks} then need to be linked to the class of test functions and in order to obtain an approximate solution to the SPDE.

In practice, the implementation in R-INLA takes this approximation one step further by requiring n test functions in order to obtain a finite dimensional approximation to the SPDE. Specific details can be found in Lindgren, Rue, and Lindström (2011), but briefly, $\phi_k = (\kappa^2 - \Delta)^{\alpha/2} \psi_k$ is used with $\alpha = 1$. Substituting these test functions into Equation (10.17) along with the approximation shown in Equation (10.18) gives a set of n equations which may be solved. These equations characterize the elements of that approximation, including a sparse precision matrix for the GMRF distributed over the vertices of the irregular lattice and defined by the random Gaussian weights $\{w_k\}$.

Example 10.10. *Fitting an SPDE model using R-INLA: black smoke monitoring locations in the UK*

Using the mesh set up in Example 10.9 we now create the R-INLA SPDE object that will be used as the model in the same form as seen in Chapter 6. The following R code creates the object for the UK black smoke monitoring data using the inla.spde2.matern() command, which in its simplest form would be spde = inla.spde2.matern(mesh, alpha=2) for the case where $\alpha = 2$ from Equation (10.15).

```
# Field std.dev. for theta=0
 sigma0 = 1
 # find the range of the location data
 size = min(c(diff(range(mesh$loc[,1])),
             diff(range(mesh$loc[,2]))))
# A fifth of the approximate domain width.
 range0 = size/5
 kappa0 = sqrt(8)/range0
 tau0 = 1/(sqrt(4*pi)*kappa0*sigma0)
 spde = inla.spde2.matern(mesh,
```

```
 B.tau=cbind(log(tau0), -1, +1),
 B.kappa=cbind(log(kappa0), 0, -1),
 theta.prior.mean=c(0,0),
constr=TRUE)
```

The value of kappa0 represents the prior belief of the distance at which the correlation, ρ, is expected to fall to 0.1, and is equal to $\rho = \frac{\sqrt{8\nu}}{\kappa}$ (Lindgren, Rue, and Lindström, 2011), where here $\nu = 1$. The value for the spatial standard deviation, tau0 is the square root of the spatial variance, σ^2, given in Equation (10.16); $\frac{1}{\sqrt{4\pi\kappa\tau}}$.

The model is then fit by defining a formula and then running the inla command using the SPDE object in the random effects term, f(spde).

```
formula = logbs ~ 1+ urban.rural +f(site, model=spde)
model = inla(formula, family="gaussian", data = BSdata
    ,
control.predictor = list(compute=TRUE),
control.compute = list(dic = TRUE, config=TRUE))
```

where urban.rural is an indicator variable which represents whether the monitoring site is in a rural (0) or urban area (1). Here the optional argument in the control.predictor means that predictions for any missing values, including predictions at unmonitored locations, will be stored and the first argument in control.compute means that the information required to compute the DIC will be retained. The second argument allows information to be stored to enable joint samples from the posterior to be obtained, the result of which means that predictions together with associated measures of uncertainty are 'automatically' available for all data points, including cases where data was and was not originally available.

We are interested in the posterior marginals of the latent field,

$$\pi(z_i|y) = \int \pi(z_i|\theta,y)\pi(\theta|y)d\theta, \qquad (10.19)$$

$$\pi(\theta_j|y) = \int \pi(\theta|y)\pi(\theta_{-j})d\theta, \qquad (10.20)$$

where $i = 1,...,N_S+P$ where N_S is the number of monitoring locations and P the number of predictions to be made and $j = 1,...J$ is the number of parameters in the model. With regard to spatial prediction, the SPDE-INLA algorithm provides the posterior conditional distribution of the random effects terms at all the vertices of the triangulation. Given these, there is a mapping to the response variable which allows samples of predictions to be obtained (Cameletti, Lindgren, Simpson, and Rue, 2011).

In order to produce a map displaying the spatial predictions of the model, we first need to define a lattice projection starting from the mesh object back to the grid on which the data lies and will be plotted. This can be performed using the inla.mesh.projector command. Then the posterior mean and

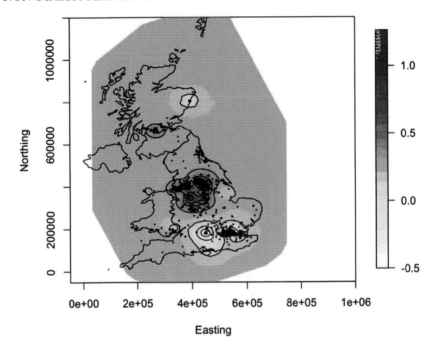

Figure 10.10: Map of predicted values of black smoke in the UK. Values are medians of posterior predicted distributions on the logarithmic scale from an SPDE–INLA model.

standard deviations can be extracted and then projected from the latent field space to the grid, using `inla.mesh.project` and then plotted as a map. The example of the result can be seen in Figure 10.10.

There are a number of different ways of building SPDE models on a mesh, performing the projection and converting the output from SPDE/R-INLA to a form that can produce maps and the package. For further details, we recommend Paula Moraga's book, Geospatial Health Data: Modeling and Visualization with R-INLA and Shiny (Moraga, 2019) and Spatial and Spatio-temporal Bayesian Models with R-INLA by Blangiardo and Cameletti (2015), both of include a number of worked examples of how to produce maps from R-INLA / SPDE models.

10.13 Non-stationary random fields

A number of approaches for dealing with non-stationary spatial random fields have been developed. The case of spatio-temporal processes is considered in Chapter 12. There one has replicates over time which, after adjusting for correlation over time, allows more scope for dealing with non-stationarity. A purely spatial process is more challenging since with only one replicate of the spatial process, estimating second-order properties such as spatial covariances is difficult. In this section, we review some of the approaches that have been developed in this situation.

10.13.1   Geometric and zonal anisotropy

Directional variogram plots are constructed by placing an origin in the spatial domain of interest, $\mathscr{S}$ from which radial lines emanate at a set of angles. For any one of those lines, the empirical variogram computed for sites within the wedge between the lines is the *directional variogram*.

One approach to dealing with geometric anisotropy is to assume the plot of the ranges on the radial direction lines form an ellipse, with the diameters of the major and minor axes determined respectively by the largest A and smallest B ranges (Webster and Oliver, 2007). Suppose as well that the major axis makes an angle φ with the horizontal axes. Rotate the horizontal axes so that it now lies along the major axes. Then inflate the diameter of the minor axes by the ratio $R = A/B$ to get a sphere in the new coordinate system.

In summary, the distance between geographic sites, $s = (s_1, s_2)$ and $s' = (s'_1, s'_2)$ is defined

$$||s - s'|| = \sqrt{(s - s')^T (s - s')} = \sqrt{\sum_k (s_k - s'_k)^2} \sqrt{\sum_k (s_k - s'_k)^2}$$

which is replaced by

$$\sqrt{(s - s')^T \zeta (s - s')}$$

in the new measure of distance where ζ is a positive definite 2×2 matrix.

Zonal anisotropy, where both the sill and the range depend on direction, proves more challenging and various methods have been suggested. The simplest is to select a small, fixed, number of zones or strata and model the field separately in each zone.

10.13.2   Moving window kriging

Moving window kriging (Haas, 1990) is perhaps the simplest approach to dealing with non-stationary data. Here, we divide the region into a number of subregions, each of which has a sufficient number of points to estimate a (stationary) variogram. The overall spatial process and its covariance structure can then be represented by a weighted average of the locally stationary processes (N. Cressie, 1986). Ordinary kriging assumes that the mean is constant over the entire region of study, but in *universal kriging* a non-constant mean is represented as a function of the location, a polynomial function of finite order, k. The assumption that $E(Z_s - Z_{s'}) = 0$ no longer holds, and the method assumes that the variogram and the order k of the polynomial are known. Unfortunately k is never known and has to be guessed, not estimated, from the data and γ has to be estimated from the residuals. Other approaches include *median polish kriging* and *intrinsic random functions of order k* (Cressie, 1986). The former involves modeling the mean term using the medians of rows and columns of a spatial grid in such a way that the resulting residual terms are stationary and thus can be used with traditional geostatistical techniques. The choice of the spatial grid is critical to this approach, and attempts are often made to define it in a meaningful way, with the precise formulation being determined by the particular application. The latter has more general model assumptions than the kriging methods, and involves estimating k and the *generalized covariance function* from k^{th} order differences (Cressie, 1993), however its use in practice is limited as it is not generally possible to estimate the covariance function and the order k of the differencing again has to be guessed, rather than estimated from the data.

10.13.3   Convolution approach

We now give a brief description of the convolution approach to modeling non-stationary fields. Calder and Cressie (2007) review this approach starting with the basic spatial process model

$$Z_s = \mu_s + m_s + v_s, \ s \in \mathscr{S},$$

where μ_s is the spatial mean and v_s is a random noise term that represents the nugget. The convolution formulation derives from the assumption

$$m_s = \mu_s + \int_{R^d} k(s,u)W_u du, s \in \mathscr{S}, \qquad (10.21)$$

where k is a kernel function and W, a general zero mean spatial process with independent increments. The spatial covariance function, which for sites s and s', is

$$C(s,s') = \int_{R^d} k(s,u)k(s',u)du,$$

must be positive definite. This model can be discretized in for discrete domains S and it can produce a variety of different non-stationary models, two of which we now describe.

A number of approaches rely on two-dimensional, non-stationary, Gaussian processes and allow spatial dependence to vary with location (Higdon, 1998; Higdon, Swall, and Kern, 1999; Higdon, 2002). In this case, W in Equation (10.21) will be a white noise process giving,

$$\int_C W_s ds \sim N(0, \tau^2 \, | \, C \, |),$$

for every C where $|\,C\,|$ is the area of subregion C and $\tau > 0$ is a constant. Moreover, $k(s,u) = k(s-u)$ has the form of the Gaussian probability density function

$$k(s) = \frac{1}{2\pi} exp\left\{ -\frac{1}{2} s^T s \right\}.$$

As a result m_s would have the usual isotropic, squared exponential, correlation function,

$$\rho(h) = exp\{-h^T h\}. \tag{10.22}$$

The above representation can be generalized by using a smoothing kernel, denoted by k_s, which depends on spatial location s. Higdon et al. (1999) chose a bivariate Gaussian kernel for their application:

$$k_s(s) = \frac{1}{2\pi} \mid \Sigma_s \mid^{-1/2} exp\left\{-\frac{1}{2}s^T \Sigma_s^{-1} s\right\},$$

where Σ_s is a function of location s. The one standard deviation ellipsoids of concentration for this kernel become ellipsoids whose major and minor axes vary in direction and length from one location to another, along with the degree of smoothing induced by the kernel over regions of the spatial domain (Paciorek and Schervish, 2006).

Fuentes (2002a, 2002b) proposes another approach where now m in Equation 10.21 represents a weighted average of locally isotropic stationary processes that are uncorrelated with each other. The geographical region is divided into well-defined subregions, each of which has a locally isotropic stationary process.

More precisely,

$$m_s = \sum_{i=1}^{k} V_{is} w_{is},$$

for $i = 1, \cdots, k$, that is, where $Cov(V_{is}, V_{js}) = 0$ for $i \neq 0$. The geographical region is divided into k well-defined subregions $A_1, \ldots, A_k$ and (V_{is}) is a local isotropic stationary process in a subregion A_i. The weights, w_{is} come from a positive kernel function centered at the centroid of A_i.

The covariance between any two locations s_1 and s_2 in the geographical region can be written as

$$\begin{aligned} Cov(m_s, m_{s'}) &= \sum_{i=1}^{k} w_{is} w_{is'} cov(V_{Is}, V_{Is'}) \\ &= \sum_{i=1}^{k} w_{is} w_{is'} C_{\theta_i}(\mid h \mid) \end{aligned}$$

depends only on the distance $\mid h \mid$ due to the isotropic stationarity. Since θ_i can change from subregion to subregion, $Cov(m_s, m_{s'})$ can depend not just on that distance but also on s and s'. Thus, the process m_s is non-stationary.

Wind direction plays an important role in the spread of air pollutants over a geographical region. Vianna-Neto, Schmidt, and Guttorp (2014) extend the convolution approach to accommodate wind direction in the kernel function of the convolution approach. They analyze the effect of wind direction on the concentration of ozone levels observed at sites located in the north-eastern region of the USA. In Chapter 12 we discuss other approaches that use covariate information in the covariance structure of spatial processes.

10.14   Summary

This chapter contains the basic theory of spatial processes and a number of approaches to modeling point-referenced spatial data. The reader will have gained an understanding of the following topics:

- Visualization techniques needed for both exploring and analyzing spatial data and communicating its features through the use of maps;
- Exploring the underlying structure of spatial data and methods for characterizing dependence over space;
- Second-order theory for spatial processes, including the covariance. The variogram for measuring spatial associations;
- Stationarity and isotropy;
- Methods for spatial prediction, using both classical methods (kriging) and modern methods (Bayesian kriging);
- Non-stationarity fields.

10.15   Exercises

Exercise 10.1. This exercise relates to units of measurement.

(i) The US ozone standard set in about 1997 was set at 0.08 (ppm, parts per million). Why did it not contain another decimal place?

(ii) The 1997 standard was changed to the more restrictive upper limit of 0.075 (ppm). Why not set this to be 75 (ppb – parts per billion) instead, to give it a simpler form?

(iii) Ground level ozone particulate concentrations $PM_{2.5}$ are measured in units of μgm^{-3} (micrograms per meter cubed). These distributions of these measurements are highly right skewed, and that has led some statistical analysts to transform these measurements as $y = \log(PM_{2.5})$. What units of magnitude should be attached to y? Why?

(iv) For levels of particulates, y, risk assessments are commonly made with $\Delta y = 10~\mu gm^{-3}$ while the log transform $y' = \log(y)$ is often employed in statistical analysis to get $\alpha \exp(\beta y')$ for the concentration response function (CRF). Would the units of measurement used for y matter when looking at the effect of such a change in the CRF? In other words, what would happen if the US EPA were to change their measurements from $10~\mu gm^{-3}$ to 10,000 milligrams m^{-3}?

Exercise 10.2. This exercise is about measuring distance on the earth's surface, as one must do in developing variogram models when large geographical domains are involved. The central problem stems from the fact that the lines of longitude are not parallel, unlike the lines of latitude.

(i) Approximately how many kilometers is a degree of latitude on the Earth's surface?

(ii) Given a circle of radius r centered at the origin, and two points on that circle, P_1 and P_2, find a formula for the distance between them along the arc of that circle between them.

(iii) Repeat the first calculation, but this time for two points on the Earth's surface, whose coordinates are given in latitude and longitude.

(iv) Use your formula to calculate the distance in kilometers between Whitehorse and Toronto (both in Canada), using the latitudes and longitudes provided by Google Maps. How does this compare to the naive result you would get if you assumed a degree of longitude was about the same as a degree of latitude in size in
Kilometers?

Exercise 10.3. Produce a map as shown in Figure 10.5 for another state or area.

Exercise 10.4. (i) What adverse effects on human populations does cadmium have in sufficiently high concentrations?

(ii) Using the R gstat library, perform a trend and spatial distribution analysis for the cadmium concentrations in the Meuse River flood plain.

Exercise 10.5. (i) For any $N_S \times 1$ random vector $\mathbf{W}$, prove that its covariance matrix $Cov(\mathbf{W})$ must be positive definite.

(ii) Suppose Z is a second order stationary process and $\mathbf{Z}$, a $N_S \times 1$ process vector over points s_i, $i = 1, \ldots, N_S$. Show that Equation (10.2) implies that $Cov(\mathbf{Z})$ must be positive definite.

(iii) Show that $C(h) = \sigma(\exp - \| h \|)$, $h \in \mathscr{R}^{\in}$ is positive definite. *Hint:* Find two zero mean random vectors $\mathbf{U} \ \mathbf{V}$ of dimension 2 such that $C(\mathbf{U}, \mathbf{V}) = C(h)$.

Exercise 10.6. In the example of mapping temperatures in California, kriging models with a constant mean term (ordinary kriging) and with a mean term including the location (x and y).

(i) Extract the temperatures for a different day and repeat the example, re-fitting the kriging models. What differences do you see in the spatial pattern, compared to that seen in Figure 10.7?

(ii) Fit variograms using the data in the example and for the other date(s) you have chosen. What do you conclude? Is there any other information that would you like to include in the mean term before fitting the spatial component of the model?

(ii) Repeat the analyze including elevation in the mean term of the model. Do you see any changes in either the variogram or the resulting maps?

Exercise 10.7. Give a theoretical example of a spatial field that is intrinsically stationary, but not second order stationary.

Exercise 10.8. Perform a Bayesian analysis of the lead data seen in Example 10.1 and display your predictions on a map (for example using get_stamenmap() within ggmap).

Exercise 10.9. Determine explicitly the form of the matrix ζ in Section 10.13 which is required to correct for geometric anisotropy.

Exercise 10.10. Prove the assertion in Equation 10.22.

Exercise 10.11. Using NIMBLE and R-INLA

(i) Fit a spatial model to the European NO$_2$ concentrations and produce a map of the spatial effects from the model using both NIMBLE and R-INLA.

(ii) Use the results from this model to produce a map of the probabilities that concentrations exceed 40 μgm^{-3}.

(iii) Land-use regression uses information on factors that might affect levels of pollution at the locations of monitoring sites. By choosing a suitable selection of factors, fit a model that estimates the effects of those factors and fits a spatial model to the residuals.

(iv) Under what circumstances could this model be used for predicting concentrations at unmonitored locations?

Chapter 11

Modeling temporal data: time series and forecasting

11.1 Overview

Modeling time series data and the temporal processes that generate them is of paramount importance in environmental epidemiology, where we find several areas of application. These include modeling underlying patterns in exposures, for example to air pollution, as well as temporal patterns in health outcomes. Predictions may be made both within the time frame of the given data and in the future, the latter of which is known as *forecasting*. An example of forecasting in environmental processes is where urban areas produce 24-hour ahead forecasts of air pollution levels (Dou, Le, and Zidek, 2012). This chapter contains a background to the study of temporal processes, which replaces space, the subject of Chapter 10, as the domain of interest whilst drawing on many of the concepts from the previous chapter.

This chapter begins by giving a general perspective on the role of time series in environmental epidemiology. Then we turn to exploratory and mainly classical methods for handling temporal data, notably on how to separate low and high frequency components of a process that evolves over time and also on characterizing dependence in the series. Next, we describe dynamic linear models (DLMs) and how to perform Bayesian inference for this class of models. Finally, we show how Bayesian methods can be used for incorporating temporal dependence into health effect analyzes.

11.2 Time series epidemiology

One of the areas in which time series methods are most extensively used in environmental epidemiology is in assessing the short-term effects of changes in air pollution on health outcomes. In this case, the data commonly takes the form of daily measurements of one, or more, pollutants that are related to daily counts of mortality or morbidity. The outcomes are likely to exhibit temporal correlation, that is, there is likely to be a high degree of dependence between values of the process, Z_t, especially within short periods of time. This is not necessarily because the outcome, for example, the number of daily deaths, is causally related to the number the day before, as might be the case with a contagious disease, but because the underlying risk factors,

DOI: 10.1201/9781003352655-11

such as temperature and pollution tend to be highly correlated day-to-day. The values of Z_t are then not mutually independent and this must be taken into account in any analysis that involves them. Classical time series composition and analysis is primarily interested in modeling the behavior of the response variable, rather than its relationship with a set of explanatory variables. However, the methods can be extremely valuable in understanding the nature of any temporal dependence which might manifest itself for example in model residuals and thus in constructing suitable models. There are many comprehensive texts on the subject of time series and forecasting, and only a brief review is presented here. For a more complete treatment of the subject see Harvey (1993), West and Harrison (1997), Diggle (1991), Hamilton (1994), Chatfield (2013) and Chatfield (2000).

11.2.1   Confounders

In addition to the possible effects of the exposure of interest, counts of mortality or morbidity will depend on a set of other risk factors, that is, confounders, and if the influence of these factors is not adequately accounted for then the estimated exposure – mortality association may be biased. Confounding may induce long-term trends, seasonal variation, over-dispersion and short-term temporal correlation. Confounders may include meteorological conditions such as temperature, humidity, wind speed and rainfall. In addition to measured confounders, there may also be unmeasured factors. When modeling, these are often represented by proxy variables such as functions of calendar time and variables that indicate the day of the week.

11.2.2   Known risk factors

The health problems that result from exposure may be felt immediately, that is on the same day (Moolgavkar, 2000), after a lag of one or two days (Peters et al., 2000) or from continued exposure over preceding weeks or from long-term exposure over several decades (Elliott et al., 2007). The choice between different lags is a longstanding research problem without consensus with regard to which should be used. Numerous approaches have been suggested, including selecting the lag that is associated with the most significant effect (Lumley and Sheppard, 2000) or the one that minimizes an objective criterion (such as the AIC). Alternatively, results for multiple lags have been presented, for example by Burnett et al. (1994). An alternative approach is to use transfer function models which considers an instantaneous effect, and it propagates a proportion of such effect to future times. The shape of this propagation depends on the chosen transfer function. The advantage is that one does not need to fix a given lag, as the estimation of the lag of the effect is data-driven (Alves, Gamerman, and Ferreira, 2010). Example 11.18 revisits the analysis of the effect of carbon monoxide on counts of infant deaths described in Alves et al. (2010). More recently, Freitas, Schmidt, Cossich, Cruz, and Carvalho (2021) proposed a spatio-temporal model to investigate the association between minimum temperature and the log-relative risk of dengue across neighborhoods of Rio de Janeiro. The novelty of their model is that the parameters of the transfer function model varied spatially, allowing the impact of temperature on the log-risk to change across space.

In studies of the short-term effects of environmental hazards, such as air pollution, it is commonly the case that risk factors will be related to meteorological covariates. These might include temperature (Mar, Norris, Koenig, and Larson, 2000), humidity (Lee et al., 2000), precipitation (Spix et al., 1993), and pressure (Vedal, Brauer, White, and Petkau, 2003). Temperature can play a central role as it drives part of the seasonal variation typically present in health data, where higher counts of morbidity and mortality are observed during cold periods. Although meteorological data are routinely available, including them in an epidemiological analysis requires a number of decisions including which lag should be used and the exact nature of the shape of their relationship with health, that is, can it be presented by a linear relationship or is something more complex required?

11.2.3   Unknown risk factors

Unknown risk factors may result in long-term trends and seasonal variation in time series studies and large-scale spatial trends, for example north to south gradients, in spatial studies. As they cannot be added to regression models in the same way as known factors, allowing for the influence of unknown risk factors is less straightforward than for known, measured, factors. In early temporal studies, Schwartz, Slater, Larson, Pierson, and Koenig (1993) and Spix et al. (1993) modeled seasonal variation with pairs of sine and cosine terms at different frequencies, and long-term trends with parametric functions such as cubic polynomials of calendar time. Other early approaches modeled these factors with indicator variables (Verhoeff, Hoek, Schwartz, and van Wijnen, 1996) which, as with parametric functions, may be overly restrictive and lack the necessary flexibility to model excessive variation in mortality. For example, the sinusoidal terms force the peak in mortality to occur at the same time each year, while the monthly indicator variables do not allow for within month variation. More recently, these unmeasured risk factors have been represented using smooth functions of calendar time, which can be more flexible than fixed parametric alternatives. Such functions have been implemented using parametric and non-parametric methods, including regression splines (Daniels, Dominici, Zeger, and Samet, 2004) and smoothing splines (Dominici, Samet, and Zeger, 2000).

Categorical, or indicator, variables are often used as proxies for factors that may be confounded with the relationship of interest. These may include variables for 'day of the week' (Kelsall, Zeger, and Samet, 1999), for times of influenza epidemics (Peters et al., 2000) and public holidays (Schwartz, 2001). In spatial studies, where the relative risk (Chapter 2, Section 2.3.1) is driven by differences in health counts between different areas, confounding variables might for example represent the effects of socio-economic deprivation which has been shown to be a strong predictor of both health (Kleinschmidt et al., 1995) and air pollution (Elliott et al., 2007).

11.3   Time series modeling

In modeling time series data, as with spatial data seen in Chapter 10, we distinguish between the underlying temporal and measurement processes. Although time is a continuous measure over $\mathcal{T}$, data will only be collected at N_T discrete points in time, $T \in \mathcal{T}$ where these points are labelled $T = \{t_0, t_1, \ldots, t_{N_T}\}$. Note that time, unlike space, does have a natural ordering.

The underlying process is not directly measurable, but realizations of it can be obtained by taking measurements, possibly with error at times in T. One way of expressing the random field is as a combination of the overall trend together with a spatial structure, for example

$$
\begin{aligned}
Y_t &= Z_t + v_t \\
Z_t &= \mu_t + \gamma_t \\
\mu_t &= \sum_{j=1}^{J} \beta_j f_j(X_t),
\end{aligned}
\qquad (11.1)
$$

where v_t is measurement error, μ_t is the mean of the underlying process, modeled as a function of covariate information which might include time itself with associated coefficients β and γ_t is a process with temporal structure.

For clarity of exposition, in the following introduction to classical time series methodology, we assume that measurement error is not present, that is, $Y_t = Z_t$ in Equation (11.1). We return to the hierarchical modeling approach in Section 11.7.

Classical time series modeling aims to decompose the variation in the series into:

- Trend – long-term movements in the mean.
- Seasonality – annual cyclical fluctuations.
- Cycles – other cyclical variations, at different frequencies, which can be greater than or less than a year.
- Residuals – other random or systematic fluctuations.

Formally, the trend, μ_t, of a time series is defined as the expectation of the set of random variables Z_t, that is $\mu_t = E(Z_t)$. It is the long-term change in the underlying process and indicates the general pattern of rise or fall of the outcome variable. A simple linear trend, $\mu_t = \alpha + \beta t$ is often referred to as a *deterministic* or *global* trend. Alternatively, a *local* trend can be modeled that evolves through time, allowing the parameters to be dependent on time, $\mu_t = \alpha_t + \beta_t$, including a recursive equation of the parameters, for example, $\alpha_t = \alpha_{t-1} + \beta_t + \omega_{t1}$ and $\beta_t = \beta_{t-1} + \omega_{t2}$, where ω_{t1} and ω_{t2} are independent evolution errors. This follows the structure of dynamic linear models (see Section 11.7).

After modeling the trend, seasonality and cyclic components, there may still be autocorrelation in the residual term, due to short-term dependencies in the data. These dependencies over time can be explicitly modeled, and details of models for this purpose are given in Example 11.8.

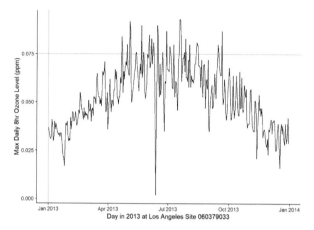

Figure 11.1: Daily concentrations of ozone (ppm) at the EPA monitoring site 060379033 in Los Angeles. The horizontal line is plotted at the current for 8 hour regulatory standard of 0.075 (ppm).

Example 11.1. *Ground level ozone concentrations*

Ozone is a colorless gas produced through a combination of photochemistry, sunlight, high temperatures, oxides of nitrogen, NO_x, emitted by motor vehicles. Levels are especially high during morning and evening commute hours in urban areas. It is one of the criteria pollutants regulated by the US Clean Air Act (1970) because of a substantial body of literature that shows a strong association with human morbidity, notably respiratory diseases such as asthma, emphysema, and chronic obstructive pulmonary disorder (COPD) (EPA, 2005). Periods of high ozone concentrations can lead to acute asthma attacks leading to increased numbers of deaths, hospital admissions and school absences. High levels of ozone concentrations can also lead to reduced lung capacity.

Figure 11.1 shows daily concentrations of ozone measured at sites located in the geographical region of Los Angeles, California. Clear seasonal patterns can be observed due to the higher temperatures in summer.

Figure 11.2 depicts the same series at the hourly level, but restricted to the so-called 'ozone season', which is taken to be 1 May–30 Sep. Here a clear 24-hour daily cycle can be seen along with a period of missing data. The latter is likely due to the monitoring systems being checked each night by the injection of a calibrated sample of air. If the instrument reports the ozone incorrectly, an alert is sounded and that instrument is taken off-line until it is repaired. This can lead to gaps in the series, as seen around hour 1100.

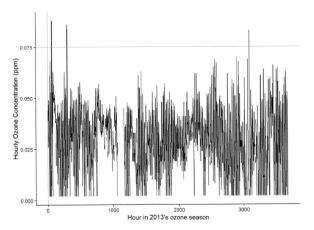

Figure 11.2: Hourly concentrations of ozone at the Los Angeles ozone (ppm) monitoring site 840060370113 during the summer ozone season 1 May–30 Sep 2013. The horizontal line is plotted at the current 8-hour regulatory standard of 0.075 (ppm).

This example shows the existence of regular, systematic or low frequency, patterns together with irregular components. The regular components include trends over time and periodic components, for example, 24-hour cycles and day of the week effects, while the irregular components are randomly distributed around the regular patterns.

11.3.1   Low-pass filtering

In some cases, like that in Example 11.1, there is a well established scientific foundation on which to build a model for the regular components, and in such cases analysis reduces to estimating the model parameters (Huerta, Sansó, and Stroud, 2004) by standard statistical methods. In other cases, exploratory analysis will be needed to identify these components. This will begin with estimating the trend by smoothing the data. There are a number of methods for doing this including moving averages (Section 2.6) fitting locally linear models and Shumway's 19 day symmetrically weighted moving average, $\sum_{-9}^{9} \psi_j y_{i-j} / \bar{y}$ (where the weights, $\psi_0, ..., \psi_9$, are symmetric and sum to one). These methods are called low-pass filters since they do not allow the irregular variation to 'pass' through them.

Example 11.2. *Low-pass filtering of carbon monoxide levels using the moving average*

Carbon monoxide (CO) is commonly called the 'silent killer' and when inhaled in large quantities it causes death by asphyxiation with minimal symptoms that include tiredness and dizziness. As it is inhaled, it passes through the

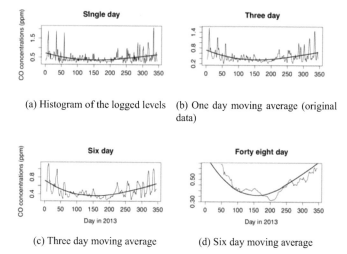

(a) Histogram of the logged levels (b) One day moving average (original data)

(c) Three day moving average (d) Six day moving average

Figure 11.3: Moving averages of the daily maximum eight-hour moving average of carbon monoxide (CO) concentrations (ppm) at a site in New York during 2013. The panels show: (a) the one (original data); (b) three; (c) six and (d) forty-eight day moving averages. To help visualize the underlying trend in the process, a smooth loess curve has been added. Regular components of the time series are seen in the results for six and forty-eight day results.

lung's gas exchange membrane into the blood stream, where it binds tightly to hemoglobin to form carboxyhaemoglobin (COHb) in the red blood cells. Oxygen is thus blocked from binding to the hemoglobin distribution throughout the body. Concern about the effects of CO has made it one of the criteria pollutants regulated by the US Clean Air Act. It is therefore subject to air quality regulations, which require that the eight-hourmoving daily average level of CO concentrations must remain below 9 ppm. Figure 11.3 shows daily average CO levels for an EPA monitoring site in New York State (Site ID:340130003) during 2013. In addition to showing the original data, which is essentially a one-day moving average, different levels of smoothing are shown (three, six and forty-eight day moving averages). In each case, a locally linear smoother known as loess is added to the plots to help identify longer term trends.

The smoothed six-day version shows a pattern of cyclical episodes of CO concentrations, each of about twenty-four days duration. Using a forty-eight-day moving average smooths out the bumps to reveal a longer cycle of about six months in duration, one that dips to its minimum in the summer months. with higher levels of CO in the winter months.

Example 11.3. *Moving average smoothers in epidemiological studies of air pollution*

A moving average approach was used by Mazumdar, Schimmel, and Higgins (1982), utilizing a 15-day moving average when analyzing daily counts of death in winters in London, UK in the 1960s. This took into account long wavelength patterns in the data, but rather than using density estimation, the weights dropped from 1 to 0 between the seventh and eighth day, which created distortions in the smoothed data. Moving averages were also used by Kinney and Ozkaynak (1991) who investigated the relationships between daily death counts (all cause, respiratory and cardiovascular) and levels of five pollutants (O_x, SO_2, NO_2, CO and KM, a measure of optical reflectance) together with temperature variables in Los Angeles County during the period 1970–79. They explored the temporal structure of any associations between mortality and the pollutants (and temperature) by pre-whitening the data and then examining the cross-correlations. The pre-whitening consisted of transforming both the input and output series using a filter designed to remove all the autocorrelation in the individual variables, in this case an AR(2) function and 365 day differencing was applied to each variable, leaving residuals that had little autocorrelation. They then used multiple regression to assess the effect of the short-term changes in the pollutants on the different outcomes, after subtracting weighted 19-day moving averages from each variable, including the outcome. In both these examples, the data were assumed to be Gaussian, which may have been plausible in large cities such as London with mean daily deaths of almost 300 (Schwartz and Marcus, 1990) and Los Angeles with mean daily deaths of 152, but most studies of air pollution and health involve far fewer daily counts and whilst filtered Gaussian data is still Gaussian, this is not generally the case for other distributions, such as the Poisson.

Given the somewhat arbitrary choice of smoothing functions such as loess, to remove long-term time trends or the number of degrees of freedom when fitting spline functions, it is important that sensitivity analysis is performed to assess the possible effects. This is particularly true where decisions have to be made as to which data should be included in the analysis. Schwartz (1994b), for example, presents results from several models using different smoothers. Different sets of outliers are excluded, for example, very hot or very humid days and different temperature variables, for example, mean daily or nightly minima. Although it is good practice to present the results from a number of different possible models, only a small selection can be presented and if they are not nested or have any common structure, then it is difficult to make sensible comparisons between the different models, in addition to the theoretical issues of testing between non-parametric models of this type.

11.4   Modeling the irregular components

After modeling the regular features of a temporal process, that is, trend, seasonality and cycles, we need to consider the random or irregular components. This has been a central focus of classical temporal process modeling. Such modeling was typically based on a single long record of measurements, for example, levels of ash in the atmosphere following a volcanic eruption. This contrasts with longitudinal data analysis, in which there are replicates of short times series of measurements arising from different subjects, for example, patients. These two modeling paradigms have evolved in very different ways.

11.4.1   Stationary processes

The concept of stationarity in time series analysis is similar to that in spatial analysis, as seen in Chapter 10. A time series is said to be stationary if the distributional structure of Y_t is unaffected by a shift in time. *Strict stationarity* means that for any choice of h, and times $t_1 < \ldots < t_k$, the joint probability distribution of $(t_1, \ldots, t_k)$ is identical to that of $(t_1 + h, \ldots, t_k + h)$. Therefore, if a process is stationary, observations from any time period can be used to make inference about the overall underlying structure.

A weaker assumption is one of *weak* or *second order* stationarity where the mean, $E(Y_t) = \mu_t$ is constant for all t, and the autocovariance function denoted for any two times t, t' by $\rho_{tt'}$ is defined by $\rho_{tt'} = Cov(Y_t, Y_{t'}) = E\left[(Y_{t'} - \mu_{t'})(Y_t - \mu_t)\right]$ depends only on elapsed time between t and t' and not their actual location, for example, $\rho_{1,5} = \rho_{11,15}$. This on its own would not imply strict stationarity.

11.4.2   Models for irregular components

A number of models have been developed for the irregular components of temporal components, and here we present a few examples of both stationary and non-stationary processes. In these examples, $Var(Y_t) = \sigma_t^2$ and for simplicity, we restrict to a discrete time domain of $T = t_1, \ldots, t_{N_T}$ for our exposition.

Example 11.4. *White noise*

$$Y_t = W_t \sim (\mu_W, \sigma_W^2), \tag{11.2}$$

where W_t are independent and identically distributed, usually with $\mu_W = 0$.

Example 11.5. *A random walk*

$$Y_t = Y_{t-1} + W_t, \tag{11.3}$$

where W_t come from a white noise process. Thus $\mu_t = t\mu_W$ and $\sigma_t^2 = t\sigma_W^2$. Hence, Y cannot be stationary. Examples of the use of such a model include modeling the logarithm of the ratio of a stock's closing price for tomorrow over that for today. Commonly it is used in process modeling for convenience since few parameters are needed to describe it (Huerta et al., 2004).

Example 11.6. *Autoregressive processes*

These process models capture local dependence in time through a Markov like model. They do not capture long memory processes where dependence can persist over days or even centuries, as described in Example 11.11.

The simplest autoregressive process is the AR(1). It is Markovian in nature: given Y_{t-1} and Y_{t+1}, Y_t is independent of all other responses, past and future. It is defined at time t as

$$Y_t = \alpha_1 Y_{t-1} + W_t,$$

where $\alpha_1 = \rho_{t-1,t}$ for all t, that is, it is a stationary process if $|\alpha_1| < 1$. The W_t are a set of realizations of a white noise process.

This model extends to the multivariate autoregressive process denoted by MAR(1):

$$\mathbf{Y}_t = \alpha_1 \mathbf{Y}_{t-1} + \mathbf{W}_t.$$

Example 11.7. *Moving average processes*

The independent, random elements, W_t, in the AR models can represent shocks to a system such as a weather system that produces extreme cold. These systems may take time to subside, leading to moving average processes. In the case of the second order, MA(2) this takes the form

$$Y_t = W_t + \beta_1 W_{t-1} + \beta_2 W_{t-2}.$$

Example 11.8. *ARMA processes*

An ARMA(p, q) process combines an AR(p) process and an MA(q) process. For example, an ARMA(1,1) would be

$$Y_t = \alpha_1 Y_{t-1} + W_t + \beta_1 W_{t-1}.$$

Example 11.9. *Inference for ARMA processes*

Ergodicity suggests that for a weakly stationary, temporal process measured with additive measurement error, we can use the following method of moments estimators:

$$\hat{\mu}(t) \equiv \frac{\sum_{t=1}^{T} Y_t}{T}$$

$$\hat{C}(\tau) = \frac{\sum_{t=1}^{T-\tau}(Y_{t+\tau} - \hat{\mu}(t))(Y_t - \hat{\mu}(t))}{T}.$$

Example 11.10. *Backshift operators*

The backshift operator is defined as $BW_t = Y_{t-1}$ for any stochastic process indexed by time $t \in T$. Thus, for an AR(1) process, we have $Y_t = \alpha BY_t + W_t$ or $w_t = (1 - \alpha B)Y_t = \phi(B)Y_t$. Thus, $Y_t = \phi(B)^{-1}W_t$ in terms of the white noise process w_t. Another example is the MA(1) moving average process of order 1 where now $Y_t = W_t + \beta W_{t-1} = (1 + \beta B)W_t = \theta(B)w_t$. Finally, combining these operators gives us the ARMA model $Y_t = \phi(B)^{-1}\theta(B)W_t$, a combination of the AR and MA models. This is a common way of representing the autoregressive process in terms of the innovations process w_t.

Example 11.11. *Long memory processes*

A long memory process is one whose temporal auto-correlation decays more slowly over time than one for an autoregressive process (Craigmile, Guttorp, and Percival, 2005).

If $d = 2$, the standard binomial expansion of $(1 - B)$ where B is a backshift operator would be

$$
\begin{aligned}
(1-B)^2 &= \binom{2}{0} + \binom{2}{1}(-B) + \binom{2}{2}(-B)^2 \\
&= \frac{2}{0!} + \frac{2 \cdot 1}{1!}(-B)\frac{2!}{2!}(-B)^2.
\end{aligned}
\tag{11.4}
$$

The same expansion as expressed in Equation 11.4 can be used when we replace 2 by d. When d is a fraction, then the series cannot terminate and has an infinite number of terms. This is what gives the process its very long memory.

Given the data, many approaches have been developed for determining and fitting process model including the method of moments, least squares, likelihood based and Bayesian methods. These have been implemented in the various software packages. The breadth of this subject is much too great for a comprehensive treatment here, and instead the reader is referred to one of the many excellent books now available on time series.

11.5   The spectral representation theorem and Bochner's lemma

Many time series processes which are indexed by integer valued time points can be expressed in terms of the sum of sine and cosine terms. Bochner's lemma tells us the covariance function of weakly stationary series can be characterized by these trigonometric functions.

To state that theorem requires a brief review of some important basic concepts. We first recall the notion of positive definiteness for covariance matrices described in Section 10.7. Such matrices are symmetric and satisfy the inequality

$$\sum_i \sum_j a_i a_j C(t_i - t_j) > 0,$$

for any vectors of constants $a_1 : a_m$ and time points $t_1 : t_m$, where $u_1 : u_m$ stands for $(u_1, \ldots, u_m)$ where in general the notation $a : b$ means $a, a+1, \ldots, b$. Thus, $r_{a:b}$ denotes the vector $(r_a, r_{a+1}, \ldots, r_m)$ and so on.

We also need some basic ideas from the theory of complex numbers, starting with the imaginary number $i = \sqrt{-1}$. This is the number, which, when squared, gives -1 and is the number on which the complex number system is built. A complex number $z = x + iy$ has both a real component x and an imaginary one y. To visualize imaginary numbers, you can plot z in the complex plane as a point, (x, y) just like you would plot a point in R^2. A close relative of z is its complex conjugate $\bar{z} = x - iy$. Straightforward algebra shows that $z\bar{z} = x^2 + y^2$, the distance square from the origin $(0, 0)$ to (x, y) in the complex plane. The complex number, represented by the point $w = (cos(\theta), sin(\theta)) = cos(\theta) + isin(\theta)$, lies on the rim of a unit circle in the complex plane: $w\bar{w} = 1$. When θ goes from 0 radians to 2π radians, w goes through one revolution around the unit circle, that is, one cycle or a frequency of 1. It turns out that w has a remarkable representation, $w = \exp\{i\theta\}$. In fact, if $w_i = \theta_i$, $i = 1, 2$ we can compute $w_1 w_2$ as $\exp\{i(\theta_1 + \theta_2)\}$, showing why the exponential function representation is so important. We can bring the temporal dynamic into this representation by letting $\theta = 2\pi\omega t$. Thus, as time advances one unit, from t to $t + 1$, the exponential is advanced around the unit circle in the complex plane from $\exp\{i2\pi\omega t\} \exp\{i2\pi\omega t\} \exp\{i2\pi\omega 1\} = \exp\{i2\pi\omega(t+1)\}$.

This appealing idea also turns out to be of fundamental importance for the theory being considered here. We start by examining the *spectral representation theorem* for weakly stationary processes. A simple example might start with a completely deterministic process $\varepsilon_t = cos(2\pi\omega_0 t)$. Since in general $sin(x)$ is an odd function, that is $sin(-x) = -sin(x)$, this process can be rewritten as

$$\varepsilon_t = \frac{cos(2\pi[\omega_0]t) + isin(2\pi[\omega_0]t)}{2} + \frac{cos(2\pi[-\omega_0]t) + isin(2\pi[-\omega_0]t)}{2}$$

$$= \sum_{\omega=-\omega_0}^{\omega_0} \exp\{i(2\pi[\omega]t)\} dU(\omega), \tag{11.5}$$

where U denotes the cumulative distribution function (CDF) that puts half of the probability on each of ω_0 and $-\omega_0$. This is a somewhat complicated way of expressing the cosine, but it demonstrates how a function can be represented as the weighted sum of two processes that move on the unit circle in the complex plane. The key to the success of the representation was a discrete distribution whose probability mass function $dU(\omega) = u(\omega)$ is symmetric around, $\omega = 0$ which results in the sine terms cancelling out, thus eliminating the imaginary number i. This could be extended to allow u to include additional frequencies.

$$\varepsilon_t = \sum_{\omega=-\omega_0}^{\omega_M} \exp\{i(2\pi[\omega]t)\} dU(\omega). \tag{11.6}$$

The previous paragraphs combined with Exercise 11.6 show how we could construct a weakly stationary random process, in the case of a power spectrum with a finite number of frequencies or to include a random component.

A simple version of the spectral representation theory says that all weakly stationary processes over continuous time, ε_t, may be presented by

$$\varepsilon_t = \int_{-\infty}^{\infty} e^{i\omega t} \, dU(\omega), \tag{11.7}$$

where U is a complex-valued process with orthogonal increments, meaning for example that if $\omega_1 < \omega_2 < \omega_3 < \omega_4$ then

$$E\left[U(\omega_2) - U(\omega_1)\right]\overline{\left[U(\omega_4) - U(\omega_3)\right]} = 0.$$

In other words, any weakly stationary process can be represented as a sum of cosines and sines with random coefficients, that is, amplitudes. A similar representation holds for discrete time and even when 'time' is replaced by 'space'.

11.5.1   The link between covariance and spectral analysis

Spectral analysis is the study of processes over their frequency domain, and it aims to determine the contribution of each frequency to the variance of the process. In other words, it looks for where the 'power' driving the process is concentrated.

As seen in Section 11.4.1 the covariance function characterizes stationarity. Bochner's lemma provides a link between the spectral representation of a time series and the covariance.

Lemma 1. (Bochner) If C is a positive definite covariance function for a stationary process, then there exists a spectral distribution function $F(\omega)$, $-1/2 \le \omega \le 1/2$ such that

$$C(\tau) = \int_{-1/2}^{1/2} \exp\{2\pi i \omega \tau\} dF(\omega), |\tau| = 0, 1, \ldots . \tag{11.8}$$

The spectral CDF in this lemma can have a probability density function called the spectral density function under conditions given in the following Corollary.

Corollary 1. $\sum_{\tau=-\infty}^{\tau=\infty} |C(\tau)| < \infty$ implies $dF(\omega) = f(\omega)d\omega$.

Note that as in the case of the spectral representation theorem, symmetry is required, that is, f must be symmetric about 0 to avoid imaginary numbers.

Bochner's theorem extends to continuous time and spatial processes in a natural way. It is of practical value since it can be used to construct temporal (and spatial) covariance functions simply by specifying f, otherwise finding a legitimate covariance function is difficult. When F is discrete, being concentrated on a countable set $\{\omega_i\}$, the integral in Equation (11.8) becomes a sum of *sin* and *cos* terms for a weakly stationary process; and the spectral distribution relates to the random measure in the spectral representation theorem as follows:

$$E[dU(\omega)d\overline{U(\omega)}] = dF(\omega). \tag{11.9}$$

A large value of $dF(\omega)$ corresponds in an informal sense with the size of the amplitudes attached to the sines and cosines. A similar result is found when the process is indexed by discrete time, except the integral in Equation (11.7) is taken over $[-\pi, \pi]$ instead.

Spectral representation theory points to the need to estimate the spectral distribution in order to learn about recurring events and their frequency. Equation (11.6) points to a method for computing that estimate when a finite number of frequencies in the spectrum contribute most of the variability in the process, as reflected in Bochner's lemma. Let us assume the process has been detrended and the resulting residuals ε_t are weakly stationary. For simplicity, these are assumed to be observed without error. In this case, Equation (11.6) suggests the inversion of the relationship between ε_t and $U(d\omega)$ and after some refinement, this idea leads to the estimate of the spectral mass function $I(\omega)$ (Chatfield, 2013), which when plotted against ω is sometimes called the periodogram. Studying this estimate or Bayesian versions of it can indicate unanticipated frequencies, for example a twice a day twelve-hour cycle in urban ozone concentrations in addition to the obvious twenty-four-hour cycle (Huerta et al., 2004). Such a discovery can then be turned into a sine–cosine temporal mean model for the ozone field.

11.6   Forecasting

The negative health impacts of environmental hazards, such as criteria air pollutants, has led to the need in some urban areas for forecasts of future levels of pollution. These are used to inform planning of activities for susceptible individuals, for example California's South Coast Air Quality Management District provides online a detailed map of forecasts in the region around Los Angeles.

This section introduces the classical theory of forecasting temporal processes. Two general approaches are described; the first uses available data to estimate coefficients in a forecasting model and then applies that model, while the second exploits autocorrelation in the temporal process to forecast future values.

11.6.1   Exponential smoothing

Following Chatfield (2013), we begin by describing the exponential smoothing model. When there is no trend or seasonality the next value is predicted from the observations to date,

$$\hat{Y}_{t+1} = c_t \hat{Z}_t + \ldots + c_1 \hat{Z}_1, \tag{11.10}$$

where $c_i = \alpha(1 - 1\alpha)^{i-1}$ with $0 < \alpha < 1$ which means that the most recent observation gets the most weight. Equation (11.10) implies

$$\hat{Y}_{t+1} = c_t \hat{Z}_t + (1 - \alpha)\hat{Y}_t. \tag{11.11}$$

An extension to this idea is at the heart of the Holt–Winters (HW) approach. Suppose $g(t)$, $t > 0$ is a differentiable function that is observed at unit intervals

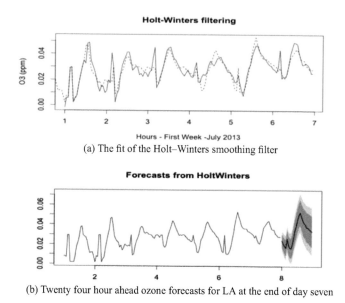

(a) The fit of the Holt–Winters smoothing filter

(b) Twenty four hour ahead ozone forecasts for LA at the end of day seven

Figure 11.4: Ozone concentration (ppm) levels at the Los Angeles site with ID 840060370113 for the first week of July 2013 with forecasts for following 24 hours.

$t = t_0, t_1, \ldots$, with $t_{i+1} = t_i + 1$, $i = 1, \ldots, I$, where I is the total number of segments that the function is split into. Then

$$g(t_{i+h}) \approx g(t_i) + h g'(t_i). \tag{11.12}$$

This gives a predictor for g h time steps ahead based on the present level $g(t_i)$ and the slope $g'(t_i)$. The HW approach extends Equation (11.11) by building upon the concept in Equation (11.12) and treating $\hat{Y}_t = S_t$ as the current 'level' of the process. So S_t is replaced by $S_t + T_t$ where T_t represents a fitted trend, $T_t = \rho(S_t - S_{t-1}) + (1 - \rho)T_{t-1}$, which is a weighted combination of the previous trend and change in the level. The l step ahead forecast is then $\hat{Y}_{t+l} = S_t + lT_t$. Further extensions to the HW method can incorporate seasonality.

Example 11.12. *Forecasting ozone levels*

We return to Example 11.1 with the objective of forecasting ozone concentrations for the next twenty-four hours. These forecasts are based on measured concentrations in Los Angeles from the first week of July 2013. We first fit the Holt–Winters model and see the results in the upper panel of Figure 11.4. The twenty-four-hour ahead forecast on day eight is seen in the lower panel.

11.6.2 ARIMA models

The second approach to forecasting exploits auto-correlation in the temporal process to forecast future values. This approach requires that we first determine the autocorrelation in the process series. This can be assessed using the *autocorrelation function* (ACF), which is equal to ρ_τ. When plotted against lag τ, it is known as the correlogram. Recall that for stationary temporal processes Y_t, $t > 0$, the autocorrelation is $\rho_\tau = Corr(Y_t, Y_{t-\tau}) = Cov(Y_t, Y_{t-\tau})/Var(Y_t)$ for all $t > \tau$ and $\tau > 0$.

When the process is non-stationary, the correlogram can be used as a diagnostic tool (Chatfield, 2013). For example, an increasing trend will be seen as a slowly declining ACF. A periodic series will induce a similar periodic pattern in the correlogram. This diagnostic role is an important one and should be part of any preliminary data analysis.

The *partial auto-correlation* (PACF) also plays a key role in the initial analysis of a temporal series. Consider the autoregressive temporal process model as seen in Example 11.6; this is a Markov model in the sense that given Y_{t-1}, Y_t will be independent of all previous observations from Y_{t-2} to Y_1. In this case, the correlogram will show a lag 2 effect. This arises as the correlation between Y_{t-2} and Y_t comes from their mutual association with Y_{t-1}. The partial ACF eliminates this spurious correlation by computing the autocovariance function between Y_{t-2} and Y_t conditional on Y_{t-1}, that is $E[(Y_{t-2}-\mu)(Y_t-\mu) \mid Y_{t-1} = y_{t-1}]$. Therefore, in practice, both the ACF and PACF need to be studied as a part of a preliminary data analysis.

One way of incorporating autocorrelation in forecasting involves pre-filtering the process to remove the (estimated) regular components, leaving a stationary process for the (estimated) residuals. An ARMA(p, q) process model might then be fit to these residuals and these models then used to forecast future, as yet unobserved residuals. These forecasts can be combined with the estimated future values of the regular components, that is, the trend and seasonality, to get forecasts of the process.

However, finding the regular components can often prove problematic. The Box–Jenkins provides an approach to this problem, which involves differencing the temporal series, until weak stationarity is obtained. The first difference of a series is $Y_t(1) = Y_t - Y_{t-1}$, the second $Y_t(2) = Y_t(1) - Y_{t-1}(1) = Y_t - 2Y_{t-1} + Y_{t-2}$, etc ... An ARMA model is then fit to the result and forecasts made. These forecasts are then integrated back to the original non-stationary process . This is known as an integrated ARMA (ARIMA) process.

11.6.3 Forecasting using ARMA models

Consider the simple case where the process is given by $Y_t = \beta t + \varepsilon_t$, $t = 1, 2, \dots, T$. An analyst recognizing the trend could estimate β in order to get the series of estimates $\hat{\varepsilon}_t = Y_t - \hat{\beta}t$. If these represent a stationary process then an ARMA model could be fit giving the forecast $\hat{\varepsilon}_{T+1}$ and thus the one step ahead forecast, $\hat{Y}_{T+1} = \hat{\beta}(T+1) + \hat{\varepsilon}_{T+1}$. However, if the analyst did not recognize the trend, they might begin by taking the first order difference $\nabla^1 Y_t = Y_t - Y_{t-1} = \beta + \varepsilon_t^*$, where $\varepsilon_t^* = \varepsilon_t - \varepsilon_{t-1}$, $t = 2, 3, \dots, T$. The trend would now have been eliminated and if the ε_t^* comprise a stationary process, an ARMA model might be fit to get the series $\hat{\varepsilon}_t^*$, $t = 2, \ldots, T + 1$, which includes the forecast. Just as in the case of continuous time $g(t) = \int_{t-1}^{t} g'(u)du + g(1)$, and so here we have $\hat{Y}_2 = \hat{\varepsilon}_2^* + Y_1$ etc... The ARMA would give a model for the ε_t^* that includes both autoregressive and moving average components. Finally, we can adapt this same idea to deal not only with trend as above, but also with seasonality.

In general, an ARIMA(p, d, q) model represents the dth difference in the process series as an ARMA process. The seasonal version is based on differences $\nabla^d Y_t$ that give d – step seasonal differences, resulting in a d-differenced series. This approach can deal with regular components, that is, trends, seasonality, etc., without the need to model them explicitly. The ARMA parameters would be estimated for the differenced series and predictions made. Forecasts on the original scale can then be reconstructed by 'integrating' the differences.

Example 11.13. *Forecasting volcanic ash*

Volcanic ash is not a substance that is commonly encountered in environmental epidemiology, however it can be widely distributed by winds and it can be a significant health hazard. A study of the Mount St. Helens volcanic eruption in May and June 1980 reports thirty-five deaths due to the initial blast and landslide. Others are reported to have died from asphyxiation from ash inhalation (Baxter et al., 1981). The respirable portion of the ash was found to contain a small percentage of crystalline free silica, a potential pneumoconiosis hazard, and a number of acute health effects were found in those visiting emergency rooms including asthma, bronchitis and ash-related eye problems.

Hickling, Clements, Weinstein, and Woodward (1999) reported that the ash plume of the relatively small Mount Ruapehu eruption of June 1996 in New Zealand extended over several hundred kilometers. A comparison of rates of respiratory disease, stroke and ischemic heart disease in the three-month period following the blast with the same time period over the previous seven years showed evidence of acute health impacts. For example, a relative risk of RR = 1.44 was found for acute bronchitis.

Figure 11.5 shows the time series of volcanic ash and 11.6 the ACF and PACF. From the plot of the time series a complex pattern can be seen which is the result of eruptions occurring at random times. The large spikes suggest the possibility of moving average components, this is a way that the ARMA process has of incorporating shocks that abate over the period following their occurrence.

There are no obvious regular components in the series that would induce autocorrelation, so we turn to analysis of the ACF and PACF. The correlogram in the left-hand panel of Figure 11.6 points to a significant autocorrelation at lag three and the possibility of an ARMA(0,3) model to capture the persistence in the ash level following a shock, and hence an MA(3) component

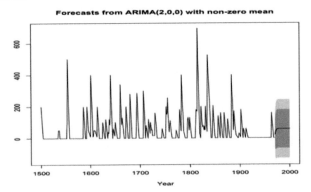

Figure 11.5: Forecasting future atmospheric levels of volcanic ash. The forecast using an ARIMA(2,0,0) is shown on the right-hand side of the plot.

or a mixture of an AR and MA model, might be considered. The PACF plot in the right-hand panel of the figure suggests a significant lag 2 effect, suggesting an ARMA(2,0) model.

The lack of obvious regular components, together with the correlogram plots, suggests the ARIMA approach differences may be used to achieve a stationary process. The `auto.arima` function in the R `forecast` library gave the following results (using the BIC criterion).

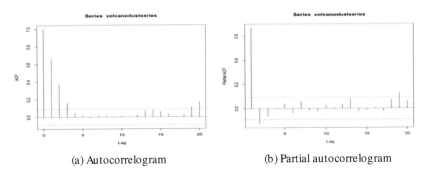

(a) Autocorrelogram   (b) Partial autocorrelogram

Figure 11.6: The autocorrelogram (ACF) and partial autocorrelogram (PACF) plots for data on volcanic ash. Panel (a) shows the ACF and suggests an MA(3) model would capture the persistence of the ash in the atmosphere for three periods. Panel (b) suggests that some of that persistence might be spurious correlation in an AR(2) model.

```
ARIMA(2,0,0) with non-zero mean

Coefficients:
ar1         ar2         intercept
 0.7533     -0.1268        57.5274
(0.0457)    (0.0458)      (8.5958)

sigma^2 estimated as 4870:   log likelihood=-2662.54
AIC=5333.09    AICc=5333.17   BIC=5349.7
```

This analysis suggests that differencing is not needed and that an AR(1) process model would be sufficient. The AIC criterion suggested an ARIMA(1,0,2) instead, this one including an MA(2) component to represent the shock. The earlier results seen in the ACF and PACF analyzes point to the ARMA(2,0,0) model and we can now use this to forecast future ash levels. The results of this can be seen in Figure 11.5.

11.7   State space models

The state space or dynamic linear modeling approach has its roots in the celebrated Kalman-Bucy filter. A Bayesian version of this was developed in the 1970s (P. J. Harrison and Stevens, 1971) and the method has been developed extensively since. It now provides a flexible and general tool for temporal and spatio-temporal modeling (J. Harrison, 1999). The review in this section about DLM's is based on Schmidt and Lopes (2019).

11.7.1   Normal Dynamic Linear Models (DLMs)

Assume that $\{Y_t, t \in T\}$ is a stochastic process observed at discrete time, such that $T = \{0, \pm 1, \pm 2, \pm 3, \ldots\}$. Let D_t be the set of information available at the time t. Thus D_t includes the observation Y_t, and covariates observed at time t (if any), and all previous information D_{t-1}. A normal dynamic linear model (NDLM) decomposes a univariate time series Y_t as the sum of two components, an overall time-varying trend, $\mathbf{F}_t'\mathbf{Z}_t$, and an error component, v_t, that follows a zero mean normal distribution with variance V_t. The latent k-dimensional vector $\mathbf{Z}_t$ is known as the *state vector* at time t and it evolves smoothly with time. More specifically, a NDLM is specified by the following equations:

$$
\begin{aligned}
Y_t &= \mathbf{F}_t'\mathbf{Z}_t + v_t, & v_t &\sim N(0, V_t) & (11.13)\\
\mathbf{Z}_t &= \mathbf{G}_t\mathbf{Z}_{t-1} + \omega_t, & \omega_t &\sim N(0, \mathbf{W}_t), & (11.14)\\
\mathbf{Z}_0 &\sim N(\mathbf{m_0}, \mathbf{C_0}), & & & (11.15)
\end{aligned}
$$

where $\mathbf{Z}_0$ is the initial information, $\mathbf{m_0}$ and $\mathbf{C_0}$ are known k-dimensional mean vector and $k \times k$ covariance matrix, respectively; $\mathbf{F}_t$ is a k-dimensional column vector of covariates, $\mathbf{G}_t$ is a $k \times k$ matrix, known as the *evolution* matrix, and $\mathbf{W}_t$ is a $k \times k$ covariance matrix describing the covariance structure among the components of $\mathbf{Z}_t$. Equations (11.13) and (11.14) are known as the *observation* and *system*, or *state*, equations, respectively. Usually, it is further assumed that v_t and ω_t are independent and mutually independent, and independent of $\mathbf{Z}_0$. Note that, given $\mathbf{Z}_t$, Y_t is conditionally independent of past observations.

A NDLM is completely specified through the quadruple $\{\mathbf{F}_t, \mathbf{G}_t, V_t, \mathbf{W}_t\}$. If it is further assumed that $V_t = V$ and $\mathbf{W}_t = \mathbf{W}$, $\forall t \in T$ this is known as the constant model.

Example 11.14. *First order polynomial model or time-varying level model*
The simplest NDLM is defined by the quadruple $\{1,1,V,W\}$, such that $y_t = \mu_t + \varepsilon_t$, and $\mu_t = \mu_{t-1} + \omega_t$, with $v_t \sim N(0,V)$, and $\omega_t \sim N(0,W)$. Here, $Z_t = \mu_t$ and $k = 1$. The ratio W/V, known as the signal-to-noise ratio, plays an important role in determining the behavior of the time varying level μ_t. As $W/V \to 0$, the first order model tends to a constant mean model, and as $W/V \to \infty$ the model reduces to a pure random walk. This model is suitable for short term forecast as it can be shown that the forecast function is constant.

Example 11.15. *Linear trend*
A linear trend model can be defined by assuming that $y_t = \mu_t + \varepsilon_t$, $\mu_t = \mu_{t-1} + \beta_{t-1} + \omega_{1t}$ and $\beta_t = \beta_{t-1} + \omega_{2t}$, where β_t is the slope of the local level μ_t. In this case, $\mathbf{Z}_t = (\mu_t, \beta_t)'$ and the NDLM is defined by the quadruple $\{\mathbf{F}, \mathbf{G}, \mathbf{V}, \mathbf{W}\}$, where $\mathbf{F}' = (1\ 0)$,

$$\mathbf{G} = \begin{pmatrix} 1 & 1 \\ 0 & 1 \end{pmatrix} \text{ and } \mathbf{W} = \begin{pmatrix} W_{11} & W_{12} \\ W_{12} & W_{22} \end{pmatrix},$$

for some known values of W_{11}, W_{12}, W_{22} and V. If $W_{22} = 0$ the model results in a constant trend model.

Example 11.16. *Fourier representation of seasonality*
A seasonal structure can be accommodated by a Fourier representation of seasonality. Assuming the period of seasonality is m, then $\mathbf{F}' = (1\ 0)$,

$$\mathbf{G} = \begin{pmatrix} \cos(2\pi/m) & \sin(2\pi/m) \\ -\sin(2\pi/m) & \cos(2\pi/m) \end{pmatrix},$$

and $\mathbf{W} = \text{diag}(W_1, W_2)$. For example, for monthly data with an annual cycle, $m = 12$.

Forward learning: the Kalman filter In a Bayesian NDLM, from Equations (11.13)–(11.15), the posterior distribution of any parameters at time t is based on all available information up to time t, D_t. One aspect of the sequential Bayesian learning in dynamic models is that the posterior distribution for the parameters at time $t-1$, $p(\mathbf{Z}_{t-1}|D_{t-1})$, when propagated through the system equation (11.14) becomes the prior distribution of the parameters at time t, $p(\mathbf{Z}_t|D_{t-1})$. Should $\mathbf{Z}_t$ be time-invariant, this step would vanish and $p(\mathbf{Z}_t|D_{t-1}) = p(\mathbf{Z}_{t-1}|D_{t-1})$. As is standard in Bayesian sequential learning, the prior at time t is then combined with the likelihood $p(Y_t|\mathbf{Z}_t)$ from the observation equation (11.13) to produce both predictive density $p(Y_t|D_{t-1})$ and posterior density $p(\mathbf{Z}_t|D_t)$.

The resultant distributions for each step described above depend on the distribution of the initial information $\mathbf{Z}_0|D_0 \sim N(\mathbf{m}_0, \mathbf{C}_0)$ and the knowledge or not of the observational variance V_t and the variance of the evolution noise, $\mathbf{W}_t$. We modify slightly the definition of the NDLM in equations (11.13) and (11.14) to accommodate the more general case when V is unknown but follows an inverse gamma prior distribution, and the distribution of the noise component follows a normal distribution conditional on the value of V, that is, $\omega_t \mid V \sim N(\mathbf{0}, V\mathbf{W}_t^*)$. The results that follow are based on Theorem 4.3 in West and Harrison (1997).

Let $\phi = 1/V$ be the observational precision. Define, at time $t = 0$, a normal-gamma prior distribution for $p(\mathbf{Z}_0, \phi|D_0)$ by $\mathbf{Z}_0|D_0, V \sim N(\mathbf{m}_0, V\mathbf{C}_0^*)$, and assume $\phi|D_0 \sim Ga(n_0/2, n_0 S_0/2)$. The derivation is done by induction, by assuming that $\mathbf{Z}_{t-1}|V, D_{t-1} \sim N(\mathbf{m}_{t-1}, V\mathbf{C}_{t-1}^*)$ and $\phi|D_{t-1} \sim Ga(n_{t-1}/2, n_{t-1}S_{t-1}/2)$. It can be shown that the steps above are given by (West and Harrison, 1997, p. 109–110):

- *Evolving the state:* The prior distribution of $\mathbf{Z}_t$ is given by $\mathbf{Z}_t|V, D_{t-1} \sim N(\mathbf{a}_t, V\mathbf{R}_t^*)$ where $\mathbf{a}_t = \mathbf{G}_t\mathbf{m}_{t-1}$ and $\mathbf{R}_t^* = \mathbf{G}_t\mathbf{C}_{t-1}^*\mathbf{G}_t' + \mathbf{W}^*$. Therefore, $\mathbf{Z}_t|D_{t-1} \sim t_{n_{t-1}}(\mathbf{a}_t, S_{t-1}\mathbf{R}_t^*)$. Here $t_\nu(\mu, \sigma^2)$ denotes a Student's t distribution with ν degrees of freedom, location μ and scale σ^2.

- *Predicting the next observation:* The one-step ahead forecast is given by $Y_t|V, D_{t-1} \sim N(f_t, V Q_t^*)$ where $f_t = \mathbf{F}_t'\mathbf{a}_t$ and $Q_t^* = 1 + \mathbf{F}_t'\mathbf{R}_t^*\mathbf{F}_t$. Therefore, $Y_t|D_{t-1} \sim t_{n_{t-1}}(f_t, S_{t-1}Q_t^*)$.

- *Updating the variance:* $\phi|D_t \sim Ga(n_t/2, n_t S_t/2)$, where $n_t = n_{t-1} + 1$, and $n_t S_t = n_{t-1}S_{t-1} + (Y_t - f_t)^2/Q_t^*$.

- *Updating the state:* The posterior distribution of $\mathbf{Z}_t$ given the information at time t, is given by $\mathbf{Z}_t|V, D_t \sim N(\mathbf{m}_t, V\mathbf{C}_t^*)$, with $\mathbf{m}_t = \mathbf{a}_t + \mathbf{A}_t(Y_t - f_t)$ and $\mathbf{C}_t^* = \mathbf{R}_t^* - \mathbf{A}_t\mathbf{A}_t'Q_t^*$, where $\mathbf{A}_t = \mathbf{R}_t\mathbf{F}_tQ_t^{-1}$. Therefore, $\mathbf{Z}_t|D_t \sim t_{n_t}(\mathbf{m}_t, S_t\mathbf{C}_t^*)$.

These recursions are commonly known as *Kalman recursions* or simply *the Kalman filter algorithm* (see, for instance, West and Harrison (1997)). If interest lies on forecasting the process h steps ahead, based on the information up to time D_t, the forecast distribution, $y_{t+h}|D_t$, can be obtained through the Kalman filter. It can be shown that $y_{t+h}|D_t \sim t_{n_t}(f_t(h), Q_t(h))$, with $f_t(h) = \mathbf{F}_{t+h}'\mathbf{a}_t(h)$, $Q_t(h) = \mathbf{F}_{t+h}'\mathbf{R}_t(h)\mathbf{F}_{t+h} + S_{t+h}$, $\mathbf{a}_t(0) = \mathbf{m}_t$, and $\mathbf{R}_t(0) = \mathbf{C}_t$.

Backward learning: the Kalman smoother

The Kalman filter is one of the most popular algorithms for the sequential update of hidden/latent states in dynamic systems. However, in the above form, it only
provides posterior distribution of a given state $\mathbf{Z}_t$ conditionally on the past observa-
tions, $Y_1,\ldots,Y_t$, $p(\mathbf{Z}_t|D_t,V)$. For simplicity, we are omitting the dependence on the
state variances $\mathbf{W}_1^*,\ldots,\mathbf{W}_n^*$. In many instances, however, one may want to obtain the
posterior distribution of the states given the whole set of observations, $Y_1,\ldots,Y_n$, that
is $p(\mathbf{Z}_1,\ldots,\mathbf{Z}_n|V,D_n)$; for instance, to understand the dynamics driving observations
as opposed to simply forecasting its future values.

Full joint distribution of states

By the Markov property of Equations (11.13)–(11.15), this joint posterior can be
rewritten as

$$p(\mathbf{Z}_1,\ldots,\mathbf{Z}_n|V,D_n) \quad = \quad p(\mathbf{Z}_n|V,D_n)\prod_{t=1}^{n-1}p(\mathbf{Z}_t|\mathbf{Z}_{t+1},V,D_t). \quad (11.16)$$

First, the forward learning scheme of the previous section (Kalman filter) is run to
obtain $p(\mathbf{Z}_t|V,D_t)$, for $t=1,\ldots,n$. Then, an analogous backward learning scheme
(Kalman smoother) is run to obtain $p(\mathbf{Z}_t|\theta_{t+1},V,D_t)$, for $t=n-1,\ldots,1$. More pre-
cisely, another (backwards) application of Bayes' theorem leads to

$$p(\mathbf{Z}_t|\mathbf{Z}_{t+1},V,D_t) \quad \propto \quad f_N(\mathbf{Z}_{t+1};\mathbf{G}_t\mathbf{Z}_t,V\mathbf{W}_t^*)f_N(\mathbf{Z}_t;\mathbf{m}_t,V\mathbf{C}_t^*)$$
$$\propto \quad f_N(\mathbf{Z}_{t+1};\widetilde{\mathbf{m}}_t,V\widetilde{\mathbf{C}}_t^*), \quad (11.17)$$

where $\widetilde{\mathbf{m}}_t = \widetilde{\mathbf{C}}_t^*(\mathbf{G}_t'\mathbf{W}_t^{-1}\mathbf{Z}_{t+1}+\mathbf{C}_t^{*-1}\mathbf{m}_t)$ and $\widetilde{\mathbf{C}}_t^* = (\mathbf{G}_t'\mathbf{W}_t^{*-1}\mathbf{G}_t+\mathbf{C}_t^{*-1})^{-1}$, for $t=$
$n-1,n-2,\ldots,1$. In practice, for some models, it may be better to use the Sherman-
Morrison-Woodbury (Golub and Loan, 1996) formulae for evaluating $\mathbf{C}_t^*$. From the
Kalman filter, $V|D_n \sim IG(n_n/2,n_nS_n/2)$, so it follows that $\mathbf{Z}_n|D_n \sim t_{n_n}(\widetilde{\mathbf{m}}_n,S_n\widetilde{\mathbf{C}}_n^*)$
and

$$\mathbf{Z}_t|\mathbf{Z}_{t+1},D_t \sim t_{n_n}(\widetilde{\mathbf{m}}_t,S_n\widetilde{\mathbf{C}}_t^*), \quad (11.18)$$

for $t=n-1,n-2,\ldots,1$.

Marginal distributions of the states

Similarly, it can be shown that the marginal distribution of $\mathbf{Z}_t$ is

$$\mathbf{Z}_t|D_n \sim t_{n_n}(\overline{\mathbf{m}}_t,S_n\overline{\mathbf{C}}_t^*), \quad (11.19)$$

where, for $t=n-1,n-2,\ldots,1$, $\overline{\mathbf{m}}_t = \mathbf{m}_t + \mathbf{C}_t^*\mathbf{G}_{t+1}'\mathbf{R}_{t+1}^{*-1}(\overline{\mathbf{m}}_{t+1}-\mathbf{a}_{t+1})$ and $\overline{\mathbf{C}}_t^* =$
$\mathbf{C}_t^* - \mathbf{C}_t^*\mathbf{G}_{t+1}'\mathbf{R}_{t+1}^{*-1}(\mathbf{R}_{t+1}^*-\overline{\mathbf{C}}_{t+1}^*)\mathbf{R}_{t+1}^{*-1}\mathbf{G}_{t+1}\mathbf{C}_t^*$.

Full conditional distributions of the states

Let $\mathbf{Z}_{-t} = \{\mathbf{Z}_1,\ldots,\mathbf{Z}_{t-1},\mathbf{Z}_{t+1},\ldots,\mathbf{Z}_n\}$ and $t=2,\ldots,n-1$, it follows that the full
conditional distribution of $\mathbf{Z}_t$ is

$$p(\mathbf{Z}_t|\mathbf{Z}_{-t},V,D_n) \quad \propto \quad f_N(Y_t;\mathbf{F}_t'\mathbf{Z}_t,V)f_N(\mathbf{Z}_{t+1};\mathbf{G}_{t+1}\mathbf{Z}_t,V\mathbf{W}_{t+1}^*)$$
$$\times \quad f_N(\mathbf{Z}_t;\mathbf{G}_t\mathbf{Z}_{t-1},V\mathbf{W}_t^*) = f_N(\mathbf{Z}_t;\mathbf{b}_t,V\mathbf{B}_t^*), \quad (11.20)$$

where $\mathbf{b}_t = \mathbf{B}_t^*(\mathbf{F}_t Y_t + \mathbf{G}_{t+1}' \mathbf{W}_{t+1}^{*-1} \mathbf{Z}_{t+1} + \mathbf{W}_t^{*-1} \mathbf{G}_t \mathbf{Z}_{t-1})$ and $\mathbf{B}_t^*(\mathbf{F}_t \mathbf{F}_t' + \mathbf{G}_{t+1}' \mathbf{W}_{t+1}^{*-1} \mathbf{G}_{t+1}$
$+ \mathbf{W}_t^{*-1})^{-1}$. The endpoint parameters $\mathbf{Z}_1$ and $\mathbf{Z}_n$ also have full conditional distribu-
tions $N(\mathbf{b}_1, V\mathbf{B}_1^*)$ and $N(\mathbf{b}_n, V\mathbf{B}_n^*)$, respectively, where $\mathbf{b}_1 = \mathbf{B}_1^*(\mathbf{F}_1 y_1 + \mathbf{G}_2' \mathbf{W}_2^{*-1} \mathbf{Z}_2 +$
$\mathbf{R}^{*-1}\mathbf{a}_1)$, $\mathbf{B}_1^* = (\mathbf{F}_1 \mathbf{F}_1' + \mathbf{G}_2' \mathbf{W}_2^{*-1} \mathbf{G}_2 + \mathbf{R}^{*-1})^{-1}$, $\mathbf{b}_n = \mathbf{B}_n^*(\mathbf{F}_n y_n + \mathbf{W}_n^{*-1} \mathbf{G}_n \mathbf{Z}_{n-1})$ and
$\mathbf{B}_n^* = (\mathbf{F}_n \mathbf{F}_n' + \mathbf{W}_n^{*-1})^{-1}$. Again,

$$\mathbf{Z}_t | \mathbf{Z}_{-t}, D_t \sim t_{n_n}(\mathbf{b}_t, S_n \mathbf{B}_t^*) \qquad \text{for all } t. \qquad (11.21)$$

Full posterior inference

When the evolution variances $\mathbf{W}_1^*, \ldots, \mathbf{W}_n^*$ are unknown, closed-form analytical full
posterior inference is infeasible and numerical or Monte Carlo approximations are
needed. Numerical integration, in fact, is only realistically feasible for very low dimensional settings. Markov Chain Monte Carlo methods have become the norm over
the last quarter of a century for state space modelers. In particular, the full joint
of Equation (11.16) can be combined with full conditional distributions for V and
$\mathbf{W}_1^*, \ldots, \mathbf{W}_n^*$. This is the well known *forward filtering, backward sampling (FFBS)*
algorithm of Carter and Kohn (1994) and Frühwirth-Schnatter (1994). The FFBS
algorithm is commonly used for posterior inference in Gaussian and conditionally
Gaussian DLMs. The main steps needed to fit DLM's with known variance evolution, using the software R, are in the package dlm, detailed in Petris, Petrone, and
Campagnoli (2009). The online resources provide a code of the FFBS algorithm
written for NIMBLE and RStan.

Integrated likelihood

Another very important result of the sequential Bayesian updating scheme de-
picted above is the derivation of the marginal likelihood of $\mathbf{W}_1^*, \ldots, \mathbf{W}_t^*$ given
$Y_1, \ldots, Y_n$. Without loss of generality, assume that $\mathbf{W}_t = \mathbf{W}$ for all $t = 1, \ldots, n$, where
n is the sample size, and that $p(\mathbf{W})$ denotes the prior distribution of $\mathbf{W}$. In this case,

$$p(Y_1, \ldots, Y_n | \mathbf{W}) = \prod_{t=1}^{n} p(Y_t | D_{t-1}, \mathbf{W}), \qquad (11.22)$$

where $Y_t | D_{t-1} \sim t_{n_{t-1}}(f_t, S_{t-1} Q_t^*)$. Therefore, the posterior distribution of $\mathbf{W}$,
$p(\mathbf{W}|D_n) \propto p(D_n | \mathbf{W}) p(\mathbf{W})$, can be combined with $p(V|\mathbf{W}, D_n)$ to produce the joint
posterior of $(V, \mathbf{W})$:

$$
\begin{aligned}
p(V, \mathbf{W}|D_n) \quad &\propto \quad p(D_n | \mathbf{W}) p(V|\mathbf{W}, D_n) p(\mathbf{W}) \\
&= \quad \left[\prod_{t=1}^{n} p(Y_t; f_t, S_{t-1} Q_t^*, n_{t-1}) \right] p(V; n_n/2, n_n S_n/2) p(\mathbf{W}).
\end{aligned}
$$

In words, Gaussianity and linearity, leads to a posterior distribution for V and
$\mathbf{W}$ by integrating out all state space vectors $\mathbf{Z}_1, \mathbf{Z}_2, \ldots, \mathbf{Z}_n$. If M independent Monte
Carlo draws $\{(V, \mathbf{W})^{(1)}, \ldots, (V, \mathbf{W})^{(M)}\}$ are obtained from $p(V, \mathbf{W}|D_n)$, then M inde-
pendent Monte Carlo draws from $p(\mathbf{Z}_1, \ldots, \mathbf{Z}_n | D_n)$ are easily obtained by repeating

the FFBS of Equation (11.16) (or Equation (11.17)) M times. This leads to M independent Monte Carlo draws from $p(\mathbf{Z}_1, \ldots, \mathbf{Z}_n, V, \mathbf{W}|D_n)$, hence there is no need for iterative Markov chain Monte Carlo (MCMC) schemes.

Example 11.17. *A NDLM to describe daily maximum levels of ozone*

This example analyzes maximum daily levels of ozone observed at a monitoring site located in Aberdeen in the UK. The sampling period is between 1 March–30 November 2017. The dataset was obtained from the openair package in R. We fit a DLM with $\mathbf{F}_t = (1, wind, temp)_t'$ and $\mathbf{G} = \mathbf{I}_3$, where $wind_t$ and $temp_t$ denote, respectively, the average wind speed and temperature at day t. Model specification is complete after assigning prior distributions to the observation variance V and elements of the diagonal evolution covariance matrix $\mathbf{W}$. Inference is performed using the integrated likelihood previously described. And a sample from the posterior distribution of the states is obtained through FFBS using composition sampling. The FFBS sampler is implemented using Nimble's custom sampler feature. The full analysis of this time series, including prior specification of the parameters and the implementation of the code in NIMBLE, is described on the online resources.

11.7.2 Dynamic generalized linear models (DGLM)

The DLM was extended by West, Harrison, and Migon (1985) to the case wherein observations belong to the exponential family. Assume that observations y_t are generated from a dynamic exponential family (EF), defined as

$$p(y_t|\eta_t, \phi) = \exp\{\phi[y_t\eta_t - a(\eta_t)]\}b(y_t, \phi), \qquad (11.23)$$

where $a(.)$ and $b(.)$ are known functions, η_t is the canonical parameter and ϕ is a scale parameter, usually time invariant. We denote the distribution of y_t as $EF(\eta_t, \phi)$. Let $\mu_t = E(y_t|\eta_t, \phi)$ and $g(.)$ be a known link function assumed at least twice differentiable, which relates the linear predictor with the canonical parameter, that is

$$g(\mu_t) = \mathbf{F}'\mathbf{Z}_t, \qquad (11.24)$$

where $\mathbf{F}$ and $\mathbf{Z}_t$ are vectors of dimension k. Following the parameterization of the exponential family in equation (11.23) it follows that the mean and variance of y_t are, respectively, given by $E(y_t|\eta_t, \phi) = \mu_t = \frac{da(\eta_t)}{d\eta_t} = \dot{a}(\eta_t)$ and $V(y_t|\eta_t, \phi) = V_t = \phi^{-1}\ddot{a}(\eta_t)$.

Usually, in practice, assuming $g(.)$ to be the natural link function provides good results (West et al., 1985). Some examples, where the link function is suggested by the definition of the canonical function, include the log-linear Poisson and logistic-linear Bernoulli models. The state parameters, $\mathbf{Z}_t$, evolve through time via a Markovian structure, that is

$$\mathbf{Z}_t = \mathbf{G}\mathbf{Z}_{t-1} + \omega_t, \quad \omega_t \sim N(\mathbf{0}, \mathbf{W}). \qquad (11.25)$$

Lastly, ω_t is the disturbance associated with the system evolution with covariance structure $\mathbf{W}$, commonly a diagonal matrix which can vary over time. The initial information of the model is denoted by $\mathbf{Z}_0$, and its prior distribution is defined through a k-variate normal distribution, that is, $\mathbf{Z}_0|D_0 \sim N(\mathbf{m}_0, \mathbf{C}_0)$, where D_0 denotes the initial information set. Typically, we assume that the components of $\mathbf{Z}_0$ and ω_t are independent for all time periods.

Posterior inference West et al. (1985) specify only the first and second moments of ω_t. They perform inference taking advantage of conjugate prior and posterior distributions in the exponential family, and used linear Bayes' estimation to obtain estimates of the moments of $\mathbf{Z}_t|D_t$. This approach is appealing as no assumption is made about the shape of the distribution of the disturbance component ω_t. However, we are limited to learn only about the first two moments of the posterior distribution of $\mathbf{Z}_t|D_t$. The assumption of normality of ω_t allows us to write down a likelihood function for $\mathbf{Z}_t$ and all the other parameters in the model. Inference procedure can be performed using Markov chain Monte Carlo algorithms. However, care must be taken when proposing an algorithm to obtain samples from the posterior distribution of the state vectors $\mathbf{Z}_t$. See Schmidt and Lopes (2019) for a review on different proposals to obtain samples from the posterior distribution of the parameters in the model.

Example 11.18. *Dynamic GLMs for daily counts of carbon monoxide on counts of infant deaths in São Paulo, Brazil*

This dataset was analyzed by Alves et al. (2010) and is related to daily counts of deaths of infants under 5 years old due to respiratory causes in São Paulo, Brazil. The sampling period is from 1 January 1994, until 31 December 1997. We fit a simplified version of the model fitted in Alves et al. (2010),

$$
\begin{aligned}
Deaths_t \mid \lambda_t &\sim Poisson(\lambda_t), \quad t = 1,2,\cdots, \\
\log(\lambda_t) &= \alpha_t + E_t + \delta_1 temperature_t + \delta_2 Humidity_t \\
&\quad + \delta_3 \cos\left(\frac{2\pi t}{365}\right) + \delta_4 \sin\left(\frac{2\pi t}{365}\right) + \delta_5 \cos\left(\frac{4\pi t}{365}\right) \\
&\quad + \delta_6 \sin\left(\frac{4\pi t}{365}\right) \\
E_t &= \rho E_{t-1} + \beta CO_t \\
\alpha_t &= \alpha_{t-1} + \omega_t, \quad \omega_t \sim N(0, W).
\end{aligned}
$$

The model includes a time varying intercept, α_t, the contemporaneous effect of temperature, humidity. The component E_t captures lagged effects of CO; ρ is the memory effect and *beta* the contemporaneous effect of CO on the logarithm of λ_t.

Let $\Theta = (\delta_1, \delta_2, \delta_3, \delta_4, \alpha_0, W, \rho, \beta)'$ be the parameter vector to be estimated. We assign independent, zero-mean normal prior distributions with relatively large variances for δ_j, $j = 1,2,3,4$, α_0 and β. Note that β captures the instantaneous effect of CO on the log of λ_t. The memory parameter ρ lies on the interval $(-1,1)$, however, values of $\rho \in (-1,0)$ provide shapes of the transfer function that have a geometric decay with alternating signs; for this reason we constrain ρ to lie on the $(0,1)$ interval, as these values provide shapes of the transfer function with geometric decay. See the online resources for a detailed analysis of this example.

11.8 Summary

The chapter contains the theory required for handling time series data, and the reader will have gained an understanding of the following topics:

- That a temporal process consists of both low and high frequency components, the former playing a key role in determining long-term trends while the latter may be associated with shorter-term changes;
- Techniques for the exploratory analysis of the data generated by the temporal process, including the ACF (correlogram) and PACF (periodogram);
- Models for irregular (high frequency) components after the regular components (trend) have been removed;
- Methods for forecasting, including exponential smoothing and ARIMA modeling;
- The state space modeling approach, which sits naturally within a Bayesian setting and provides a general framework within which a wide class of models, including many classical time series models, can be expressed;
- Implementing time series processes within a Bayesian hierarchical framework.

11.9 Exercises

Exercise 11.1. Give a direct proof that the random process in Equation (11.5) is weakly stationary.

Exercise 11.2. Find a recursive relation for the autocorrelation function of an AR(2) process.

Exercise 11.3. For a white noise process indexed by discrete time, find the spectral density function.

Exercise 11.4. For a random walk process, find the mean and variance as a function of time.

Exercise 11.5. This exercise explores the effect of the regular component of a temporal process if hidden in the irregular component.

(i) A statistician observes without error a process $Y_t = a + bt, t = 0,1,2,\ldots T$ without realizing it is deterministic. Find a theoretical formula for an estimate of the autocorrelation for this process. In particular, show how the sum of the geometric series $\sum_{i=t}^{n} x^i$ can be used to find the first and second 'sample' moments you need for this exercise.

(ii) What conclusions can you draw from this exercise about the possible effects of the deterministic component on the computed autocorrelation of a time series?

Exercise 11.6. Perform the same kind of analysis as in Exercise 11.5 for another deterministic function for example, a periodic function.

Exercise 11.7. Given a stationary series, prove that if the autocovariances are all positive, then the mean of the process will be estimated with greater variance than if all the autocovariances are null.

Exercise 11.8. Obtain the autocorrelation function of an ARMA(1,1) process, writing it as an MA(∞).

Exercise 11.9. Show how an AR(2) process can be represented as a dynamic linear model.

Exercise 11.10. We will call a stationary temporal process Y_t, $-\infty < t, \infty$ L2 continuous if for every t, $\lim_{h \to 0} E[Y_{t+h} - Y_t]^2 = 0$. Show that Y_t is L2 continuous if and only if the covariance function $C(t)$ is continuous at $t = 0$. Extend this result to L2 differentiability. This exercise shows that the 'smoothness' of a process is determined by the smoothness of the covariance function.

Exercise 11.11. Show that a Gamma prior, $\tau_w \sim Ga(a, b)$ combined with a normal likelihood, $[\gamma_t | \gamma_{t-1}, \tau_2] \sim N(\gamma_{t-1}, \tau_w)$, to give a Gamma posterior, paying particular attention to the form of the updated parameters.

Exercise 11.12. When modeling PM_{10} in London using a spatio-temporal model, Shaddick and Wakefield (2002) considered a range of models including a single-site, temporal only, model using a random walk, RW(1), process within a Bayesian hierarchical model. The data for the examples in that paper are available in the online resources for the book.

(i) Replicate the analysis in the paper by fitting a RW(1) model to these data using R – INLA and NIMBLE and compare the results from the two approaches.

(ii) Repeat the analysis using different models for the underlying temporal process: (i) RW(2), (ii) AR(1) and (iii) AR(2). What do you conclude about the appropriateness of these models for representing the temporal structure of this data? Which one would you choose and why?

Chapter 12

Bringing it all together: modeling exposures over space and time

12.1 Overview

In recent years, there has been an explosion of interest in spatio-temporal modeling and there have been a number of noteworthy publications in this field, including Le and Zidek (2006), Cressie and Wikle (2011) and Banerjee et al. (2015). However, none of these are specifically concerned with environmental epidemiology, where interest is in the relationship between human health and spatio-temporal processes of exposures to harmful agents. This might be, for example, the relationship between deaths and air pollution concentrations or future climate simulations, the latter of which may involve 1000s of monitoring sites that gather data about the underlying multivariate spatio-temporal field of precipitation and temperature. Although the main concern may be the effects on human health, there may be other effects, for example acid precipitation and its negative impact on the flora and fauna in addition to those related to human health.

12.2 Strategies

There are many ways in which space and time can be incorporated into a statistical model, and we now consider a selection. One must first choose the model's space-time domain. Is it to be a continuum in both space and time? Or a discrete space with a finite number of locations at which measurements may be made?

Time is obviously different from space. For one thing, it is directed, whereas any approach to adding direction in space is bound to be artificial. A major challenge in the development of spatio-temporal theory has been combining these fundamentally different fields in a single modeling framework. Much progress has been made in this area over the last three or four decades to meet the growing need in applications of societal importance, including those in epidemiology.

As seen in Chapter 11 there are competing advantages to using finite (discrete) and continuous domains. Indeed, a theory may be easier to formulate over a continuous domain, but practical use may entail projecting them onto a discrete domain. Time is regarded as discrete because measurements are made at specified, commonly equally spaced, time points. The precise methodology will be determined by

DOI: 10.1201/9781003352655-12

the nature of the data that is available over space, for example is it point-referenced or collected on a lattice?

Some general approaches to incorporating time are as follows:

Approach 1: Treat continuous time as another spatial dimension, for example, spatio-temporal kriging (Bodnar and Schmid, 2010). There is extra complexity in constructing covariance models compared to purely spatial process modeling (Fuentes, Chen, and Davis, 2008) and possible reductions in the complexity based on time having a natural ordering (unlike space) are not realized.

Approach 2: Represent the spatial fields as vectors, $\mathbf{Z}_t : N_S \times 1$, and combine them across time to get a multivariate time series.

Approach 3: Represent the time series as vectors, $\mathbf{Z}_s : 1 \times N_T$, and use multivariate spatial methods, for example, cokriging.

Approach 4: Build a statistical framework based on deterministic models that describe the evolution of processes over space and time.

Approach 1 may appeal to people used to working in a geostatistical framework. Approach 2 may be best where temporal forecasting is the inferential objective, while Approach 3 may be best for spatial prediction of unmeasured responses. Approach 4 is an important new direction that has promise because it includes background knowledge through numerical computer models. For further details about this approach, see Section 15.3.

If the primary aim is spatial prediction, then you would want to preserve the structure of the spatial field. However, if the primary interest is in forecasting, this would lead to an emphasis in building time series models at each spatial location. The exact strategy for constructing a spatio-temporal model will also depend on the purpose of the analysis. A regulator may need to estimate the effect of ambient levels of an environmental hazard on human health. This would be expressed as a concentration response function (CRF) (see Section 13.5.1) that relates the levels of ambient concentrations to health outcomes. That function would indicate the potential beneficial effect of reductions in ambient levels. An environmental epidemiologist might wish to plug a process model into an exposure response function (ERF) where it is the predicted exposures rather than ambient levels. Predicting personal exposures means that both ambient and indoor sources, for example, carbon monoxide from a poorly maintained gas heater, would be represented and thus give a truer exposure profile (Shaddick, Lee, Zidek, and Salway, 2008; Zidek, Meloche, Shaddick, Chatfield, and White, 2003; Zidek, Shaddick, White, Meloche, and Chatfield, 2005). Interest may lie in forecasting an ambient measurement twenty-four hours ahead of time. Or to spatially predict such levels at unmonitored sites to get a better idea of the exposure of susceptible school children in a school far from the nearest ambient monitor. In deciding how to expand or contract an existing network of monitoring sites in order to improve prediction accuracy or to save resources, a spatio-temporal model will be required together with a criterion on which to evaluate the changes you recommend. This last topic is the subject of Chapter 14.

12.3 Spatio-temporal models

A spatial-temporal random field, $Z_{st}, s \in \mathscr{S}, t \in \mathscr{T}$, is a stochastic process over a region and time period. This underlying process is not directly measurable, but realizations of it can be obtained by taking measurements, possibly with error. Monitoring will only report results at N_T discrete points in time, $T \in \mathscr{T}$ where these points are labelled $T = \{t_1, \ldots, t_{N_T}\}$. The same will be true over space, leading to a discrete set of N_S locations $S \in \mathscr{S}$ with corresponding labelling, $S = \{s_1, \ldots, s_{N_T}\}$.

If the temporal aspect is incorporated into the structure of Equation (10.1), then Z_{st} can be represented as a space-time random field, which can again be expressed in terms of a hierarchical model such as that introduced in Section 7.5 for the measurement and process models

$$
\begin{aligned}
Y_{st} &= Z_{st} + v_{st} \\
Z_{st} &= \mu_{st} + \omega_{st}
\end{aligned}
\qquad (12.1)
$$

where v_{st} represents independent random measurement error. The term μ_{st} is a spatio-temporal mean field (trend) that is often represented by a model of the form $\mu_{st} = x_{st}\beta_{st}$. For many processes, this mean term represents the largest source of variation in the responses. Over a broad scale it might be considered as deterministic if it can be accurately estimated, for example, as an average of the process over a very broad geographical area. However, where there is error in modeling, μ_{st} the residuals ω_{st} play a vital role in capturing the spatial and temporal dependence of the process.

The spatio-temporal process modeled by ω can be broken down into separate components representing space, m, time, γ and the interaction between the two, κ (Cressie and Wikle, 2011).

$$
\omega_{st} = m_s + \gamma_t + \kappa_{st}.
\qquad (12.2)
$$

The first two of these can be modeled using models seen in Chapters 10 (space) and 11 (time). In this example, **m** would be a collection of zero mean, site-specific deviations (spatial random effects) from the overall mean, μ_{st}, that are common to all times. For time, γ would be a set of zero mean time-specific deviations (temporal random effects) common to all sites. The third term κ_{st} in Equation (12.2) represents the stochastic interaction between space and time. For example, the effect of latitude on temperature depends on the time of year. The mean term, μ_{st} may constitute a function of both time and space, but the interaction between the two would also be manifest in κ_{st}. This would capture the varying intensity of the stochastic variation in the temperature field over sites, which might also vary over time. In a place such as California the temperature field might be quite flat in summer but there will be great variation in winter. It is likely that there will be interaction acting both through the mean and covariance of the model.

Many variations of the models in Equations (12.1) and (12.2) have been published for specific applications, including ones that take a multi-resolution approach where terms corresponding to stochastic subregional blocks of medium level resolution and then micro-level models for local levels (Reinsel, Tiao, Wang, Lewis, and Nychka, 1981; Sahu et al., 2006; Caselton and Zidek, 1984; Schumacher and Zidek, 1993).

Example 12.1. *Effect of wildcat drilling in Harrison Bay, Alaska*

Here $N_T = 2$ and $t = 1, 2$ represent times before and after the startup of exploratory drilling in Harrison Bay, Alaska, the Beaufort Sea oil field having already been established. Interest in this case was on human welfare rather than human health, namely on the effect of such drilling on the food chain of the indigenous people who lived in that area. Clearly the risk of this drilling would depend on how wind and sea currents carried the plume of drilling mud which is used to lubricate the drill stem as it digs into the earth. Experts were asked to independently draw boundaries of what they saw to be the zones of equitable risk. There was surprising agreement amongst the experts. This led in the end to a model of the form

$$Y_{st} = Z_{st} + v_{st}, \ t = 1, 2, \ s \in S \quad (12.3)$$
$$Z_{st} = \mu_{st} + \omega_{st}, \quad (12.4)$$
$$\mu_{st} = \mu + \beta_s + \gamma_t x_t$$
$$\beta_s \ ind \sim \ N(0, \sigma_\beta^2),$$

where the dummy variable is $x_t = I\{t = 2\}$ and b_s puts s into its zone of equitable risk. This simple model was chosen, in part because of its simplicity; it resulted in a paired t-test like analysis to detect change. However, to allow full account for uncertainty, random effects are assigned to the risk zones. The spatial domain S consisted of a geographic grid superimposed on the risk zones. The eventual design was based on that knowledge that the National Oceanic and Atmospheric Agency (NOAA), which was overseeing the project, would prefer a simple method of analysis for assessing the impact. The Bayesian elements were used to find the expected value of the uncertain non-centrality parameter for the test. This depended on the subset S that was to be selected, and so was optimized to find the optimal design. That led to maximizing the contrast in the field, with the optimal sites distributed between low and high risk zones. That in turn led to a theoretical paper that generalized this approach (Schumacher and Zidek, 1993).

Example 12.2. *Modeling pollution fields*

It has long been recognized that particulate air pollution is associated with adverse health impacts in humans. Thus, it is now a criteria air pollutant that is regulated to ensure air quality. Of particular concern is $PM_{2.5}$, consisting of small particles formed from gaseous emissions, for example, from the burning of wood. Both their mass μgm^{-3} and their counts ppm are considered important since a large number of tiny particles in the PM$_{2.5}$ mix, for example those of size less than 1 micron in diameter, can penetrate deeply into the lung.

Primary interest lies in the spatial prediction of the PM$_{2.5}$ field. However, in general a spatio-temporal modeling approach is preferable since the quasi replicates of the spatial field over time enables better parameter estimation. Sahu et al. (2006) used the following model for the underlying spatio-temporal mean term,

$$\mu_{st} = \beta_0 + \beta_1 p_s + \beta \alpha_s \times p_s + \sum_{l=2}^{12} \zeta_l u_{tl}, \qquad (12.5)$$

where the dummy $u = I\{t$ is in month m$\}$ tells us the month in which the time (week) $t = 1, \ldots, 52$ is located. Although in some ways an appealing and simple way of handling seasonality when temporal replicates are available, it comes at a cost of eleven degrees of freedom. These are used in estimating the set of the $\{\zeta_l\}$ coefficients. Here p_s denotes human population density while α_s is a rural–urban indicator function. The process model used by Sahu et al. (2006) was,

$$Z_{st} = \mu_{st} + \omega_{st}, + p_s v_{st} \qquad (12.6)$$

where the sum of the last two terms is thought of as representing a spatially varying temporal trend. To complete the model description for this example, we need a covariance structure and here Sahu et al. (2006) assumed that space and time are separable (see Subsection 12.3.1) and they used the exponential covariance functions for both.

12.3.1   Separable models

In most applications, modeling the entire spatio-temporal structure will be impractical because of high dimensionality. A number of approaches have been suggested to deal with this directly, and we now discuss the most common of these, that of assuming that space and time are *separable* (Gneiting, Genton, and Guttorp, 2006). This is in contrast to cases where the space-time structure is modeled jointly, which are known as *non-separable* models.

Separable models impose a particular type of independence between space and time components. It is assumed the correlation between Z_{st} and $Z_{s't}$ is $\rho_{ss'}$ at every time point, t while the correlation between Z_{st} and $Z_{t's}$ is $\rho_{tt'}$ at all spatial time points s.

The covariance for a separable process is therefore defined as

$$Cov(Z_{st}, Z_{s't'}) = \sigma^2 \rho_{ss'} \rho_{tt'}$$

for all $(s,t), (s',t') \in \mathscr{S} \times \mathscr{T}$.

Expressed in matrix form, for Gaussian processes, we get the Kronecker product for the covariance matrix,

$$\mathbf{\Sigma}^{Tp \times Tp} = \sigma^2 \rho_T^{N_T \times N_T} \otimes \rho_S^{N_S \times N_S}. \tag{12.7}$$

where ρ_1 is the between row temporal autocorrelations and ρ_2 is the between column spatial correlations.

Example 12.3. *Kronecker products*

The Kronecker product is an operation on two matrices of arbitrary size, resulting in a block matrix. It is a generalization of the outer product from vectors to matrices.

For matrices $\mathbf{A} : n \times m$ and $\mathbf{B} : p \times q$ their Kronecker product is defined as $\mathbf{A} \otimes \mathbf{B}$ as the linear operator acting on $\{Z : m \times q\}$ as follows:

$$(\mathbf{A} \otimes \mathbf{B})\mathbf{Z} = \mathbf{A}\,\mathbf{Z}\,\mathbf{B}' \tag{12.8}$$

From this definition, properties of the product can be easily proven. The following are examples:

$$\begin{aligned}
(\mathbf{A} \otimes \mathbf{B})(\mathbf{C} \otimes \mathbf{D}) &= (\mathbf{AC} \otimes \mathbf{BD}) & (12.9)\\
(\mathbf{A} \otimes \mathbf{B})' &= \mathbf{A}' \otimes \mathbf{B}' & (12.10)\\
(\mathbf{A} \otimes \mathbf{B})^{-1} &= \mathbf{A}^{-1} \otimes \mathbf{B}^{-1}, & (12.11)
\end{aligned}$$

$$\text{if } \mathbf{A} \text{ and } \mathbf{B} \text{ are non-singular}$$

The model shown in Equation 12.7 assumes temporal correlations are the same at every site. Likewise, the spatial correlations are the same at every point in time. These are strong assumptions which greatly simplify things but they do seem to be reasonable in a lot of applications, for example through cross-validation yields good results (Le and Zidek, 2006). Due to the reduction in computational burden that comes with this approach, the majority of work on space-time modeling tends to be based on analyzing the temporal and spatial aspects separately, and then to combine the chosen models in a single separable model.

Example 12.4. *Spatial prediction for daily levels of particulate matter*

L. Sun, Zidek, Le, and Ozkaynak (2000) use the approach suggested by Le, Sun, and Zidek (1997) to develop a spatial predictive distribution for the space-time field of daily ambient PM_{10} in Vancouver, Canada. For simplicity, they analyzed each of the monitoring sites separately and chose a single, AR(1), model to represent the temporal structure. They recognize the possibility that spatial correlation between sites might 'leak' into the lagged values of the series, due to modeling each site univariately. This would not have happened if a multivariate auto-regression was used, but such an approach may be infeasible with numerous monitored and unmonitored sites. They then used the de-trended residuals to obtain posterior distributions of the covariance matrix, which was then extended to include unmonitored sites using a semi-parametric approach for the spatial covariance of hourly ozone levels (Sampson and Guttorp, 1992), and allowed the parameters of the model to vary as functions of time of day.

Example 12.5. *Modeling wind velocity*

Haslett and Raftery (1989) modeled wind velocity measurements in Ireland using a combination of kriging and ARMA time series models to predict values at gauged sites that have short runs of data. They use kriging estimates of the variance of the random field, using an exponential model for the covariance-distance relationship. They built space-time models by linking models for the observed data, Y, directly at each of the sites through a spatially correlated set of innovations whose covariance structure was derived from the underlying continuous spatial process, which was assumed to be realized independently at each t. They then combine the spatial and temporal aspects in a model of the form

$$
\begin{aligned}
Y_{st} &= \mu_s + \nabla^{-d}\phi(B)^{-1}\theta(B)\omega_{st} \qquad (12.12) \\
\mathbf{m}_t &= (m_{t1}, \dots, m_{tN_S})' \sim N_{N_S}(0, \sigma_m^2\Sigma_s)
\end{aligned}
$$

where the matrix Σ_s represents the spatial correlation, and does not depend on time. ∇^{-d} is the Binomial expansion of $(1 - B)^{-d}$, where B is the backshift operator as described in Chapter 11, Section 11.4.2, and d can have non-integer value, leading to fractional differencing and long memory processes. It is noted that in Equation 12.1, the observed data is modeled directly, that is there is a measurement error term in level one.

Example 12.6. *Winter temperature*

In an early Bayesian application Handcock and Wallis (1994) to consider the spatio-temporal modeling of winter temperature data, but their approach was to carry out separate spatial analyzes in each year using a Gaussian random field model. The mean and covariance parameters of this model were then examined temporally and found to be stable, which they concluded was justification for the use of a simple model that essentially treated spatial and temporal aspects separately. They developed a stationary spatio-temporal random field for mean temperature using eighty-eight weather stations in the northern U.S. They first developed a Gaussian random field map using a Bayesian kriging approach as a function of latitude, longitude and elevation, examining variograms in different directions to look for anisotropy. Having produced a spatial structure, they consider the yearly temperatures by examining each site separately, fitting AR(1) models and finding that only three out of the eighty-eight were significant, leading to the conclusion that there was little evidence of short-term temporal dependency. They then examined long-term dependency using ARIMA models with non-integral or fractional differencing, as discussed in Example 12.5, finding little evidence of long memory dependence and also, that the spatial structure was changing over time.

Example 12.7. *Models with cyclical variance*

Recall that the general hierarchical model involves first and foremost a process model. The relationship between measurements and the process is described in the measurement model. In addition, there is the parameter model, which in a Bayesian framework will contain the prior distributions assigned to all unknown parameters. Hence, the model parameters are random quantities and can be assigned spatial and temporal distributions. For example, consider the process model

$$Z_{st} = \mu + \beta_s cos(2\pi\omega t) + v_{st}, \; s \in S, \; t = 1, \dots N_T \tag{12.13}$$

with μ constant, $v_{st} \; ind \sim N(0, \sigma_v^2)$ and $\beta = (\beta_1, \dots, \beta_p) \sim N_{N_s}(0, \Sigma_\beta)$. It has the unusual property that the process's marginal variance $Var(Z_{st}) = \Sigma_\beta cos^2(2\pi\omega t) + \sigma_v^2$ variance is cyclical. Huerta et al. (2004) use a more complex version of such a model that has been used and criticized for a variety of reasons (Dou, Le, and Zidek, 2007). Amongst other things, models such as these have wiggly credibility bands around the path of the process over time $Z_{st}, \; t = 0, 1, \dots, T$ for a fixed s. Such a band may seem unnatural, depending on the context and nature of the prior distribution on the process amplitudes β. That distribution could represent the modeler's epistemic uncertainty (see Chapter 3) about the size of β. In that case, it would be expected to shrink to zero in the future as increasing amounts of data become available over time and knowledge about β increases in certainty. More likely β would also include aleatory uncertainty in nature to allow for things like fluctuating wind directions, for example. In any case, careful thought needs to be given in selecting the parameter model in a Bayesian context to ensure that the aleatory uncertainty about a process is preserved as the epistemic uncertainty is resolved (see Chapter 3).

12.3.2 *Non-separable processes*

Non-separable processes will often be more difficult to understand than when separation processes can be assumed for space and time, and as a consequence modeling is often complex. In particular, dealing with the Kronecker products (see Example 12.3) that define the covariance poses technical challenges if the wrong approach is taken.

To illustrate, consider the simple problem of showing that $(\mathbf{A}\otimes\mathbf{B})^{-1}=\mathbf{A}^{-1}\otimes\mathbf{B}^{-1}$. This problem proves to be very difficult if we ignore the algebraic roots of the Kronecker product as a linear operator (see below) and instead use the matrix definition, which for simplicity in the case of 2×2 matrices is the 4×4 matrix given by:

$$\begin{pmatrix} a_{11} & a_{12} \\ a_{21} & a_{22} \end{pmatrix} \otimes \begin{pmatrix} b_{11} & b_{12} \\ b_{21} & b_{22} \end{pmatrix} = \begin{pmatrix} a_{11}\mathbf{B} & a_{12}\mathbf{B} \\ a_{21}\mathbf{B} & a_{22}\mathbf{B} \end{pmatrix} \qquad (12.14)$$

Another example, also very relevant to the development of spatio-temporal models, is the separable case for Gaussian processes. This is based on matrix multiplication.
    Suppose that

$$\mathbf{Z} = \begin{pmatrix} z_{11} & z_{12} \\ z_{21} & z_{22} \end{pmatrix} = \begin{pmatrix} \mathbf{z}_1 \\ \mathbf{z}_2 \end{pmatrix}$$

In this case, what is $(\mathbf{A}\otimes\mathbf{B})\mathbf{Z}$? The answer obtained by using the matrix definition of the product employs the idea of vectorizing the matrix $\mathbf{Z}$ more precisely to define,

$$vec(\mathbf{Z})^{4\times 1} = \begin{pmatrix} \mathbf{z}_1^T \\ \mathbf{z}_2^T \end{pmatrix}$$

Then we can show that

$$(\mathbf{A}\otimes\mathbf{B})vec(\mathbf{Z}) = vec(\mathbf{AZB}') \qquad (12.15)$$

However even in this simple case the technicalities are relatively complex. A much better approach that avoids use of the vec operator treats the Kronecker product as a linear operator.
    So why is all this important for modeling spatio-temporal Gaussian processes? There, the domain where measurements will be taken is $(s,t)\in \mathscr{S}\times\mathscr{T}$ where $\mathscr{S}\times\mathscr{T}$ denotes what is called the 'product space' of $\mathscr{S}$ and $\mathscr{T}$. Over that domain, responses for a separable Gaussian process can be represented by a random matrix with a matrix normal distribution (see Appendix A):

$$\mathbf{Z}^{N_S\times N_T} \sim N_{N_S\times N_T}[\mu,\sigma^2\rho_S\otimes\rho_T]$$

So if the temporal auto correlation matrix were known, we could easily reduce the process to another with independent replicates over time as follows.

$$\mathbf{Z}^* = (\mathbf{I}\otimes\rho_T^{-1/2})\mathbf{Z} \sim N_{N_S\times N_T}[(\mathbf{I}\otimes\rho_T^{-1/2})\mu,\sigma^2\rho_S\otimes\mathbf{I})]$$

Even if ρ_T is unknown, in some cases it may be possible to estimate it well, for example, when it has a simple parametric form and there are many time points.

12.4   Dynamic linear models for space and time

Here, we extend the state space model for the temporal setting introduced in Section 11.7 to the spatio-temporal setting. As before the key elements are the measurement and process models in the linear Gaussian situation where for $t \in T$ $\mathbf{Y}_t : N_S \times 1$ denotes the measurement sequence and $\mathbf{Z}_t : N_S \times 1$, the process sequence:

$$\begin{aligned} \mathbf{Y}_t &= \mathbf{F}_t^T \mathbf{Z}_t + v_t, v_t \sim N[\mathbf{0}, V_t] \\ \mathbf{Z}_t &= \mathbf{G}_t \mathbf{Z}_{t-1} + w_t, \quad w_t \sim N[\mathbf{0}, \mathbf{W}_t] \end{aligned}$$

where $\mathbf{F}_t : p \times N_S$, $\mathbf{G}_t : p \times p$, $V_t : N_S \times N_S$, and $\mathbf{W}_t : p \times p$ are known. Generally $\mathbf{F}_t$ is called the 'design matrix', v_t the observational error, $\mathbf{G}_t$ the state matrix and ω_t, the evolution error with evolution covariance matrix $\mathbf{W}_t$. To finish the DLM's specification we need

$$[\mathbf{Z}_0|\mathbf{Y}_0] \quad \sim \quad N[\mathbf{m}_0, \mathbf{C}_0]$$

The model is implemented by applying the forward filtering – backward sampling algorithm (J. Harrison, 1999).

Example 12.8. *Modeling hourly ozone concentrations using DLMs*

The DLM has been applied to model hourly ozone concentrations in both Mexico City and Chicago (Huerta et al., 2004; Dou, Le, and Zidek, 2010; Dou et al., 2012). We now describe a version of the DLM that was developed to represent the daily cycles in the levels of ozone concentrations in urban areas (Huerta et al., 2004). The model recognizes the need to reflect both aleatory and epistemic uncertainty, as discussed in Example 3.5 and its sequel. It does this by incorporating in the measurement model's random residual terms m_{st} of spatial (but not temporal) correlation. More precisely $Cov(\mathbf{m}_t) = \sigma_y^2 \exp(-\mathbf{D}/\lambda_y)$, where $\mathbf{m}_t = (m_{s_1 t}, \dots, m_{s_{N_S} t})$ and $\mathbf{D}$ denotes the intersite distance matrix. The data and process models for the DLM are then defined by

$$\begin{aligned} \text{Data model: } Y_{st} &= Z_{1t} + S_{1t} Z_{2st} + S_{2t} Z_{3st} + v_{st} \\ \text{Process models:} & \\ Z_{1t} &= Z_{1(t-1)} + \gamma_t^1 \\ Z_{jst} &= Z_{js(t-1)} + \gamma_{jst}^2, \ j = 2, 3 \end{aligned}$$

The twelve and twenty-four-hour ozone cycles are captured by, $S_{jt}(a_j) = cos(\pi jt/12) + a_j sin(\pi jt/12)$, $j = 1, 2$ while the Z_{jst}, $j = 2, 3$ are random amplitudes. The model parameters are the processes in the model. The first Z_{1t} depends only on time and plays the key role of establishing the baseline level. It evolves according to a random walk model and with an innovation term distributed as $\gamma_t^1 \sim N(0, \sigma_y^2 \tau_y^2)$. The remaining two coordinates of the trivariate vector valued process $\mathbf{Z}_t$, that is the amplitudes Z_{jst}, $j = 2, 3$, evolve according to a random walk like the first coordinate. Their innovation terms are allowed to be spatially dependent, that is letting $\gamma_{jt}^2 = (\gamma_{j1t}, \dots, \gamma_{jsN_St}^2)$,

$Cov(\gamma_{jt}^2) = \sigma_y^2 \tau_j^2 \exp(-\mathbf{D}/\lambda_j)$. Finally, the parameters $\tau_j^2, \tau_y^2, \lambda_j$ are specified in advance. We could have added another term to capture the effect of covariates such as temperature, but for simplicity that is ignored here.

The model was initially applied over Mexico City (Huerta et al., 2004) to model a sequence of measurements made at ten sites. Both spatial prediction and temporal forecasting were performed.

The promise of the DLM approach led to its application (by the second author and his co-investigators) in regions in the eastern United States. Approximately 300 sites were involved and measurements were made over the so-called ozone season of about 120 days (2880 hours) during the summer. Interest was in spatial prediction to rural areas which have few ozone sites, despite the importance of the pollutant's effects on human welfare, crops, forests and both flora and fauna in general. It soon became obvious that the extension of the DLM developed for Mexico City would not work in our application. There, the models involved nearly 1.7 million parameters due to the large number of monitoring sites and measurements over time. We found that with even substantial computational power, only a maximum of ten sites could be handled for data covering the entire ozone season.

Thus, in the end, an investigation was undertaken for urban areas with ten sites to explore the possibility of using the method in those domains. There the method worked quite well, although we did discover some unusual features, one of which has been previously discussed involving Equation 12.13, that the sinusoidal character of the mean function induces wiggly posterior credibility bands around the inferred process due to the random amplitudes in the model. In other words, the degree of uncertainty expressed by those bands varies cyclically over time. That uncertainty would be a combination of aleatory and epistemic uncertainty so this effect would be muted as the amount of available data increased. Finally, the random walk (non-stationary) model used in this model to reduce the overall number of parameters in the model leads to posterior credibility bands that increase in width as time increases–even when conditioning on the full set of measurement collected over all those time points. This would seem to be an argument against use of the random walk model in Bayesian dynamic modeling (Dou et al., 2012).

12.5 An empirical Bayes approach

Dealing with large amounts of spatio-temporal data will often mean that implementing DLMs can be computationally prohibitive. One possible solution to this difficulty is to consider an empirical Bayes approach, known as the Bayesian spatial predictor (BSP) (Le and Zidek, 2006). An empirical comparison of the BSP and DLM is given in Example 12.9, but first we review the theory behind the approach.

To align our description of the BSP model with that in Le and Zidek (2006) entails a slight modification in our notation. In the BSP model, the responses are represented as elements of a random matrix, where the columns rather than rows represent spatial sites. Each gauged site (a location at which there is a monitor) $s \in S$ has a vector of k responses corresponding to a number of different exposures, meaning this is a multivariate model. A gauged site therefore has k 'quasi-sites' where measurements could be made, but gauges may not have been installed to measure all responses at that site. Therefore, the number of columns in the response matrix would be $N_S \times k$ where the number of rows would be N_T.

For expository simplicity, we will describe the univariate case where $k = 1$. However, we emphasize the importance of multivariate responses. There may be several responses of interest at each site and even when interest focuses on a single response, it can be advantageous to incorporate other responses, so that strength can be borrowed from them through their stochastic dependence. Also, even with a univariate response it can sometimes be desirable to group its successive realizations over time in blocks, thus creating a multivariate Gaussian field. For instance, we could put hourly responses into blocks of length 24 hours and make the t's represent days. This strategy means avoiding the challenging issue of modeling fine scale temporal dependence.

In applications some sites will not have been monitored or 'gauged' in the terminology of Le and Zidek (2006), for the entire period $t \in T$ and they will be labelled with a u, standing for 'ungauged'. Others will have had monitors from the beginning when $t = 1$ and they are labelled with a g. In general, startup times will be staggered, with some starting very recently. Commonly, even after a site is gauged, it does not monitor all the responses of interest, leading to a complex pattern of non-random blocks of missing data in both ungauged and gauged sites. Therefore, we need notation to distinguish between the observed and missing responses at gauged sites, leading to labels g_o and g_m.

With that background we may now describe the process as through a response matrix:

$$\mathbf{Z}^{N_T \times N_S} = \left[\mathbf{Z}^{[u]}, \left(\begin{array}{c} \mathbf{Z}^{[g_1^m]} \\ \mathbf{Z}^{[g_1^o]} \end{array} \right), \cdots, \left(\begin{array}{c} \mathbf{Z}^{[g_k^m]} \\ \mathbf{Z}^{[g_k^o]} \end{array} \right) \right] \qquad (12.16)$$

where:

- m means no measurement for this response;
- g means the site is gauged, and it also stands for the total number of ungauged sites to reduce the notational burden;
- u means an ungauged site and also the total number of ungauged sites;
- $N_S = u + g$.

Equation 12.16 shows the staircase pattern in the data matrix once the gauged sites have been reordered from newest to oldest (from left to right).

Both the measurement or process models may incorporate factors and covariates. We will call factors things the experimenter controls, for example rural–urban in the selection of sites. Covariates would be the predictors or potential confounders that may co-vary with the response of interest.

The design matrix $\mathbf{X}$ in the BSP model contains just those covariates that are common to all sites, and they may be discrete or continuous. A discrete example would be a binary (present or absent) and continuous ones would be things like 'temperature' measured at the airport, or 'degree of visibility', when the domain of interest is an urban area. The BSP conditions on the design matrix and treats it as a constant.

But there is a second type of covariate that is site-specific, for example hourly concentrations of NO_x (oxides of nitrogen) X_{st} when hourly ozone concentrations $Y_{st} = Z_{st}$ (assuming no measurement error) are the responses of interest. The BSP can handle this case because it is a multivariate model that would first model the joint distribution $[Y_{st}, X_{st}]$ and then use the conditional distribution $[Y_{st} \mid X_{st} = x_{st}]$ in the analysis of the health effects of ozone. BSP does not explicitly allow for site-specific factors such as elevation, for example, but it can be adapted for use in that context.

For expository simplicity, assume just one covariate X_t over the domain of interest, one that is treated as a constant $X_t = x_t$. The BSP measurement model is then for $s \in S$ and $t \in T$

$$Z_{st} = x_t \beta_s + \omega_{st} = x_t \tilde{\beta}_0 + x_t \tilde{\beta}_s + \omega_{st} \qquad (12.17)$$

for time t and site s. Here the non-site-specific $\tilde{\beta}_0$ can be fitted by classical methods when there are lots of data so that the estimate has a small standard error. Removing the effect of, $x_t \hat{\beta}_0$ or 'prefiltering' in the parlance of BSP theory, is thus like removing a constant from the random response. We can rewrite the model as

$$Z_{st}^* = Z_{st} - x_t \hat{\beta}_0 = x_t \tilde{\beta}_s + \omega_{st}$$

leaving the uncertain site-specific coefficient, $\tilde{\beta}(s)$, as a random site effect from the point of view of a frequentist or an uncertain fixed parameter from that of a Bayesian. For really smooth random fields, it can nearly be zero for all sites. In vector form, we have $\mathbf{Z}_t^* = x_t [\tilde{\beta}_{s_1}, \dots, \tilde{\beta}_{s_{N_s}}] + \omega_t$.

The BSP's distributional assumptions are:

$$\begin{cases} Z \mid \beta, \Sigma \sim N(\mathbf{X}\beta, \mathbf{A} \otimes \Sigma) \\[2mm] \beta \mid \Sigma, \beta_0, F \sim N(\beta_0, F^{-1} \otimes \Sigma) \\[2mm] \Sigma \sim GIW(\Theta, \delta) : \text{Generalized inverted Wishart} \end{cases} \qquad (12.18)$$

Here $\mathbf{A}$ is assumed to be known, so that by a simple transformation, it can without loss of generality be taken to be the identity matrix. In practice, a plug-in estimate may be used during the pre-filtering stage of the analysis. For instance, for long temporal aggregates such as monthly averages: $\mathbf{A} \approx I_n$ $\mathbf{A} \approx I_n$ sometimes achieved by removing a single low frequency temporal component across all sites. The generalized inverted Wishart (GIW), which allows different degrees of freedom for different steps in the staircase, extends the standard Wishart distribution $\Sigma \sim IW(\Psi, \delta)$. The latter, which is the multivariate version of the σ^2 scaled chi-squared distribution, can be used in the absence of a staircase data pattern. However, the GIW allows much more flexibility by allowing the response vector coordinates to be grouped into blocks with different degrees of uncertainty to represent different levels of uncertainty.

With g denoting the number of gauged or partially gauged sites, we get the following posterior distribution:

$$[\mathbf{Z}^u \mid D, \mathscr{H}] \quad \sim \quad \left[Y^{[u]} \mid \mathbf{Z}^{[g_1^m, \dots, g_g^m]}, D, \mathscr{H} \right] \times$$

$$\prod_{j=1}^{g-1} \left[\mathbf{Z}^{[g_j^m]} \mid \mathbf{Z}^{[g_{j+1}^m, \dots, g_g^m]}, D, \mathscr{H} \right] \times \left[\mathbf{Z}^{[g_g^m]} \mid D, \mathscr{H} \right]$$

Each factor is a matrix-t distribution (see Appendix A). The mean, covariance, and degrees of freedom are functions of $\mathscr{H}$ and D. Thus, the posterior is completely characterized given $\mathscr{H}$ since all the hyperparameters that determine the priors are in $\mathscr{H}$. The EnviroStat package uses an empirical Bayes approach and estimates those hyperparameters through a maximum likelihood approach.

Example 12.9. *A comparison of the DLM and BSP approaches*

In this example, we compare the results of using the DLM and BSP approaches when modeling ozone concentrations in the Chicago area (Dou, 2007).

This example involves two different approaches to spatio-temporal modeling, the first is the dynamic linear modeling (DLM) approach where coefficients can change over time and the second is the Bayesian spatial predictor (BSP) approach which uses an empirical Bayes within Bayes approach to minimize computation times where many of the sites are involved (Le and Zidek, 2006).

A total of twenty-four hourly ozone concentration monitoring sites were selected in the Chicago area, treating fourteen of them as gauged and keeping ten as validation (ungauged) sites. These can be seen in Figure 12.1. Application of the BSP in compact geographical regions, like this case study, usually begins by pre-filtering; that is, fitting a regional (not site-specific) trend (Li, Le, Sun, and Zidek, 1999). More precisely, that would mean fitting $\tilde{\beta}_0$ in Equation 12.17 and subtracting the estimated trend from the series of measurements to get detrended residuals. Pre-whitening those residuals by fitting a time series model results in a second set of residuals. This could mean for example fitting a stationary time series model such as AR(2), in this case with coefficients that are constant across the region. Often the temporal dependence in the resulting residuals are negligible and the A in Equation 12.18 is approximately equal to the identity.

However, that does not work in this case, since space and time are not separable. Here, fitting factors 'month' and 'weekday – weekend' followed by the fitting of an AR(2) model may yield residuals with greatly reduced spatial correlation compared with the original process (Dou et al., 2010). This has been referred to as 'correlation leakage' (Li et al., 1999) and it makes spatial prediction difficult. So an alternative approach was used, one that takes advantage of the multivariate model built into the BSP approach. Vectors of

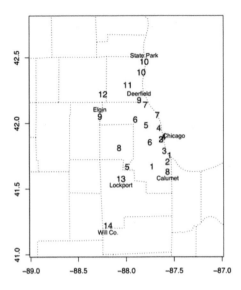

Figure 12.1: Locations of fourteen gauged and ten ungauged validation hourly ozone concentration monitoring sites in the Chicago area, whose data were used in a comparison of the DLM and BSP approaches.

consecutive hourly concentrations in each day were used as the responses and a multivariate model was used for these vectors with 'month' and 'weekday – weekend' as the explanatory factors. Preliminary analysis pointed to the use of just two consecutive hours per day, meaning that the resulting vectors were separated by twenty-two hours and hence are uncorrelated. For example, if we wished to predict the 11 AM hourly concentration at an ungauged site based on the measurements at the gauged sites, we would put the 10 AM and 11 AM responses in the response bivariate vectors and make spatial predictions based on both 10 AM and 11 AM responses at the gauged sites, thus borrowing strength across both time and space for spatial prediction.

The DLM and BSP were empirically compared in two different contexts, the first using two hour vector responses, and the second five (Dou et al., 2010). In these contexts, the BSP yields superior empirical spatial prediction performance in terms of the mean squared prediction error (MSPE). Table 12.1 shows results obtained by Dou (2007).

In Figure 12.2 we show the spatial predictions of values at Site 10 made by the two methods in Figure 12.2. As Site 10 is in proximity to gauged sites, both predictors do quite well. These find that overall, the BSP is more accurate and its 95% credibility bands are narrower than those of the DLM, again reflecting the findings reported elsewhere (Dou et al., 2010).

Table 12.1: The mean square prediction error $(\sqrt{ppb})^2$ at Chicago's ungauged sites comparing the multivariate BSP and the DLM. In all cases but that of the eighth ungauged site, the BSP predictions are more accurate than those of the DLM.

Ungauged Site	MSPE (DLM)	MSPE (BSP)
1	1.79	1.16
2	1.55	1.61
3	1.80	1.30
4	1.46	0.94
5	1.92	1.03
6	1.85	0.99
7	1.60	0.97
8	2.62	2.67
9	1.63	1.01
10	0.87	0.38

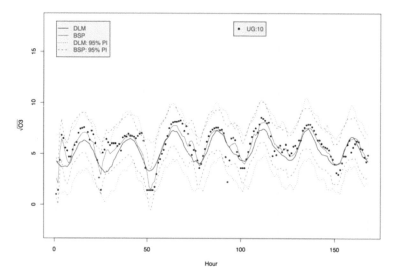

Figure 12.2: Spatial predictions of hourly ozone levels at the validation Site 10. The DLM and BSP approaches were used and their 95% credibility intervals are shown. The gray solid line represents the latter, which tends to track the observations at the validation site rather better than the DLM method. Note that the validation site lies in close proximity to the gauged sites. Both of the credibility bands tend to be too wide, the dashed 95% band for the BSP tending to be the narrower of the two, as can be seen near hour 50.

Overall, the BSP enjoys computational advantages over the DLM, and it outperforms the latter based on empirical assessments made in this example and elsewhere (Dou et al., 2010). While the DLM was originally designed for temporal modeling, the BSP can also be used as a temporal forecasting methodology. Another empirical comparison of the two methods (Dou et al., 2012), also comes out in favor of the BSP for forecasting hourly ozone concentrations at least in the near future. However, the BSP does require preliminary data analysis in the form of pre-filtering and pre-whitening, or equivalently the estimation of the covariance **A** in the distribution model. It also requires the assumption of separability of time and space, although that assumption can be side-stepped, as seen in this example by resorting to multivariate response vector modeling.

The DLM is powerful, flexible and intuitive. However, finding good hyperparameter estimates can be challenging. Computation times are long. It took 10 days for 3000 MCMC iterations running C code on dual processors, whereas BSP took about four hours for the same sort of calculation. The posterior variance conditional on all the data increases over time due to the random walk model used for the model coefficients, and the resulting credibility bands tend to have a wobble induced by the random amplitude coefficients multiplying the sines and cosines in the model. It is difficult to assess the distribution of aleatory and epistemic uncertainty (see Chapter 3) as the amount of data increase, nor can we assess its degree of correlation leakage, if any.

12.6   A spatio-temporal model for downscaling using R-INLA

Air pollution constitutes the highest environmental risk factor in relation to health. In order to provide the evidence required for health impact analyzes, to inform policy and develop potential mitigation strategies comprehensive information is required on the state of air pollution. Information on air pollution traditionally comes from ground monitoring (GM) networks but these may not be able to provide sufficient coverage and may need to be supplemented with information from other sources (e.g. chemical transport models; CTMs). However, these may only be available on grids and may not capture micro-scale features that may be important in assessing air quality in areas of high population. Therefore, it needs to be acknowledged that measurements from ground monitors and estimates from SAT or CTMs are fundamentally different quantities, with the latter is subject to uncertainties and biases arising from errors in inputs and possible model misspecification. In addition, the information they provide will be available at different geographical scales, that is point locations vs. grid cells, an issue termed the 'change of support problem' by (Gelfand et al., 2001), and a model will be required that can align the different sources in the spatial (and possibly temporal) domains.

One approach to linking data at different resolutions is to use spatially varying coefficient models, often referred to as *downscaling* models. In a downscaling model, the parameters in the calibration equation are allowed to vary continuously over space (and potentially time) allowing predictions to be made at the point level thus allowing local, sub-grid cell variation. Examples of downscaling in this setting include (van de Kassteele et al., 2006), who modeled PM_{10} concentrations over Western Europe using information from both satellite observations and a CTM; (McMillan, Holland, Morara, and Feng, 2010) who modeled $PM_{2.5}$ in the North Eastern U.S. using estimates from the Community Multiscale Air Quality (CMAQ) numerical model; (van Donkelaar et al., 2016) modeled annual average $PM_{2.5}$ calibrating ground measurements against estimates from both satellite remote sensing and CTMs; (Kloog et al., 2014) who modeled $PM_{2.5}$ in the Northeastern U.S. using satellite – based aerosol optical depth (AOD); and (Berrocal, Gelfand, and Holland, 2010a) and (Zidek, Le, and Liu, 2012a) who modeled ozone in the Eastern U.S. (Eastern and Central in the case of Zidek et al.) using estimates from CMAQ and a variant of the MAQSIP (Multiscale Air Quality Simulation Platform) model, respectively.

Here, we show an example of calibration between data sources that are available at different levels of support, namely ground monitors at point locations and estimates from CTMs on grid cells. Set within a Bayesian hierarchical framework, the coefficients of calibration equations are allowed to vary continuously over space and time, enabling downscaling where ground monitoring data is sufficient to support it. We are specifically interested in the implementation of complex models for larger scale problems that may result in difficulties when attempting to use the methods for implementation proposed in the above examples, especially those using Markov Chain Monte Carlo. Here, we use the integrated nested Laplace approximations (INLA) (Rue et al., 2009) as described in Chapter 6. that allow high-resolution estimates of exposures to air pollution to be produced, together with associated measures of uncertainty.

The model calibrates information from gridded covariates, $X_{r\ell t}$, against ground measurements, Y_{st}, with both fixed and spatially and temporarily varying random effects for both intercepts and covariates,

$$Y_{st} = \tilde{\beta}_{0st} + \sum_{p \in P} \beta_p X_{p\ell_{pst}} + \sum_{q \in Q} \tilde{\beta}_{qst} X_{q\ell_{qst}} + \varepsilon_{st} \qquad (12.19)$$

where $\varepsilon_{st} \sim^{iid} N(0, \sigma_\varepsilon^2)$. Here, ℓ_{ps} (and ℓ_{qs}) denote the grid cell in grid p (and q) containing the point location s. The set of R covariates contains two groups, $R = (P, Q)$, where P have fixed effects, β_p, and Q are assigned spatio-temporally varying random effects, $\tilde{\beta}_{pst}$.

This is an example of statistical calibration and downscaling is based on estimating relationships between measurements, Y_{st}, available at a discrete set of locations $s \in S = \{s_1, \ldots, s_{N_S}\}$ and time points $t \in T = \{t_1, \ldots, t_{N_T}\}$ and a set of covariates $X_{r\ell t}$, $r = 1, \ldots, R$, for example CTMs, satellite remote sensing, land use indicators, and topography, on grids of N_{L_r} cells $\ell \in \{\ell_1, \ell_2, \ldots, \ell_{N_{L_r}}\}$ at time t.

The spatio-temporally varying coefficients $\tilde{\beta}_{0st}$ and $\tilde{\beta}_{qst}$, $q \in Q$, take the form

$$\begin{aligned} \tilde{\beta}_{0st} &= \beta_0 + \beta_{0st}, \\ \tilde{\beta}_{qst} &= \beta_q + \beta_{qst}, \end{aligned}$$

where β_{0st} and β_{qst} provide temporal and spatial adjustments around fixed effects β_0 and β_q, respectively. For clarity of exposition, the following description is restricted to the coefficients associated with a single covariate, that is $\hat{\beta}_{st}$. In time, $\beta_t = (\beta_{1t}, \beta_{2t}, \ldots, \beta_{Nst})$ is assumed to evolve as a first-order autoregressive process

$$\beta_t = \rho \beta_{t-1} + \omega_t$$

where $\omega_t = (\omega_{1t}, \omega_{2t}, \ldots, \omega_{Nst})$ are assumed to be independent and identically distributed draws from a stationary, isotropic, zero-mean Gaussian random field, $\omega_t \sim N(0, \sigma_\omega^2 \Sigma)$, with Matérn covariance function

$$Cov(\omega_{s_i t_i}, \omega_{s_j t_j}) = \delta_{ij} \frac{\sigma_\omega^2}{2^{v-1}\Gamma(v)} (\kappa \|s_i - s_j\|)^v K_v (\kappa \|s_i - s_j\|) \qquad (12.20)$$

where δ_{ij} is the Dirac delta function, K_v is the modified Bessel function of the second kind, σ_ω^2 is the overall variance, v controls the smoothness of the spatial process, κ controls the strength of the distance/correlation relationship and $\|\cdot\|$ is Euclidean distance. Moreover, ω_{st} is modeled as being separable over space and time with the covariance structure is constructed using a Kronecker product (Cameletti et al., 2011).

Gaussian priors, $N(0, 1000)$, are assigned to each of the fixed effects β_0, β_p and β_q. For the spatio-temporal random effects, the smoothness parameter is fixed, $v = 1$ as in (Lindgren, Rue, and Lindström, 2011). Penalized Complexity (PC) priors are used for the variance of the observations (σ_ε^2; such that $\mathbb{P}(\sigma_\varepsilon > 1) = 0.1$) as well as the range parameters (κ_p; such that $\mathbb{P}(\kappa_p < 0.1) = 0.1$), variances, ($\sigma_{\omega p}^2$; such that $\mathbb{P}(\sigma_{\omega p} > 1) = 0.1$) and the autocorrelation parameters (ρ_p; such that $\mathbb{P}(\rho_p > 0) = 0.9$) of the spatio-temporal processes ((D. Simpson, Rue, Riebler, Martins, and Sørbye, 2017; Fuglstad, Simpson, Lindgren, and Rue, 2018)).

12.6.1   Approximating the continuous spatio-temporal field

In typical downscaling applications, the spatial processes governing the coefficients are modeled as Gaussian random fields (GRFs). The field is defined by the covariance matrix and performing inference with numerous monitoring locations over many time points may be computational challenging using traditional methods of performing Bayesian inference (e.g. MCMC) as large, dense, linear systems must be solved at each iteration. This poor computational scaling with the size of the data is known as the 'big N' problem. A number of methods specifically tailored to scaling up inference in spatial and spatio-temporal problems have been proposed over the past decade, and some of the most broadly used methods use a specially constructed finite-dimensional Gaussian random field that trades off scalability with accuracy (Cressie and Johannesson, 2008; Katzfuss, 2017; Lindgren, Rue, and Lindström, 2011). A review of recent methods, as well as information about their performance on a simple spatial model, can be found in (Heaton et al., 2018).

Here, we propose representing the continuous field by an approximation based on an (irregular) triangulation. A triangulation is a partition of a domain of interest into a collection of connected non-overlapping triangles. The triangles of a triangulation

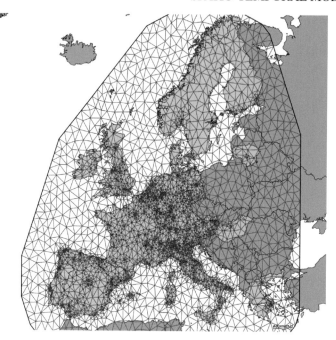

Figure 12.3: Mesh over Western Europe with red dots denoting the locations of ground monitors.

are formed by points given in the domain of interest. This will allow us to control the smoothness of the process, by allowing it to vary more quickly over space where there is data and less so when there is less data, therefore focussing the computational effort and thus enabling downscaling where the data is sufficient to support it. In the case of air pollution this may be more appropriate, as this allows us to define a denser set of triangles where data are dense spatially and less where is it is more sparse. Furthermore, we use Delaunay triangulation which places constraints on the maximum angle size and the triangulation to be convex (Hjelle and Dæhlen, 2006). An example of such a mesh can be seen in Figure 12.3, where we define the mesh to be more dense in urban areas but less dense in the rural and unpopulated areas.

Once a triangulation of the domain has been defined, the spatial field can be approximated using,

$$\omega_{st} = \sum_{k=1}^{n} \phi_{ks} w_{kt} \qquad (12.21)$$

where n is the number of vertices (or nodes) of the triangulation, $\{\phi_{ks}\}$ are a set of piecewise linear basis functions that are one at vertex k and zero at all other vertices, and $\{w_{kt}\}$ are a set of stochastic weights. The weights w_{kt} are assigned a zero-mean multivariate Gaussian distribution $\boldsymbol{w}_t \sim N(0, \Sigma)$.

Here, we follow (Lindgren, Rue, and Lindström, 2011) and select the distribution of the weights such that we approximate the GRF by a Gaussian Markov random field (GMRF). A GMRF is a discretely indexed GRF, $Z \sim N(0, \Sigma)$ and if one can be found that best represents our GRF then we will be able to take advantage of efficient computation, as typically, the inverse of the covariance matrix, $Q = \Sigma^{-1}$ will be sparse, due to a conditional independence property, in which $Z_i \perp\!\!\!\perp Z_j | Z_{-ij} \iff Q_{ij} = 0$ (where Z_{-ij} denotes Z with the ith and j^{th} elements removed) (Rue and Held, 2005). The structure of the precision matrix of this process is defined by the triangulation of the domain and the set of bases functions used. In order to ensure the Markov structure that is required for a GMRF, the set of basis functions should be piecewise linear,

$$\phi_{ks} = 1 \qquad \text{at vertex } k \qquad\qquad (12.22)$$
$$0 \quad \text{at all other vertices} \qquad\qquad (12.23)$$

then $w_t \sim N(0, \Sigma)$ will be a GMRF.

Furthermore, if the GRF, $\{\omega_s \mid s \in \mathbb{R}^d\}$, is assumed to have a Matérn covariance function as in Equation 12.20, then the approximation given by Equation 12.21 is a finite element method solution to the following SPDE,

$$(\kappa^2 - \Delta)^{\alpha/2}(\tau\omega_s) = \mathscr{W}_s \ s \in \mathbb{R}^d, \ \alpha = v + d/2, \ \kappa > 0, \ v > 0$$

where $(\kappa^2 - \Delta)^{\alpha/2}$ is a pseudo-differential operator, Δ is the Laplacian, κ is the scale parameter, τ controls the variance and $\mathscr{W}_s$ is spatial white noise with unit variance. Any GRF model defined with a Matérn covariance structure can be approximated by a GMRF in this way provided $v + d/2$ is integer valued. This approach can be extended to GRFs on manifolds, non-stationary and anisotropic covariance structures (Lindgren, Rue, and Lindström, 2011; Bakka et al., 2018; Krainski et al., 2018).

12.6.2 Inference

The model presented in Chapter 6, Section 6.7 can be expressed in general form as

$$\eta_i = \mathbb{E}(Y_{st}) \quad = \quad \beta_0 + \sum_{p=1}^{P} \beta_p X_{pst} + \sum_{q=1}^{Q} f_q(X_{q\ell t}), \qquad (12.24)$$

where, β_0 is an overall intercept term, the set of β_p $(p = 1, \ldots, P)$ are the coefficients associated with covariates X_{qst}, the set of functions, $f_1(\cdot), \ldots, f_P(\cdot)$ represent the random effects which can take the form of random intercepts and slopes, non-linear effects of covariates, spatial, temporal and spatio-temporal random effects.

All unknown parameters are collected into two sets: $\theta = (\beta_q, f_q)$, which contains all the parameters, and ψ, which contains all the hyperparameters that control the variability and strength of the relationships between the observations and the fixed and random effects. The set ψ contains the Gaussian noise parameter σ_ε^2, along with the variance, range parameter and autocorrelation parameter associated with the spatio-temporal random effects, $\sigma_{\omega p}^2$, κ_p and ρ_p. Assigning a Gaussian distribution to the set of parameters $\theta \sim N(0, \Sigma(\psi_2))$ results in a latent Gaussian model (LGM) as described in Chapter 6.

The aim is to produce a set of high-resolution exposures to air pollution over an entire study area in time. The marginal posterior distribution for a prediction in a particular location, s, and time, t, can be expressed as

$$p(\hat{Y}_{st}|Y) = \int \int p(\hat{Y}_{st}|\theta, \psi, Y) p(\theta|\psi, Y) p(\psi|Y) d\theta d\psi \qquad (12.25)$$

There is also interest in finding the marginal posterior densities for each ψ_k and θ_j given the observed data Y,

$$\begin{aligned} p(\psi_k|Y) &= \int p(\psi|Y) d\psi_{-k} \\ p(\theta_j|Y) &= \int p(\theta_j|\psi, Y) p(\psi|Y) d\psi. \end{aligned}$$

Here, ψ_{-k} denotes the set of parameters, ψ, with the kth entry removed. In most cases, these will not be analytically tractable and therefore approximations of the posterior distributions $p(\psi|Y)$ and $p(\theta_j|\psi, Y)$ as well as numerical integration will be needed.

The approximation for the joint posterior, $p(\psi|Y)$, is given by

$$\tilde{p}(\psi|Y) \propto \left. \frac{p(Y, \theta, \psi)}{\tilde{p}(\theta|\psi, Y)} \right|_{\theta = \hat{\theta}(\psi)}$$

where $\tilde{p}(\theta|\psi, Y)$ is a Gaussian approximation of $p(\theta|\psi, Y)$ evaluated at the mode $\hat{\theta}(\psi)$ of the distribution $\theta|\psi$. The approximation, $\tilde{p}(\psi|Y)$, is equivalent to a Laplace approximation, and it is exact if $\tilde{p}(\theta|\psi, Y)$ is Gaussian. The approximation used for the posterior, $p(\theta_j|\psi, Y)$ is given by

$$\tilde{p}(\theta_j|\psi, Y) \propto \left. \frac{p(Y, \theta, \psi)}{\tilde{p}(\theta_{-j}|\theta_j, \psi, Y)} \right|_{\theta_{-j} = \hat{\theta}_{-j}(\theta_j, \psi)}$$

where $\tilde{p}(\theta_{-j}|\theta_j, \psi, Y)$ is a Gaussian approximation of the distribution $p(\theta_{-j}|\theta_j, \psi, Y)$. The distribution $\tilde{p}(\theta_j|\psi, Y)$ is then obtained by taking Taylor expansions of $p(Y, \theta, \psi)$ and $\tilde{p}(\theta_{-j}|\theta_j, \psi, Y)$, up to third order, aiming to correct a Gaussian approximation for location errors due to potential skewness (Rue et al., 2009).

In order to estimate the marginal posterior distributions given by Equation 12.26, a set of integration points and weights are built using the distribution $\tilde{p}(\psi|Y)$. Firstly, the mode of $\tilde{p}(\psi|Y)$ is found numerically by Newton-type algorithms. Around the mode, the distribution $\log(\tilde{p}(\psi|Y))$ is evaluated over a grid of K points $\{\psi^{(k)}\}$, each with associated integration weights $\{\Delta^{(k)}\}$. If the points define a regular lattice, then the integration weights will be equal. The marginal posteriors, $p(\psi_k|Y)$, are obtained using numerical integration of an interpolant of $\log(\tilde{p}(\psi|Y))$. The marginal posteriors, $p(\theta_j|Y)$, are obtained using numerical integration

$$p(\theta_j|Y) = \sum_k \tilde{p}(\theta_j|\psi^{(k)}, Y) \tilde{p}(\psi^{(k)}|Y) \Delta^{(k)} \qquad (12.26)$$

where $\tilde{p}(\theta_j | \psi^{(k)}, Y)$ and $\tilde{p}(\psi^{(k)} | Y)$ are the posterior distributions $\tilde{p}(\psi | Y)$ and $\tilde{p}(\theta_j | \psi, Y)$ evaluated at the set of integration points $\{\psi^{(k)}\}$ while $\Delta^{(k)}$ are integration weights (Martins, Simpson, Lindgren, and Rue, 2013).

Inference of the model presented in Section 6.7 can be implemented using the R interface to the INLA computational engine (R-INLA) (Rue et al., 2012). For further details, see Rue et al. (2009).

12.6.3 Prediction

In a fully Bayesian analysis, predictions (as given by Equation 12.25) are treated as unknown parameters and posterior distributions of these quantities are estimated alongside the model parameters. This may cause computational issues particularly when predicting at a very large number of locations in time, again due to the need to manipulate large covariance matrices.

One approach would be to perform inference with predictions at a few locations simultaneously and to repeat this a number of times to obtain a full set of predictions, as used in (Shaddick et al., 2018) when predicting global air quality on a high resolution grid ($0.1^o \times 0.1^o$ resolution). However, uncertainty may be underrepresented as the joint variance between predictions is ignored. An alternative approach, which is the one taken here, is to take joint samples from the posterior distributions, $\tilde{p}(\theta | \psi, Y)$ and $p(\psi | Y)$ and use each set of samples (of the model coefficients) to create predictions using Equation 12.19, resulting in a set of joint predictions of the quantity of interest. This provides an efficient method for predicting at any required location in space and time as once the samples of the model coefficients are obtained, prediction is done using a linear combination. Summarizing the joint samples at each location will produce the marginal predictive posterior distributions required. Furthermore, full posterior distributions for other quantities of interest such as country – level annual average and population – weighted annual average concentrations or changes over time can be produced.

Although R-INLA estimates marginal posterior densities, as shown in Equation 12.26, it is possible to sample from the joint posterior distribution using the function inla.posterior.sample in the R-INLA package. In computing the approximation to the required distributions as shown in Equation 12.26 the approximated distributions at the integration points can be retained. Joint samples from the posteriors can be obtained by sampling from Gaussian approximations at the integration points for all of the parameters.

Example 12.10. *Modeling PM$_{2.5}$ in Europe by integrating ground measurements with outputs from numerical modeling*

In this example, we demonstrate the use of the model presented in Section 12.6 in modeling and mapping PM$_{2.5}$ in Europe. The study region consists of 20 countries within Europe: Austria, Belgium, Denmark, Finland, France, Germany, Greece, Hungary, Ireland, Italy, Liechtenstein, Lithuania, Luxembourg, Netherlands, Norway, Portugal, Spain, Sweden, Switzerland and the

United Kingdom. The sources of data used here can be allocated to one of four groups: (i) ground monitoring data; (ii) estimates from CTMs; (iii) other sources including land-use and topography and (iv) estimates of population counts. Ground monitoring is available at a distinct number of locations, whereas the latter three groups are available on grids and provide coverage of the entire study area with no missing data.

Annual average concentrations of $PM_{2.5}$ (measured in $\mu g/m^3$) from between 2010 and 2016 were extracted from the Air Quality e-Reporting database (European Environment Agency, 2018). The database is maintained by the European Environment Agency (EEA) and provides a comprehensive and quality-assured source of information of air quality from all national and local monitoring networks in EU Member States and other participating countries. Measurements were used if they had $\geq 75\%$ of daily coverage over a year. The locations of 3436 ground monitoring sites (for $PM_{2.5}$ and NO_2) active between 2010 and 2016 can be seen in Figure 12.4.

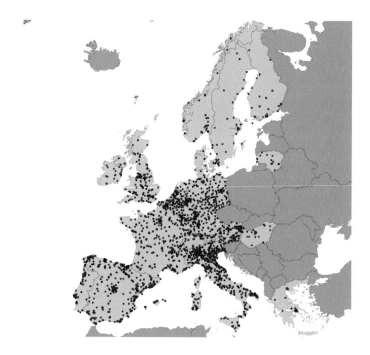

Figure 12.4: Locations of ground monitors measuring NO_2 or $PM_{2.5}$ between 2010 and 2016 in the study area. Red dots denote monitors that only measure $PM_{2.5}$ during this period, with blue dots denoting monitors only measuring NO_2 and black dots denoting monitors measuring both and $PM_{2.5}$.

Numerically simulated estimates of $PM_{2.5}$ were obtained from the MACC-II Ensemble model available on a 10 km × 10 km resolution grid at an hourly temporal resolution. In each grid cell, the Ensemble model value was defined as the median value (in μgm^{-3}) of the following seven individual regional CTMs: CHIMERE from INERIS, EMEP from MET Norway, EURAD – IM from University of Cologne, LOTOS – EUROS from KNMI and TNO, MATCH from SMHI, MOC AGE from METEO – France and SILAM from FMI (see Inness et al. (2013) and Copernicus Atmosphere Monitoring Service (2018) for details). Estimates were aggregated over time to obtain annual average concentrations of NO_2 and $PM_{2.5}$ for each grid cell.

Information on roads was extracted from the EuroStreets digital road network version 3.1, derived from the TeleAtlas MultiNet 2008 data set. The road data was classified into 'all' and 'major' roads using the classification available in EuroStreets. These were then projected on to a 100 m × 100 m resolution grid, which were also aggregated to obtain estimates on a 1 km × 1 km resolution grid, with each cell the sum of road length within the cell.

Information on land use was obtained using the European Corine Land Cover (ECLC) 2006 data set was obtained (ETC-LC Land Cover (CLC2006), 2014). This dataset covered the whole study area except Greece. For Greece, ECLC 2000 was used (ETC-LC Land Cover (CLC2000), 2013).

Information on altitude was obtained from the SRTM Digital Elevation Database version 4.1 with a resolution of approximately 90 m resolution and aggregated to obtain 100 m × 100 m and 1 km × 1 km resolution grids (Jarvis, Reuter, Nelson, and Guevara, 2008). SRTM data is only available up to 60^oN and was therefore supplemented with data from with Topo30 data. For more information, see (de Hoogh et al., 2016).

A comprehensive set of population data on a high-resolution grid was obtained from Eurostat. The GEOSTAT 2011 version 2.0.1 database provides estimates of population at a 1 km × 1 km resolution across Europe in 2011 (EUROSTAT, 2016).

We fit a model with random effects on both the intercept terms and coefficients associated with the MACC – II Ensemble CTM. We use the data which is available for multiple years by extending the model to allow spatio-temporally variation relationships between GMs and CTM using the formulation of the model given in Equation 12.19, with the relationship between the information on roads (length of all and major roads), land use (the proportion of areas that are residential, industry, ports, urban green space, built up, natural land), altitude assumed to be (fixed and) linear, with transformations of some of the covariates, notably altitude ($\sqrt{a/max(a)}$ where $a = $ altitude $- min$(altitude)), to address non-linearity. To allow for the skew in the ground measurements and the constraint of non-negativity, the square-root of the measurements are used for NO_2 and the (natural) logarithm of the measurements are used for $PM_{2.5}$.

Full posterior distributions from the final model (Model (iv)) were produced for each cell on a high-resolution grid (consisting of approximately 3.7

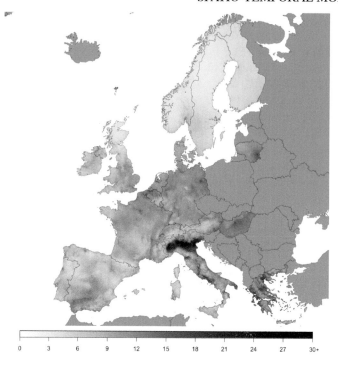

Figure 12.5: Median annual average concentrations of NO_2 and $PM_{2.5}$ (in μgm^{-3}) in 2016, by grid cell (1 km $\times$ 1 km resolution).

million, 1 km $\times$ 1 km cells) covering Western Europe. Figure 12.5 show maps of estimated annual average concentrations (at a 1km $\times$ 1km resolution) of $PM_{2.5}$ in 2016 (medians of the posterior distribution in each grid cell) respectively. One of the major advantages in using a Bayesian model is that we have posterior distributions at every point in the map and this allows us to express uncertainty and, in this case, to calculate probabilities of exceedances. These can be seen in Figure 12.6 which shows the estimated probability that the annual average $PM_{2.5}$ in 2016 exceed that of the previous WHO AQG of 10 μgm^{-3} respectively. $PM_{2.5}$ is derived from a wide range of sources, including energy production, industry, transport, agriculture, dust and forest fires, and it is known that particles can travel in the atmosphere over long distances. This can be seen in Figure 12.5 where concentrations are much more widespread with the highest observed in Northern Italy, a region with a high population and industrial activity. Figure 12.6(b) also shows that concentrations are more widespread with high probabilities of exceeding the WHO AQGs occurring in both urban and rural areas.

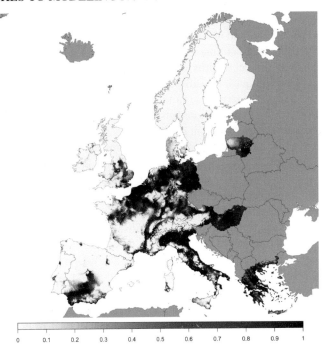

Figure 12.6: Probability that the annual average concentration of PM$_{2.5}$ (in μgm^{-3}) in 2016 exceed the WHO AQGs, by grid cell (1 km $\times$ 1 km resolution).

12.7   Approaches to modeling non-separable processes

The complexity of non-separable spatio-temporal processes, often combined with computational issues has resulted in the development of a number of different approaches to modeling them. Here we provide a brief description of a selection of the available approaches.

The problems of high-dimensionality in modeling the entire space-time structure were addressed by Mardia, Goodall, Redfern, and Alonso (1998) as well as by Wikle and Cressie (1999) who reduce the dimensionality of the mean term in the same fashion as in principle component analysis (Chatfield and Collins, 1980), to an orthonormal sequence of deterministic spatial functions. The former describe these functions as 'principal' and 'trend fields', with the trend fields being functions of the co-ordinates of the sites and the principal fields selected from kriging estimates for a set of 'normative' sites. The hierarchical model (12.1) is now expressed as,

$$
\begin{aligned}
Y_{st} &= Z_{st} + v_{st} \\
Z_{st} &= \sum_{j=1}^{p} A_{tj}\phi_j(s) + m_s \\
A_t &= HA_{t-1} + J\eta_t
\end{aligned}
\tag{12.27}
$$

where either H and/or J must be non-diagonal in order to incorporate spatial structure into the temporal component. Mardia et al. (1998) call this method the 'kriged Kalman filter' (KKF) and outline a likelihood-based estimation strategy while Wikle and Cressie (1999) give an (approximate) Bayesian estimation approach. In addition to the estimation techniques, the difference between the two approaches is that there is no measurement error term (v_{st}) in the first level of the KKF. This results in an error term consisting of two components, $v_{st} + m_s$, and as there is no attempt to incorporate the inherent variability in predicting the underlying process from the data, introducing the possibility of over smoothed estimates (Cressie and Wikle, 1998). The KKF computes $E(\sum_{j=1}^{p} a_{tj}\phi_j(s)|Z_{st})$ whereas Wikle and Cressie (1999) compute $E(Y_{st}|Z_{st})$.

Wikle, Berliner, and Cressie (1998) present a fully Bayesian hierarchical model in which they approach the problems of high dimensionality by explicitly modeling parameters lower in the hierarchy. They expand the second level of Equation 12.1 to include long-term temporal patterns, $\beta_{1s}\cos(\Omega t) + \beta_{2s}\sin(\Omega t)$. They use a vector autoregressive process (VAR) (Chatfield, 2013; Cressie, 1993) to model the dynamic aspect of the space-time interaction, A_{st}, that is $A_t = HA_{t-1} + \eta_{st}$. The updating parameter, H_t, was simplified by using a 'nearest neighbor' VAR (Cressie, 1993) in which $A_{st} = a_{st}A_{(st-1)} + bA_{s^1(t-1)} + cA_{s^2(t-1)} + dA_{s^3(t-1)} + eA_{s^4(t-1)} + \eta_{st}$, where $|s^i - s| = 1$, the four locations within distance one of s. In this form, the autoregressive parameter for the location in question, a_{st}, varies spatially, but b, c, d and e do not. Consequentially, the model has no spatial interaction between A_{st} and $A_{s't} : s \neq s'$. Estimation was achieved using MCMC which was simplified to some extent by using Gaussian error terms at each level, except for the variance hyperparameters, which were inverse Gamma.

Brown, Diggle, Lord, and Young (2001) considered the spatio-temporal modeling of radar-rainfall data in Lancashire, UK. They consider both separable and nonseparable models. In the former, they describe a state space model with observation equation $X_t = A + B_t X_t + v_t$ and second level being a first-order vector autoregressive progress, VAR(1) (Chatfield, 2013; Cressie, 1993), $A_{st} - \mu_{st} = H(A_{t-1} - \mu_{st}) + J\eta_{st}$. The covariance structure can be expressed as $\Gamma_k = H^k(H\Gamma_0 H' + JJ')$, with J influencing the purely spatial covariance, and H describing how the spatial covariance decays at larger time lags. They also fit a Gaussian density to the autoregressive parameters, A_{st}, which 'blurs' the field, allowing interaction between different sites at different time points (P. E. Brown, Karesen, Roberts, and Tonellato, 2000). If two locations, s and s' are close in space, then the values of A_{st} and $A_{s't}$ will be calculated using values from overlapping neighborhoods, leading to the outcomes being highly correlated. Fitting the model, which they achieve using the MLE, requires the covariance matrix of all the grid points not just the gauged points, making the Kalman filter difficult. Instead, they construct a complete multivariate model with the likelihood evaluated by inverting the covariance matrix. As previously mentioned, in most applications the size of the covariance matrix will prohibit using it directly, initiating the use of data reduction methods. In this particular application, the problems of dimensionality were lessened by being able to delete data points where there was no rainfall, as they added no information. The resulting covariance matrix, whilst still large (2000×2000) was then invertible.

A spatio-temporal model for hourly ozone measurements was developed by Carroll et al. (1997). The model, $Z_{st} = \mu_t + \omega_{st}$ combines a trend term incorporating temperature and hourly/monthly effects, $\mu_t = \alpha_{hour} + \beta_{month} + \beta_1 temp_t + \beta_2 temp_t^2$, which is constant over space, and an error model in which the correlation in the residuals was a non-linear function of time and space. In particular the spatial structure was a function of the lag between observations, $COV(v_{st}, v_{s't'}) = \sigma^2 \rho(d,v)$, where d is the distance between sites and $v = |t' - t|$ is the time difference, with the correlation being given by

$$\rho(d,v) = \begin{cases} 1 & d = v = 0 \\ \phi_v^d \psi_v & d \text{ otherwise} \end{cases}$$

where $\log(\psi_v) = a_0 + a_1 v + a_2 v^2$ and $\log(\phi_v) = b_0 + b_1 v + b_2 v^2$. The correlation of the random field is thus a product of two factors, the first, ψ_v^d depends on both the time and space, the second only on the time difference. Unfortunately, as N. Cressie (1997) pointed out, this correlation function is not positive definite. Using results from the model, there were occasions when $Cov(Z_{st}, Z_{s't}) > Cov(Z_{st}, Z_{st})$. This highlights a genuine lack of a rich set of functions that can be used as space-time correlation functions.

12.8 Summary

In this chapter, we have seen the many ways in which the time can be added to space in order to characterize random exposure fields. In particular, the reader will have gained an understanding of the following topics:

- The additional power that can be gained in an epidemiological study by combining the contrasts in the process over both time and space
- How to characterize the stochastic dependencies across both space and time for inferential analysis.
- General strategies for developing such approaches.
- Separability and non-separability in spatio-temporal models, and how these could be characterized using the Kronecker product of correlation matrices.
- Examples of the use of spatio-temporal models in modeling environmental exposures.

12.9 Exercises

Exercise 12.1. (i) Verify Equation 12.15 for the 2 × 2 case and show your work.

(ii) Repeat (i) for the general case.

Exercise 12.2. Verify Equation 3.5 and show your work.

Exercise 12.3. Verify Equations 12.9–12.11 and show your work.

Exercise 12.4. A simple but sometimes useful spatio-temporal, multiresolution model is built on the idea that a location s falls into the region comprised of a number of relatively homogeneous subregions. The process is determined by a deterministic regional effect plus random subregional effects. Within subregions, any residual effects can be considered white noise.

(i) Build a spatio-temporal model based on that information, assuming the space-time covariance is separable.

(ii) Determine that covariance in terms of the parameters of your model.

Exercise 12.5. Returning to Example 12.2

(i) Compute the process covariance matrix for the process at time $t = 2$.

(ii) Find a linear transformation of the process column vector $\mathbf{Y}_2 = (Z_{21}, \ldots Z_{21})'$ that makes its coordinates independent.

(iii) Determine the power function for the test of the null hypothesis of no change between times, $t = 1, 2$ and give an expression for its expected value under the Bayesian model in that example.

Exercise 12.6. Add to the process model in Equation 12.13 the measurement model $Y_{st} = Z_{st} + v_{st}$, $s = 1, \ldots, N_S$, $t = 1, \ldots, N_T$.

(i) Find the posterior predictive distributive distribution of $Z_{(n+1)s}$ for a given site s and determine what happens as n, the amount of data available increases.

(ii) What deficiencies do you see in the proposed process say where Z represents hourly temperature, t the hour of the day, and $t = 0$ is set at the time when the hourly temperature is expected to be at its maximum? What is the frequency ω in this case?

Chapter 13

Causality: issues and challenges

13.1 Overview

The topic of this chapter is of immense importance. In fact, in 2022 the King Baudouin Foundation awarded the inaugural USD 1,000,000, Rousseeuw Prize for Statistics to James Robins and a team of investigators with whom he worked. Their pioneering work for which he award was made was on the subject of causal inference, with applications in Medicine and Public Health. The second author, Zidek, had the privilege of serving on the international jury that selected the inaugural winners of the prize and thus learned much about their work as well as about its importance and impact. Like Florence Nightingale 1.5, James Robins began his career in a field of medicine. And like her, he was self-taught in statistical science. His motivation came from his discovery in the 1980s, that no theory existed for handling causal inference for longitudinal observation data. That led, according the Professor David Hand, writing in the November 2022 newsletter of the Institute of Mathematical Statistics, to a 121-page research paper, he described it as follows:

> In particular, in 1986 James (Jamie) Robins wrote a 121-page paper (Robins, 1986) describing an approach to estimating the causal effects of treatments with time-varying regimes, direct and indirect effects, and feedback of one cause on another, from observational data.

> This work was seminal, and the Robins 'g-formula' turned out to be a key for tackling such tangled causal webs. The 'g' refers to generalized treatment regimes, including dynamic regimes, in which a later treatment depends on the response to an earlier treatment.

> But that was just the beginning. It prompted several decades of intensive and focused research. Later papers by Robins and the other laureates ...

Often the aim of a study is to determine the *cause* of a disease so that we may devise treatment or prevention. There are two broad types of study in medical research: experimental and observational. In an experiment or clinical trial, we make some intervention and observe the result. In an observational study, we observe the existing situation and try to understand what is happening.

When examining the association between two variables, bias may be introduced by confounding. A confounder is a variable which is strongly associated with the response and effect of interest, which can result in spurious associations being observed between the variable of interest and a health outcome. In a randomized controlled trial, the randomization of treatment allocation is designed to eliminate, as far as possible, the effects of confounding variables. The interpretation of observational studies is more difficult than a randomized trial, as bias due to confounding may influence the measure of interest. If careful consideration is taken beforehand to identify and measure important confounders that may differ between exposure groups, these can be incorporated in the analysis and the groups can be adjusted to take account of differences in these baseline characteristics. Of course, if further factors are present and not included, these will bias the results.

Causality cannot be inferred from observational studies. Only in very rare cases have controlled experiments been used to assess the impact of an environmental hazard on human subjects, for example randomly selected, healthy subjects have jogged in exposure chambers into which varying concentrations of ozone are pumped with the outcome being a decrement in the subject's lung function. For the most part, controlled experiments of this type are not possible due to ethical and practical reasons. Therefore, observational studies are used in which the contrasts between high and low levels are used as a proxy for the treatment and non-treatment groups that would be used in a controlled trial.

The effect of an environmental hazard can be estimated using an observational study, and the risk of exposure to the hazard is often expressed using the relative risk. This shows the increase in the health outcomes that is associated with a one-unit increase in the level of an environmental hazard. This has been interpreted as predicting the degree to which lowering the level of the hazard by say one unit would reduce its health effect. For example, in their 2007 health risk assessment report, the US EPA staff used the results of published epidemiological studies of the effects when computing the expected decrease in O_3 related non-accidental mortality that would result if the ozone standards were reduced from the current levels. The implication is that there is a causal link between ozone and mortality as defined by the 'counterfactual' approach: if levels of O_3 were those specified by the proposed standard, then there would be a specified number of deaths. The argument would be compelling if it had been demonstrated that O_3 caused the deaths assumed in the calculation. However, this is not usually possible using results from observational studies. This chapter will review the roadblocks encountered in establishing that casualty.

13.2   Causality

Finding causes, however defined, is fundamental to the development of a process model. Brumback (2021) gives a comprehensive review of quest for the definition and the search for both. Attempts to define stretches at least as far back as Hume's 1753 treatise (Hume, 2011) where he states:

'We may define a cause to be an object followed by another, and where all the objects, similar to the first, are followed by objects similar to the second. Or, in other words, where, if the first object had not been, the second never had existed'.

In fact, Hume has mixed up two definitions of causation here, as noted in the Stanford Encyclopedia of Philosophy's entry entitled 'Counterfactual theories of causation.' It is the second one that has been developed in succeeding years and would support the interpretation of the concentration response function above. Elaborate theories of causality now exist and include stochastic versions with applications in the health sciences (Robins and Greenland, 1989; VanderWeele and Robins, 2012).

Suffice it to say that the counterfactual definition cannot give us a basis for arguing that high levels of O_3 cause ill health, although we have a *prima facie* case based on the fact of the observational studies used in its assessment. Given that we cannot claim a causative association between an environmental hazard and increases in adverse health outcomes, must we settle for mere association? An answer is provided by the Bradford-Hill criteria, which are a group of minimal conditions necessary to provide adequate evidence of a causal relationship, although it should be noted that none of the criteria are sufficient on their own (Hill, 1965).

Strength of association: The stronger the association between a risk factor and outcome, the more likely the relationship is to be causal.

Specificity: There must be a one-to-one relationship between cause and outcome.

Biological plausibility: There should be a plausible biological mechanism, which explains why exposures might cause adverse health effects.

Biological gradient: Change in disease rates should follow from corresponding changes in exposure (dose-response) with greater exposure leading to increase in adverse health effects.

Temporal gradient: Exposure must precede outcome.

Consistency of results: The same effect should be seen among different populations, when using different study designs and at different times.

Coherence: Does the relationship agree with the current knowledge of the natural history/biology of the disease?

Experimental evidence: Is there evidence that removal of the exposure alters the frequency of the outcome?

Analogy: Similar findings in another context may support the claim of causality in this setting.

13.2.1   Transfer of causality

Depending on what comes through the knowledge channel, a proposed process model can have two classes of covariates, some of which cause change in the process and some not. The data model, which prescribes how well the covariates are measured, may inadvertently measure the non predictors well, the other poorly. If some variables in each of these two groups are stochastically associated with one another, what we call a 'transfer of causality' can occur. The non-causative predictors can be found from the data to be predictive of the process. Some of these can turn out to be seen as confounders. We show this by means of an example.

Example 13.1. *Transfer of causality*

In this example, we see how even if causality were present, it may be difficult to attribute it to a particular exposure when there are variables, which are highly collinear. This phenomenon is called the transfer of causality. This can be described by a hypothetical example taken from Zidek, Wong, Le, and Burnett (1996).

A health count, Y, is Poisson distributed with mean $\exp\{\alpha_0 + \alpha_1 z\}$ conditional on an exposure $Z = z$ with $\alpha_0 = 0$ and $\alpha_1 = 1$, which are not known to the investigator in this simulation study. A second explanatory variable W is seen by the investigator as a possible predictor of Y. The investigator measures both of these predictors with a classical measurement error model:

$$
\begin{aligned}
Z^* &= Z + V_1 \\
X^* &= X + V_2
\end{aligned}
$$

where V_1 and V_2 are independent of each other and of Z and X. The predictors $Z \sim N(0,1)$ and $X \sim N(0,1)$ have correlation ρ, which induces the collinearity. The variances of the measurement errors U and V are σ_{V1}^2 and σ_{V2}^2, respectively. The investigator thinking both of these predictors are relevant fits a Poisson regression model with mean dependent on both Z^* and X^*, i.e $E(Y) = \exp\{\beta_0 + \beta_1 Z^* + \beta_2 W^*\}$. It turns out that the significance of the estimated coefficient $\hat{\beta}_2$ grows as the measurement error in Z and the collinearity between W and Z increases. When $\rho = 0.9$, the effect is dramatic and $\hat{\beta}_2$ dominates $\hat{\beta}_1$ when σ_{v1} reaches 0.5, which is 50% of the α_1. It is now W that appears to have the greatest effect, even though Z is the true cause of the outcome.

13.2.2   Impact of data aggregation

The aggregation of samples can lead to an issue about causality called Simpson's paradox. That discovery of the paradox goes at least as far back as Bartlett (1935), but Simpson seemed to be the one to put it on the statistical map in his famous paper (Simpson, 1951). Blyth articulated the paradox very clearly in Blyth (1972), and we base our description of the paradox in his paper.

Example 13.2. *The Blyth Example*

A doctor, 'Dr', employed a statistician, 'Stat', to assist in carrying out a medical trial. Dr told Stat that he needed to include a few subjects from a nearby center in the treatment group $\bar{C}$, in addition to those from the larger center C, where his main practice was located. Dr thus proposed total sample sizes of $11,000$ and $10,100$, respectively, in the two sites, for a total sample of $21,100$.

Table 13.1: Aggregated summary of trial results.

Outcome	$\bar{T}$	T
$\bar{S}$	5950	9005
S	5050	1095

Table 13.2: Disaggregated summary of trial results.

Outcome	C		$\tilde{C}$	
	$\bar{T}$	T	$\bar{T}$	T
$\bar{S}$	950	9000	5000	5
S	50	1000	5000	95

To the Treatment groups, he proposed to allocate, respectively 10,000 and 100. Stat recommended a randomized trial design. More precisely, a patient arriving at Dr's clinic in C was to be assigned to the treatment group T with probability 0.91 and to the control group $\bar{T}$ otherwise. As for the other site $\bar{C}$, the probabilities were to be 0.01 and 0.99 instead. These choices were motivated by practical considerations having to do with the challenge of applying the treatment.

The trial was conducted. For some patients, the outcome was deemed a 'success' S and for others a 'failure' $\bar{S}$. Dr tabulated his results and presented them to the statistician in Table 13.1.

Seeing the results, Stat complained that Dr should have discontinued the study much earlier. The T was not nearly as good as $\bar{T}$. But Dr defended his conclusion, since the disaggregated results showed that quite the opposite was true, as seen in the Table 13.2.

Blyth notes that this paradox cannot be explained away by the small sample size. To make his point, he presents his findings in a different display in Table 13.3. That table presents just the success rates for the disaggregated trial data. [(iii)] Blyth argues the same disaggregation results could well have been obtained as seen in Table 13.3 based on a much larger sample. The issue remains, is T better than $\bar{T}$?

Blyth's closing argument where Blyth invokes, effectively an infinite sample size, demonstrates the Berliner process model approach as seen in Chapter 4. That interpretation points to a further step in a selection process that yields an additional

Table 13.3: Disaggregated summary of trial results.

Outcome	C		C	
	$\bar{T}$	T	$\bar{T}$	T
S	5%	10%	50%	95%

stratum to an already stratified sample. In other words, the investigator produced a sample with just the strata T vs $\bar{T}$ and C vs $\bar{C}$. The added stratum would correspond to the subpopulations of those for whom T and $\bar{T}$ would be successful vs those for whom they would not be successful. Nature provides the (unknown) selection probabilities for these associated selection processes. This overall allocation yields the sample totals seen in Table 13.2. The potential population available for the experiment may well have measurable attributes Z of potential interest to the experimenters. Available knowledge could be used to model relationships among the Z's while the data can provide the information needed to fit those models, to yield additional information about the value of the new treatment.

The Blyth example, although hypothetical, is realistic. While working abroad in a government research lab, the second author, Zidek, was consulted about an issue that had arisen in connection with a multi-center clinical trial. The clinicians in the various centers held strong views about the potential benefit of a new treatment compared to a placebo. But those views differed dramatically from one site to another. Consequently, the proposed randomization plans differed from one center to another, leading to a situation like that in the Blyth example. Knowing about the possibility of the trial leading to a paradoxical result, Zidek pointed out the potential interpretation difficulties that might arise after the trial was over. However, the final result is unknown to the authors.

That consultation led Zidek to a theoretical inquiry. Its overarching goal was the degree of control over the sample selection protocols. In other words, the degree centers in a multi-center trial should be allowed latitude in choosing their randomization protocols. More specifically, given a 2×2 table of selection probabilities as described above, could a confounder exist that would lead to a Simpson-disaggregaton, hereafter abbreviated as SDis? If so, how extreme could the confounding problem be? (Zidek, 1984).

To answer those questions, Zidek went directly to the sample-selection process, and we now describe the results. But new notation is required. For any event A, let $\bar{A}$ represent its complement. Further, for any two events, AB would represent their intersection. We will let $pr(A)$ to represent the probability of an event A. Finally: S and $\bar{S}$ will represent, respectively, 'success' and 'failure'; C and $\bar{C}$ the first (Dr's major center) and second subpopulation group, respectively. Thus, for example, $pr(T|C)$ would be the probability that nature selects a random subject located in center C into the 'treatment' group. And $pr(\bar{T}C)$ would be the probability of being selected into the group of subjects selected in the center C and also into the treatment group.

In this new notation, we can rewrite the large-sample version of Blyth's tables. First, we get Table 13.4. For example, $pr(S)$ would denote the marginal (overall) marginal probability of a 'success', and $pr(T)$, the overall marginal probability of assignment to the treatment group. Finally, we expand the marginal probabilities to get a replacement for Blyth's Table 13.2 and get Table 13.5.

Table 13.4: Aggregated summary of trial results.

Outcome	$\bar{T}$	T	
$\bar{S}$	$pr(\bar{S}|T)$	$pr(\bar{S}|\bar{T})$	$[\bar{S}]$
S	$pr(S|T)$	$pr(S|\bar{T})$	$pr(S)$
	$pr(T)$	$pr(\bar{T})$	

Table 13.5: Disaggregated summary of trial results.

	C		$\bar{C}$	
	$\bar{T}$	T	$\bar{T}$	T
$\bar{S}$	$pr(\bar{S}|\bar{T}C)$	$pr(\bar{S}|TC)$	$pr(\bar{S}|\bar{T}\bar{C})$	$pr(\bar{S}|T\bar{C})$
S	$pr(S|\bar{T}\bar{C})$	$pr(S|T)$	$pr(S|\bar{T})$	$pr(S|T)$
	$pr(\bar{T}C)$	$pr(TC)$	$pr(\bar{T}\bar{C})$	$pr(T\bar{C})$

Armed with our new notation, we can represent Blyth's example more abstractly. First, in Table 13.4 we may rewrite the success probabilities as

$$P_1 = pr(S|T)$$
$$P_2 = pr(S|\bar{T}).$$

Table 13.5 allows us to partition these marginal probabilities as

$$P_1 = pr(S|T) = pr(C|T)pr(S|CT) + pr(\bar{C}|T)pr(S|\bar{C}T)$$
$$= \bar{\alpha}_1 Q_1 + \alpha_1 R_1 \tag{13.1}$$

where $\alpha_1 = pr(\bar{C}|T)$, $Q_1 = pr(S|CT)$ and $R_1 = pr(S|\bar{C}T)$. A complementary representation of the data obtains for P_2, with α_2 replacing α_1. Note, for example, that Q_1 would mean the probability of success given that an individual that was in the center C and received treatment T.

We now turn to the SDis problem. Two quantities play a key role that derives from the practical problems seen in Blyth's two cities example. They are the probabilities of receiving the 'treatment' in each of the two centers participating in the trial:

$$\beta_1 = pr(T|\bar{C})$$
$$\beta_2 = pr(T|C), \text{ leading to} \tag{13.2}$$
$$\frac{\beta_1}{\beta_2} = \frac{pr(\bar{C})}{pr(C)} \times \frac{pr(\bar{C}|T)}{pr(C|T)} \tag{13.3}$$

A SDis can arise when

$$\beta_1 \neq \beta_2$$

The following identity shows the impact of unequal center selection probabilities combined with the effect of unequal 'treatment' vs 'control' selection probabilities for randomly selected subjects in each center:

$$\frac{\alpha_1}{\bar{\alpha}_1} = \theta \times \frac{\beta_1}{\beta_2} \tag{13.4}$$

$$\frac{\alpha_2}{\bar{\alpha}_2} = \theta \times \frac{\bar{\beta}_1}{\bar{\beta}_2}$$

where $\theta = pr(\bar{C})/pr(C)$, $0 < \theta < \infty$ (Zidek, 1984).

We now add constraints to restrict the randomization needed for the allocation of subjects to the 'treatment' and 'control' subgroups, thereby limiting the possibility of an SDis. In the sequel for any $u \in (0.1)$, let $\bar{u} = 1 - u$. Using the notation in Equation 13.1 and in Zidek's paper (Zidek, 1984), define an SDis as follows.

Definition 5. (Controlled SDis) A Controlled SDis at levels $0 \leq \gamma_2 \leq \gamma_1 \leq 1$ is defined to be an SDis with

$$P_1 = (1 - \alpha_1)Q_1 + \alpha_1 R_1$$
$$P_2 = (1 - \alpha_2)Q_2 + \alpha_2 R_2 \tag{13.5}$$

where $0 \leq P_2 < P_1 \leq 1$, $0 \leq Q_1 \leq Q_2 \leq 1$ and $0 \leq R_1 \leq R_2 \leq 1$ while

$$0 \leq \gamma_2 \leq \beta_i \leq \lambda_1 \leq l, i = 1, 2, \tag{13.6}$$

and the α's are given in Equation 13.4.

Note that in Equation 13.6, the γ's must be specified by the experimenters, and these then put limits on the α's through Equation 13.4.

Can a controlled SDis exist? The answer depends on a combination of the sizes of the P's and the γ's. The condition is surprisingly simple and depends on two key parameters:

$$\Gamma = \frac{\gamma_2/(1 - \gamma_2)}{\gamma_1/(1 - \gamma_1)}$$

$$R = \frac{P_2/(1 - P_2)}{P_1/(1 - P_1)}.$$

We get a surprisingly simple answer to the question we have raised.

Theorem 2. (Zidek) An SDis exists if and only if

$$\Gamma < R. \tag{13.7}$$

But perhaps a more important question concerns the severity of the disaggregation. For that we need some measure of severity and that is given in the following definition.

Definition 6. Maximal Simpson-disaggregation A maximal Simpson-disaggregation is one that maximizes

$$D = \frac{1}{2}(|Q_2 - Q_1| + |R_2 - R_1|), \tag{13.8}$$

the average of the resulting differences in the Q's and R's.

The next theorem answers that question. To facilitate the statement of that theorem, let D be as defined above and

$$
\begin{aligned}
m &= \min\{\bar{P}_1, P_2\}^2/(P_1\bar{P}_2), \\
M &= \max\{\bar{P}_1, P_2\} \\
\zeta &= (\Gamma \times P_2 \times \bar{P}_1)^{1/2}.
\end{aligned}
$$

Theorem 3. (Severity of the Simpson-disaggregation) Assume that inequality in Equation 13.7 holds. Then a maximal Simpson-disaggregation at levels $\gamma_1 \le \gamma_1$ exists and the maximal D-value is,

$$D = \begin{cases} \frac{1}{2}(P_1 + P_2) - \zeta & (0 \le< \Gamma \le m) \\ M(1 - \frac{\Gamma}{R}) & (m \le \Gamma < R) \end{cases}. \tag{13.9}$$

Moreover, if $P_1 \ge 1/2$, then $\alpha_2/\bar{\alpha}_2 = \bar{P}_2/(P_2 - R_2), Q1 = 1, R_1 = 0$,

$$
Q_1 = \begin{cases}
P_1 + \zeta & (m \le \Gamma < R, (0 \le< \Gamma \le m) \\
! & (m \le \Gamma < RMR, \bar{P}_1 < P_2) \\
P_1 + \Gamma\bar{P}_1/R & (m \le \Gamma < R, \bar{P}_1 \ge P_2)
\end{cases}
$$

$$
R_2 = \begin{cases}
P_2 - \zeta & (m \le \Gamma < m(0 \le< \Gamma \le m) \\
P_2(1 - \Gamma/R) & (m \le \Gamma < R, \bar{P}_1 < P_2) \\
0 & (m \le \Gamma < R, \bar{P}_1 \ge P_2)
\end{cases}
$$

We conclude this subsection with a real example, wherein the SDis plays a role.

Example 13.3. *Age-related causal effects*

von Kügelgen, Gresele and Schölkopf von Kügelgen, Gresele, and Schölkopf (2021) present a case study, in the context of AI modeling, wherein Simpson's paradox plays a key role. In the motivating application for the paper the outcome is binary, S now meaning 'dead' and $\bar{S}$, 'alive'. From the aggregated sample, the COVID-19 case fatality rate (CFR) is reported as a percentage, although as a fraction, this would correspond to an estimated probability of death. The roles of T and $\bar{T}$ in Blyth's example are played by China and Italy. Finally, the role of the confounder is played by the ten-year age group into which the subject might fall. So 'confounder' is no longer binary, $\bar{C}$ and C, as it was in the Blyth example, but instead it is the 'age' group C. So this example differs from the Blyth example. Nevertheless, the authors refer to it as a 'textbook example' of Simpson's paradox.

But the result is conceptually identical to that seen in Blyth's hypothetical example. And in their conclusion they state:

> 'for all age groups, CFRs in Italy are lower than those in China, but the total CFR in Italy is higher than that in China. ... It constitutes a textbook example of a statistical phenomenon known as Simpson's paradox.
> ...(von Kügelgen et al., 2021)'

The paper cited in Example 13.3 also includes a causal graph, which we have recreated in our own notation in Figure 13.1. It exemplifies, the power of visualization in both data science and model description. We list below, the *tikz* script we used to construct the graph. Other scripts can be found on the following website: https://dkumor.com/posts/technical/2018/08/15/causal-tikz/.

```
\documentclass[crop,tikz,convert=pdf2svg]{standalone}

% Tikz settings optimized for causal graphs.
\usetikzlibrary{shapes,decorations,arrows,calc,arrows.meta,
    fit,positioning}
\tikzset{
    -Latex,auto,node distance =1 cm and 1 cm,semithick ,
    state/.style ={ellipse, draw, minimum width = 0.7 cm},
    point/.style = {circle, draw, inner sep=0.04cm,fill,
        node contents={}},
    bidirected/.style={Latex-Latex,dashed},
    el/.style = {inner sep=2pt, align=left, sloped}
}

%\begin{document}

% The graph
\begin{tikzpicture}
    \node[state] (1) {$C$};
    \node[state] (2) [right =of 1] {$S$};
    %\node[state] (3) [right =of 2] {$Y$};
    \node[state] (4) [above right =of 1,xshift=-0.6cm,
        yshift=-0.3cm] {$T$};
```

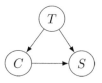

Figure 13.1: A causal diagram showing that country T is influencing both the case fatality probability S and the age demographic.

```
    \path (1) edge node[above] {
    %$\lambda_{zx}$
    } (2);
    \path (4) edge node[el,above] {
    %$\lambda_{wz}$
    } (2);
     \path (4) edge node[el,above] {
    %$\lambda_{wz}$
    } (1);
\end{tikzpicture}
\end{document}}}
```

The von Kügelgen et al. (2021) paper is strongly recommended as it contains much more than we can cover in the space we have. In particular, it includes references to other studies in which the paradox emerges and relevant sources of data. In particular, they make a remark on the importance of this 'paradox' that we now quote:

> While the previous reasoning provides a perfectly consistent explanation in a statistical sense. the phenomenon may still seem puzzling, as it defies our causal intuition-similar to how an optical illusion defies our visual intuition. Humans appear to naturally extrapolate conditional probabilities to read them as causal effects, which can lead to inconsistent conclusions and may leave one wondering: how can the disease in Italy be less fatal for the young, less fatal for the old, but more fatal for the people overall? It is for this reason of ascribing causal meaning to probabilistic statements that the reversal of (conditional) probabilities ... is perceived as and referred to as a 'paradox'.

13.3 Ecological bias

Often, health data are only available as aggregated daily counts, meaning that an ecological regression model is required. Such models answer fundamentally different epidemiological questions from individual level models, and the results should not be stated in terms of a causal link between air pollution and health. For a review, see Plummer and Clayton (1996). The use of ecological studies in this context is contentious, and has been discussed by Richardson, Stücker, and Hémon (1987); Greenland and Morgenstern (1989); Wakefield and Salway (2001). A causal relationship between air pollution and health can only be estimated from individual level data, but personal mortality or morbidity events may be unavailable for confidentiality reasons, while pollution exposures are expensive and impractical to obtain for more than a few individuals.

As such data are largely unavailable, a few researchers have attempted to estimate a link between air pollution and health by aggregating individual exposure – response models to the population level, see for example Zeger et al. (2000); Sheppard and Damian (2000); Wackernagel (2003); Wakefield and Shaddick (2006). However, such individual level models are typically non-linear, as they are based on Bernoulli observations, meaning that the aggregation cannot be done exactly. The resulting error is known as ecological bias. The description focuses on the context of a spatial ecological study, but the problem is equally applicable in time series studies (Shaddick, Lee, and Wakefield, 2013).

13.3.1 Individual level model

Consider a spatial study where the study region A is split into N subareas A_l $(A_1,\ldots,A_{N_l})$, each of which contains n_l individuals. Then for a prespecified time interval, let $Y_{il}^{(1)}$ denote a Bernoulli disease indicator variable, which is one if an individual i in the area l has the disease and zero if not. In addition, consider p exposures $\mathbf{Z}_{il} = (Z_{il1},\ldots,Z_{ilp})$ measured for these individuals and q area level covariates $\mathbf{X}_l = (X_{l1},\ldots,X_{lq})$, which are constant for all individuals within the area l. For this description, we assume that the true exposures are available and later consider the case using measurements of the true exposure, $Y_{il}^{(2)}$, which may contain error. If $(Y_{il}^{(1)}, \mathbf{Z}_{il}, \mathbf{X}_l)$ are all available, then an individual level model is given by

$$Y_{il}^{(1)} \sim \text{Bernoulli}(p_{il}) \qquad (13.10)$$

$$\ln\left(\frac{p_{il}}{1-p_{il}}\right) = \beta_0 + \mathbf{Z}_{il}'\beta_z + \mathbf{X}_l'\beta_x$$

where $\beta = (\beta_0, \beta_z, \beta)$ are the regression parameters to be estimated. If the disease in question is rare then p_{il} will be small, so $\log(p_{il}/(1-p_{il})) \approx \log(p_{il})$ and the logit link can be replaced by a log link.

13.3.2 Aggregation, if individual exposures are known

In many cases the disease indicators $Y_{il}^{(1)}$ are not known, and only the aggregate disease count for each area, $Y_l = \sum_{i=1}^{n_l} Y_{il}^{(1)}$, is available. The aim is now to aggregate the individual level model shown in Equation 13.10 up to a model for Y_l, which is known. If we initially assume that the exposures for all individuals are constant within each area, that is $\mathbf{Z}_{il} = \mathbf{Z}_l$, then $p_{il} = p_l$ meaning that the risk of disease is constant for all individuals across each area. Conditional on the exposures and covariates in this simplified case, the health model for $Y_l^{(1)}$ is given by:

$$Y_l^{(1)} \sim \text{Binomial}(n_l, p_l)$$

$$\ln\left(\frac{p_l}{1-p_l}\right) = \beta_0 + \mathbf{Z}_l'\beta_z + \mathbf{X}_l'\beta_x$$

and the individual level parameters in the model given in Equation 13.10 are the same as those in the ecological model above. In contrast, if individual exposures are not constant within an area then the aggregate counts $y_k^{(1)}$ are not Binomial as the individual Bernoulli disease probabilities are not equal. In this case, the distribution of $Y_l^{(1)}$ inherited from $Y_{il}^{(1)}$ is non-standard, and instead we focus on the mean and variance structure of $Y_l^{(1)}$. If we can assume that the individual level exposures $\mathbf{Z}_{il}$ are known and that the disease indicators $Y_{il}^{(1)}$ are independent, then

$$
\begin{aligned}
\mathbb{E}[Y_l^{(1)}|\mathbf{Z}_{il}] &= \mathbb{E}\left[\sum_{i=1}^{n_l} Y_{il}^{(1)}|\mathbf{Z}_{il}\right] \\
&= \sum_{i=1}^{n_l} \mathbb{E}[Y_{il}^{(1)}|\mathbf{Z}_{il}] \\
&= \sum_{i=1}^{n_l} p_{il}
\end{aligned}
$$

$$
\begin{aligned}
\mathrm{Var}[Y_l^{(1)}|\mathbf{Z}_{il}] &= \mathrm{Var}\left[\sum_{i=1}^{n_l} Y_{il}^{(1)}|\mathbf{Z}_{il}\right] \\
&= \sum_{i=1}^{n_l} \mathrm{Var}[Y_{il}^{(1)}|\mathbf{Z}_{il}] \qquad \text{(assuming independence)} \\
&= \sum_{i=1}^{n_l} p_{il} - p_{il}^2
\end{aligned}
$$

where again

$$
g(p_{il}) = \beta_0 + \mathbf{Z}_{il}'\beta_z + \mathbf{X}_l\beta_x
$$

Here g is typically a log or logit link function. In this case one approach would be to specify a Poisson distribution for $Y_l^{(1)}$ as they are counts with a log link, giving the model (again conditional on $\mathbf{Z}$):

$$
Y_l^{(1)} \sim \mathrm{Poisson}(\mu_l)
$$

$$
\mu_l = \exp(\beta_0 + \mathbf{X}_l'\beta_x) \sum_{i=1}^{n_l} \exp(\mathbf{Z}_{il}'\beta_z)
$$

In the above model, the individual level parameters β_z can still be estimated. However, in view of the variance function, this model should be altered to allow for under dispersion as $\mathrm{Var}(Y_l^{(1)}|\mathbf{Z}_{il}) = \mathbb{E}[Y_l^{(1)}|\mathbf{Z}_{il}] - \sum_{i=1}^{n_l} p_{il}^2$.

13.3.3   Aggregation if the individual exposures are not known

In ecological studies, the individual exposures $\mathbf{Z}_{il}$ are unknown, and only a summary measure of exposure for each area $\tilde{\mathbf{Z}}_l$ is available. Such an exposure is likely to be the population mean for the area, or be a surrogate obtained from a centrally sited monitor. In this situation, the mean and variances of $Y_l^{(1)}|\tilde{\mathbf{Z}}_l$ can be derived from the equations $\mathbb{E}[\,U\,] = \mathbb{E}[\,\mathbb{E}[U|V]\,]$ and $\mathrm{Var}\, U = \mathbb{E}[\,\mathrm{Var}\, U|V]] + \mathrm{Var}\,[\mathbb{E}[U|V]\,]$ as:

$$
\begin{aligned}
\mathbb{E}[Y_l^{(1)}|\tilde{\mathbf{Z}}_l] &= \mathbb{E}[\sum_{i=1}^{n_l} Y_{il}^{(1)}|\tilde{\mathbf{Z}}_l] \\
&= \sum_{i=1}^{n_l} \mathbb{E}[Y_{il}^{(1)}|\tilde{\mathbf{Z}}_l] \\
&= \sum_{i=1}^{n_l} \mathbb{E}[\mathbb{E}[Y_{il}^{(1)}|\mathbf{Z}_{il}]|\tilde{\mathbf{Z}}_l] \\
&= \sum_{i=1}^{n_l} \mathbb{E}[p_{il}|\tilde{\mathbf{Z}}_l] \\
&= \sum_{i=1}^{n_l} \mathbb{E}[p_{Z_k}|\tilde{\mathbf{Z}}_l] \\
&= n_l \mathbb{E}[p_{Z_k}|\tilde{\mathbf{Z}}_l]
\end{aligned}
$$

where p_{Z_k} is the disease risk in area l dependent upon the exposure distribution in area l and the observed summary measure $\tilde{\mathbf{Z}}_l$. This exposure distribution is represented by a random variable $\mathbf{Z}_l \sim f(.|\tilde{\mathbf{Z}}_l)$, and each unknown individual exposure $\mathbf{Z}_{il}$ is assumed to be a realization from this distribution. Therefore, the expectation in the above equation is with respect to the distribution $\mathbf{Z}_l|\tilde{\mathbf{Z}}_l$, and assuming a log rather than logit link as the disease risks will be small, the expectation function is given by

$$
\begin{aligned}
\mathbb{E}[Y_l^{(1)}|\tilde{\mathbf{Z}}_l] &= n_l \mathbb{E}[p_{Z_k}|\tilde{\mathbf{Z}}_l] \\
&= n_l \mathbb{E}[\exp(\beta_0 + \mathbf{x}_l'\beta_x + \mathbf{Z}_l'\beta_z)|\tilde{\mathbf{Z}}_l] \\
&= \exp(\beta_0 + \mathbf{x}_l'\beta_x)\mathbb{E}[\exp(\mathbf{Z}_l'\beta_z)|\tilde{\mathbf{Z}}_l]
\end{aligned}
\tag{13.11}
$$

where the expectation is with respect to $\mathbf{Z}_l|\tilde{\mathbf{Z}}_l$. In the last line n_l is a constant and has been absorbed into the intercept term β_0. The associated variance is given by

$$
\begin{aligned}
\mathrm{Var}(Y_l^{(1)}|\tilde{\mathbf{Z}}_l) &= \mathrm{Var}(\sum_{i=1}^{n_l} Y_{il}^{(1)}|\tilde{\mathbf{Z}}_l) \tag{13.12} \\
&= n_l \mathbb{E}[p_{Z_k}|\tilde{\mathbf{Z}}_l] - n_l \mathbb{E}[p_{Z_k}|\tilde{\mathbf{Z}}_l]^2
\end{aligned}
$$

Again p_{Z_k} is the disease risk in area l dependent upon the exposure distribution $\mathbf{Z}_l|\tilde{\mathbf{Z}}_l$. Now from the mean function (13.11), an appropriate mean model for disease counts $Y_l^{(1)}$ is given by

$$
\begin{aligned}
Y_l^{(1)} &\sim \mathrm{Poisson}(\mu_l) \tag{13.13} \\
\mu_l &= \exp(\beta_0 + \mathbf{X}_l'\beta_x)\mathbb{E}[\exp(\mathbf{Z}_l'\beta_z)|\tilde{\mathbf{Z}}_l]
\end{aligned}
$$

where again the expectation is with respect to $\mathbf{Z}_l|\tilde{\mathbf{Z}}_l$. However, this model assumes the mean and variance are equal, which from the above derivations is not true as the theoretical variance will be less than the mean. However, the naive ecological model used by the majority of studies is worse still, having the general form

$$Y_l^{(1)} \sim \text{Poisson}(\mu_l)$$

$$\mu_l = \exp(\beta_0 + \mathbf{X}_l'\beta_x)\exp(\dot{\mathbf{Z}}_l'\beta_z^*) \qquad (13.14)$$

where the difference is because the risk function is exponential, meaning that in general

$$\exp(\mathbb{E}[\mathbf{Z}_l|\tilde{\mathbf{Z}}_l]'\beta_z^*) \neq \mathbb{E}[\exp(\mathbf{Z}_l'\beta_z)|\tilde{\mathbf{Z}}_l]$$

where $\mathbb{E}[\mathbf{Z}_l|\tilde{\mathbf{Z}}_l] = \tilde{\mathbf{Z}}_l$. Therefore, adopting the naive ecological model means that you are estimating the ecological rather than individual level relationship between exposure and health, so that in general $\beta_z \neq \beta_z^*$. Therefore, the naive ecological model (13.14) uses the wrong mean function and incorrectly assumes that the variance is equal to the mean. This is known as pure specification bias. Note that pure specification bias is not a problem if either exposure is constant within an area, or the disease model is linear, as in both cases models (13.13) and (13.14) are equivalent.

13.4   Acknowledging ecological bias

There have been two major approaches for incorporating ecological bias, which were first suggested by Prentice and Sheppard (1995) and, Richardson et al. (1987) respectively. These are now described with the focus on estimating the mean function in Equation 13.13.

13.4.1   Aggregate approach

The aggregate approach assumes that personal exposures $\mathbf{Z}_{il}$ are available, but not the individual health indicators $Y_{il}^{(1)}$. A simple, but unrealistic, situation is that exposure for all individuals $\mathbf{Z}_{il}^{n_l}$ are available, which is exactly the case discussed in Section 13.3.2. In this setting, the mean and variance are given by

$$\mathbb{E}[Y_l^{(1)}|\mathbf{Z}_{il}^{n_l}] = \mu_l = \exp(\beta_0 + \mathbf{x}_l'\beta_x)\sum_{i=1}^{n_l}\exp(\mathbf{Z}_{il}'\beta_z)$$

$$Var(Y_l|\mathbf{Z}_{il}^{n_l}) = \exp(\beta_0 + \mathbf{X}_l'\beta_x)\sum_{i=1}^{n_l}\exp(\mathbf{Z}_{il}'\beta_z) \qquad (13.15)$$

$$- \exp(\beta_0 + \mathbf{X}_l'\beta_x)^2\sum_{i=1}^{n_l}\exp(2\mathbf{Z}_{il}'\beta_z)$$

Prentice and Sheppard (1995) do not make any parametric assumptions about the distribution for $Y_l^{(1)}$ (such as Poisson) and instead adopt a quasi-likelihood estimation approach based on the mean and variance above.

13.4.2   *Parametric approach*

The parametric approach was introduced by Richardson et al. (1987), and assumes that the individual exposures come from a parametric distribution. That is, we assume that $\mathbf{Z}_{il} \sim f(.|\phi_l)$, where the parameters ϕ_l will change with area l. The desired individual level model given by Equation 13.10 is the conditional model $Y_{il}^{(1)}|\mathbf{Z}_{il}, \beta \sim \text{Bernoulli}(p_{il})$, with link function $g(p_{il}) = \beta_0 + \mathbf{Z}_{il}'\beta_z + \mathbf{X}_l'\beta_x$. However, in this situation we only know that $\mathbf{Z}_{il}$ comes from a distribution $f(.|\phi_l)$, so the desired model is for $Y_{il}^{(1)}|\beta, \phi_l$, where the exposure distribution f has been averaged over. In this scenario, $Y_{il}^{(1)}|\beta, \phi_l \sim \text{Bernoulli}(p_{il}^*)$ as it is still a Bernoulli indicator, and assuming a log link p_{il}^* is given by

$$
\begin{aligned}
p_{il}^* &= \mathbb{E}[Y_{il}^{(1)}|\beta, \phi_l] \\
&= \mathbb{E}[\mathbb{E}[Y_{il}^{(1)}|\mathbf{Z}_{il}, \beta, \phi_l]|\beta, \phi_l] \\
&= \mathbb{E}[p_{il}|\beta, \phi_l] \\
&= \mathbb{E}[\exp(\beta_0 + \mathbf{Z}_{il}'\beta_z + \mathbf{x}_l'\beta_x)|\beta, \phi_l] & (13.16) \\
&= \exp(\beta_0 + \mathbf{X}_l'\beta_x)\mathbb{E}[\exp(\mathbf{Z}_{il}'\beta_z)|\beta, \phi_l] & (13.17)
\end{aligned}
$$

where $\mathbb{E}[\exp(\mathbf{Z}_{il}'\beta_z)|\beta, \phi_l]$ is the moment generating function of the exposure distribution $f(.|\phi_l)$. We now consider two cases separately, firstly we assume that the exposures $\mathbf{Z}_{il}$ are independent across individuals i, and we then look at the more realistic situation that they are correlated.

If the exposures $\mathbf{Z}_{il}$ are independent across individuals i, then from the equation above $p_{il}^* = p_l^*$ because it is the same for each individual in area l (the unknown exposures have been averaged over). Therefore, as all individuals in an area have the same risk function and the Bernoulli outcomes are independent, the resulting aggregate model for Y_l is given by

$$
\begin{aligned}
Y_l^{(1)} &\sim \text{Binomial}(n_l, p_l^*) \\
p_l^* &= \exp(\beta_0 + \mathbf{X}_l'\beta_x)\mathbb{E}[\exp(\mathbf{Z}_{il}'\beta_z)|\beta, \phi_l],
\end{aligned}
$$

which is often approximated by a Poisson distribution as the events are rare giving

$$
\begin{aligned}
Y_l^{(1)} &\sim \text{Poisson}(\mu_l) & (13.18) \\
\mu_l &= \exp(\beta_0 + \mathbf{X}_l'\beta_x)\mathbb{E}[\exp(\mathbf{Z}_{il}'\beta_z)|\beta, \phi_l]
\end{aligned}
$$

where $\mu_l = n_l p_l^*$ and n_l has been absorbed into the constant β_0. We now discuss a number of forms for $f(.|\phi_l)$.

If we assume that $\mathbf{Z}_{il} \sim N(\phi_{1k}, \Phi_{2l})$ then the moment generating function is given by $\exp(\phi_{1l}'\beta_z + \beta_z'\Phi_{2l}\beta_z/2)$. Therefore, the mean function for the Poisson model (13.18) becomes

$$
\mu_l = \exp(\beta_0 + \mathbf{X}_l'\beta_x)\exp(\phi_{1l}'\beta_z + \beta_z'\Phi_{2l}\beta_z/2)
$$

with the same results holding for the Binomial model. If (ϕ_{1k}, Φ_{2l}) are estimated from a sample, then this model differs from the naive ecological model in that it incorporates the variance matrix in the mean function as well as the mean. Note that if either the variance is zero or it does not depend on area l (so $\beta_z' \Phi_{2l} \beta_z / 2$ is merged into the intercept term), then this model is identical to the naive ecological model and pure specification bias will not be a problem. This mean function holds true for all values of β_z.

13.5   Exposure pathways

13.5.1   Concentration and exposure response functions

Concentration response functions (CRFs) are estimated primarily through epidemiological studies, by relating changes in ambient concentrations of pollution to a specified health outcome, such as mortality (see Daniels et al. (2004) for example). In contrast, exposure response functions (ERFs) have been estimated through exposure chamber studies, where the physiological reactions of healthy subjects are assessed at safe levels of the pollutant (see EPA (2005) for example). However, ERFs cannot be ethically established in this way for the most susceptible populations such as the very old and very young who are thought to be most adversely effected by pollution exposure. This paper presents a method for estimating the ERF based on ambient concentration measures.

We specifically consider the case of particulate air pollution, which has attained great importance in both the health and regulatory contexts. For example, they are listed in the USA as one of the so-called criteria pollutants that must be periodically reviewed. Such a review by the US Environmental Protection Agency led to a 2006 revision of the US air quality standards (EPA, 2004). These require that in US urban areas, daily ambient concentrations of PM_{10} do not exceed 150 μgm^{-3} more than once a year on average over three years. Concern for human health is a driving force behind these standards, as the US Clean Air Act of 1970 states they must be set and periodically reviewed to protect human health without consideration of cost while allowing for a margin of error.

Example 13.4. *The short-term effects of air pollution on health*

The majority of studies relating air pollution with detrimental effects on health have focused on short-term relationships, using daily values of aggregate level (ecological) data from a fixed geographical region, such as a city. In such studies, the association between ambient pollution concentrations and mortality is of interest for regulatory purposes, primarily because it is only ambient pollution concentrations that are routinely measured. However, personal exposures are based on indoor as well as outdoor sources, and are likely to be different from ambient concentrations (see for example Dockery and Spengler, 1981 and Lioy, Waldman, Buckley, Butler, and Pietarinen, 1990) because the population spend a large proportion of their time indoors. Therefore, to obtain more conclusive evidence of the human health impact of air pollution via an ERF, exposures actually experienced by individuals as well as any subsequent health events are required. Ideally, these would be obtained by individual level studies conducted under strict conditions, such as in randomized controlled trials, but issues of cost and adequate confounder control make them relatively rare (a few examples are given by Neas, Schwartz, and Dockery, 1999, Yu, Sheppard, Lumley, Koenig, and Shapiro, 2000 and Hoek, Brunekreef, Goldbohm, Fischer, and van den Brandt, 2002). An alternative approach is to obtain only individual level pollution exposures, which can be related to routinely available (aggregated) health and confounder data. However, such exposures are still prohibitively expensive to obtain for a large sample of the population, and consequently only a small amount of personal exposure data has been collected (see for example, Lioy et al., 1990 and Ozkaynak et al., 1996).

Form of an exposure response function (ERF)

Often the association between an environmental hazard and health outcomes is modeled using a log-linear or logistic model as seen in Chapter 2 with, in the case of Poisson regression, the log rate being modeled as a function of the levels of the hazard in question and potential covariates as seen in Equation 2.11 in Chapter 2,

$$\log \mu_l = \beta_0 + g(\beta_z Z_l) + \beta_x X_l \tag{13.19}$$

where $g(\beta_x Z_l)$ represents the effect of exposure, Z, and β_x is the effect of a covariate, X_l.

Here, we specifically consider the nature of the relationship between the exposure and the (log) rate, which is encapsulated in the function $g(\beta_z Z)$. This is the exposure response function, which is commonly represented by the form given in (2.11) with the simplification $g(x) = x$. However, this simplification that $g(x) = x$ may not be appropriate in environmental studies, because there must eventually be an upper bound on the effect that the hazard can have on health. An alternative approach is to consider a general function g that satisfies the desirable requirements of: (i) boundedness; (ii) increasing monotonicity; (iii) smoothness (thrice differentiability) and (iv) $g(0) = 0$. Note that these properties are not commonly enforced on CRFs estimated for ambient pollution concentrations using generalized additive models, as seen in Chapter 11 (see for example Daniels et al., 2004).

13.6   Personal exposure models

Exposure to an environmental hazard will depend on the temporal trajectories of the population's members, which will take individual members of that population through a sequence of micro-environments, such as a car, house or street. For background on the general micro-environmental modeling approach, see Berhane et al. (2004).

Information about the current state of the environment may be obtained from routine monitoring, for example in the case of air pollution, or through measurements taken for a specialized purpose. An individual's actual exposure is a complex interaction of behavior and the environment. Exposure to the environmental hazard affects the individual's risk of certain health outcomes, which may also be affected by other factors such as age and smoking behavior. Finally, some individuals will actually contract the health outcome of interest, placing a care and financial burden on society. Thus, for example, policy regulation on emission sources can indirectly affect mortality and morbidity and the associated financial costs. However, this pathway is complex and subject to uncertainties at every stage.

There will be uncertainty in determining which are the important pathways for the environmental hazard and which one(s) should be used in the assessment. For example, in the case of exposure to mercury, it can be found in air, sea and land. Sources include emissions from power plants, since it is found in coal. Once airborne, it can be transported over long distances and may eventually end on land through wet and dry deposition. From there it can be leached into lakes or taken up into the food chain. Levels of ambient mercury are thus determined by a variety of environmental factors, of which some like wind direction are random. These ambient levels help determine exposure through such things as food consumption, fish or shellfish (that contain a very toxic form called methyl mercury) being a primary source. Alternatively, exposure can be from breathing air containing mercury vapor, particularly in warm or poorly ventilated rooms, that comes from evaporation of liquid mercury, which is found in many places like school laboratories. In any case, exposure will depend on the micro-environments that are visited, time spent in them and the internal sources within. Clearly individual factors such as age determine the time-activity patterns that affect the levels of exposure to the hazard, for example, breast milk is a source of mercury in many micro-environments for infants. Careful consideration of the population being studied is therefore very important, especially when the intention is to apply the results more generally.

13.6.1 Micro-environments

The identification of appropriate micro-environments (MEs) and the associated estimation of levels of the environmental hazard are an essential part of linking external measurements with actual individual exposures. Figure 13.2 shows an example of a $2 \times 3 \times 24$ concentration array that highlights the path followed by an imaginary individual through time. Their activities take the individual from home, to outdoor, to indoor (at work), to outdoor, to indoor and back to home at times 5, 6, 14, 16 and 17. The sequence of personal exposures is obtained by reading the array of the highlighted cells from left to right. The choice of these micro-environments by an individual may be a reflection of the ambient conditions.

There are two types of micro-environment: closed and open. A closed micro-environment is one for which the derivation of the local concentration involves a mass balance equation. Such a micro-environment may have local sources that produce amounts of the environmental hazard, and its volume as well as other quantities are in the mass balance equation that is used to derive the resulting local concentration. In this case, the concentration to which its occupants are exposed will be increased.

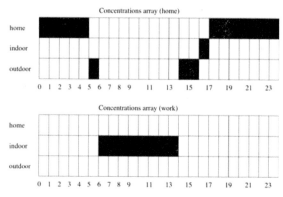

Figure 13.2: The path followed by a randomly selected individual through 24 hours of time. The $2 \times 3 \times 24$ local array categorizes their exposure to pollution at home or work and whether they are exposed to sources either in the home, (other) indoor or outdoor.

On the other hand, as air from within is exchanged with air from outside, there is a tendency for the micro-environment local concentration to adjust itself to the ambient one. In contrast, an open micro-environment is one for which there is no source and for which the local concentration is a simple linear transformation of the ambient one.

To determine local concentrations of the environmental hazard within the different micro-environments, both open and closed, requires some modeling assumptions, which themselves introduce uncertainty. Firstly, we must identify an appropriate set of micro-environments for the environmental hazard under consideration, which itself can introduce uncertainty if this is misspecified or important micro-environments are missing. In a closed micro-environment, the mass balance equation is a differential equation and may involve approximations to solve. It will also require various input data, for example air exchange rates, or rates at which local sources produce the pollutants; these will need to be estimated and so will introduce uncertainty. For an open micro-environment, the relationship between local and ambient levels and the estimation of the parameters controlling that relationship will both be subject to uncertainty.

The state of the environment only partly determines the exposure to the risk factor that is experienced by individuals. Estimating the exposure involves characterizing the link between levels of the environmental hazard and actual exposure. There are two elements to this; the first is how being in a specific environment translates into an exposure, which could involve complex modeling, and the second concerns how individuals move around through different micro-environments and thus determines cumulative exposure. This can be influenced to some extent by policy and other decision makers, albeit indirectly; for example, reporting high pollution days on local weather forecasts may encourage susceptible individuals to stay at home where possible.

Example 13.5. *Estimating personal exposures of particulate matter*

There are a number of implementations of the micro-environment framework, with early models being largely deterministic in nature (Ott, Thomas, Mage, and Wallace, 1988; MacIntosh, Xue, Ozkaynak, Spengler, and Ryan, 1994). More recently, models have incorporated levels of uncertainty into the estimation procedure (Burke, Zufall, and Ozkaynak, 2001; Law, Zelenka, Huber, and McCurdy, 1997; Zidek et al., 2005; Zidek, Shaddick, Meloche, Chatfield, and White, 2007).

In this example, we describe the use of a probabilistic exposure model known as pCnem (Zidek et al., 2005, 2007). Zidek et al. (2005) predict exposure distributions for particulate matter in London in 1997 for the subpopulation of working females. Daily data from eight PM_{10} monitoring sites were uploaded to the pCNEM site, together with maximum daily temperatures for London for 1997. Each site represents a pCNEM's exposure district, that is a geographical area surrounding it whose ambient PM_{10} level can realistically be imputed to be that of its central monitoring site. The spatial distribution of PM_{10} in London for this period has been shown to be relatively homogeneous (Shaddick and Wakefield, 2002), meaning that the boundaries of the exposure regions are less critical than might otherwise be the case.

The subpopulation considered here is that of working women who smoke, live in Brent in semi-detached dwellings that use gas as the cooking fuel and work in the Bloomsbury exposure district. Two subcases are considered, one covering the spring and the other the summer of 1997. For each of the two cases, the output from a single pCNEM run consists of a sequence of 'exposure events' for a randomly selected member of the subpopulation. That individual is composite; a different time activity is selected for each succeeding day. This composite individual better represents her subpopulation's activity patterns than any single member would do. Each event in the sequence takes place in a random micro-environment and consists of exposure to a randomly varying concentration of PM_{10} for a random number of minutes.

The output from the pCNEM model, consisting of 30 replicates generated for each of the two different cases, can be analyzed in a variety of ways. The results for daily averages appear in Figure 13.3. The working females experience high exposures for a period of about 4 days near the beginning of the year, during which a number of replicates have high levels of average daily exposure, approaching or exceeding 50 μgm^{-3}. This is still well below the standard for daily average level for PM_{10} of 150 μgm^{-3} in both the UK and the US. During August of 1997, similar peaks are seen in daily average exposures and again, there are notable extremes among the replicate values, at about or exceeding 50 μgm^{-3}.

Finally, Figure 13.4 shows the differential impact of a hypothetical 20% deflation termed 'rollback' of actual PM_{10} levels in the spring of 1997. The capacity of pCNEM to enable such 'scenario' analyzes proves to be one of

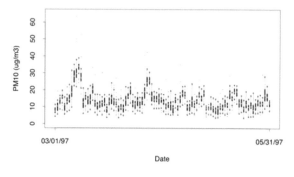

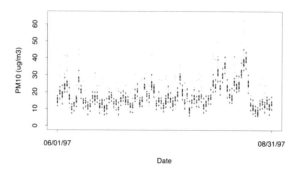

Figure 13.3: Box plots depict the estimated predictive distributions of particulate matter (PM_{10}) exposure in 1997 for a random member of a selected subpopulation of Londoners. Here, distributions are for average daily exposures. Both panels are for women who live in semi-detached Brent dwellings, work in Bloomsbury, smoke, and cook with gas. The top and bottom panels refer to spring and summer, respectively.

the program's most important features, giving regulators a way to check the impact of proposed changes on subpopulation groups. The deflated scenario values are set by the user and computed as the linear reduction, $baseline + p \times (x - baseline)$ for every hourly datum, x, for both Brent, the residential exposure district and Bloomsbury where they worked. In our example, the reduction factor and baseline were chosen somewhat arbitrarily to be p=0.8 and baseline = 15 μgm^{-3}. The result of the rollback in both summer and spring is similar, showing a reduction of a little less than 1 μgm^{-3}, although from differing baseline levels.

pCNEM, which was used for the analysis, is described in the previous example, remained freely available to online clients for use in their local areas for nearly two decades. But it had to be taken down in 2022 due to its age and lack of availability of suitable software upgrades. However, the principles involved in its creation live

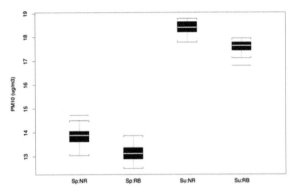

Figure 13.4: Boxplots compare the estimated predictive distributions of particulate matter (PM$_{10}$) exposure in 1997 for a random member of a selected subpopulation of Londoners. Here, distributions are for average daily exposures on spring and summer days for working females (labelled 'Sp' and 'Su' respectively) before ('NR') and after ('RB') a 20% rollback in (hourly) ambient levels. The women are smokers, use gas as a cooking fuel, live in a semi-detached dwelling in Brent and work in Bloomsbury.

on through online packages freely available from the US EPA. One of these, TRIM, is described on a freely available manual Post, Maier, and Mahoney (2007). The alternative called SHEDS is also available from the EPA Scientific Advisory Panel (2002).

13.7   Summary

This chapter contains a discussion of the differences between causality and associa-tion. It covers specific issues that may be encountered in this area when investigating the effects of environmental hazards on health. The reader will have gained an un-derstanding of the following topics:

- Issues with causality in observational studies.
- The Bradford-Hill criteria, which are a group of minimal conditions necessary to provide adequate evidence of a causal relationship;
- Ecological bias, which may occur when inferences about the nature of individuals are made based upon aggregated data;
- The role of exposure variability in determining the extent of ecological bias;
- Approaches to acknowledging ecological bias in ecological studies;
- Simpsons paradox and confounding as a roadblock to causality;

- Personal exposure and the difference between concentration and exposure response functions;
- Models for estimating personal exposures, based upon concentrations in different micro-environments.

13.8 Exercises

Exercise 13.1. For the model seen in 13.1 we are going to investigate the effect of transfer of causality with different levels of measurement error and collinearity.

(i) Write R code to perform the example shown in the text with $\alpha_0 = 0, \alpha_1 = 1$ and $Z \sim N(0,1), Z \sim N(0,1)$. Verify that with $\rho = 0.9$ the 'transfer' occurs when $\sigma_{v1} = 0.5$.

(ii) Investigate how this threshold changes with different levels of collinearity, that is different levels of ρ. Produce a graph of threshold against ρ.

(iii) Repeat the investigation performed in part (ii) for lower values of ρ. What do you conclude?

(iv) Investigate the effect that measurement error variance has in the 'transfer of causality'. What do you conclude?

Exercise 13.2. Using the model shown in Equation 13.18 if we assume that $\mathbf{Z}_{il} \sim N(\phi_{1l}, \Phi_{2l})$ mean function for the Poisson is

$$\mu_l = \exp(\beta_0 + \mathbf{X}_l^T \beta_x) \exp(\phi_{1k}^T \beta_z + \beta_z^T \Phi_{2l}.\beta_z/2).$$

Exercise 13.3. Again using the model shown in Equation 13.18, find the mean function if we assume the exposures are univariate and have distribution, $z_{il} \sim$ Gamma(ϕ_{1l}, Φ_{2l}), where (ϕ_{1l}, Φ_{2l}) represent the mean and variance of the exposure distribution.

Exercise 13.4. Return to the model shown in Equation 13.18.

(i) Why might it be difficult to use a log-normal distribution for exposures in the same way?

(ii) Show how a Taylor series expansion for $\mathbb{E}[\exp(\mathbf{Z}_{il}'\beta_z)|\beta, \phi_l]$ could be used in order to find the mean function where exposures are log-normally distributed.

Exercise 13.5. The exposures for individuals i in an area l may be correlated, for example if the exposure is spatially correlated and the exact locations of each individual are known. In this case $(Y_{il}^{(1)}, y_{jl}^{(1)})$ are still Bernoulli variables but are not independent, as the correlation in $(\mathbf{Z}_{il}, \mathbf{Z}_{jk})$ induces correlation into the health data. Therefore, the sum $Y_l^{(1)} = \sum_{i=1}^{n_l} Y_{il}^{(1)}$ is not a Binomial random variable.

(i) Find the mean and variance of $Y_l^{(1)}$.

(ii) Find the covariance of $Y_l^{(1)}$.

(iii) Under what circumstances will the covariance you found in part (iii) be zero?

Exercise 13.6. Develop an example like that in 13.2 with both multiway tables of integers and estimates in other tables of the selection probabilities for the associated cells.

Exercise 13.7. Prove Theorem 2.

Exercise 13.8. Show how Theorem 2 may be applied using an example.

Exercise 13.9. Prove Theorem 3.

Exercise 13.10. Show how Theorem 3 may be applied using an example.

Exercise 13.11. Extend Theorems 2 and 3 to cover the example in paper of (von Kügelgen et al., 2021).

Exercise 13.12. Reproduce the causal diagram in Example 13.3.

Exercise 13.13. Other examples are cited with data sources in von Kügelgen et al. (2021). Carry out assessment of the work cited in those examples and draw appropriate causal diagrams if appropriate.

Chapter 14

The quality of data: the importance of network design

14.1 Overview

The famous London fog of 1952 left no doubt about the human health risks associated with air pollution, and in particular airborne particulates. An estimated 4000 excess deaths were attributed to the fog Ministry of Health (1954), which was due to a considerable extent to coal combustion. The result was the general recognition that levels of air pollution should be regulated. This led to the Clean Air Acts of the United Kingdom (1956) and the United States (1970). These Acts set air quality standards whose enforcement required networks of monitors. By the early 1970s the UK had over 1200 monitoring sites measuring black smoke (BS) and sulfur dioxide (SO_2).

Mitigation measures, which included restrictions on the burning of coal, were successful and the levels of these pollutants declined over time. In turn, that led to the perception that the number of monitoring sites could be reduced. The process by which the sites were selected for elimination is undocumented, but empirical analysis of the results over time show that they tended be the ones at which the levels of BS were lowest Shaddick and Zidek (2014). The result was that the annual average level of BS in the UK was substantially overestimated Zidek, Shaddick, and Taylor (2014).

The analysis cited above for BS in the UK has not been repeated for other environmental monitoring networks but it is plausible that many of them were also adaptively changed over time with sites retained at locations with higher levels of the environmental hazard field Guttorp and Sampson (2010). These considerations highlight the importance of good data in statistical analysis, something that is commonly ignored by statistical analysts who use data without due regard to their quality. A primary determinant of that quality in environmental epidemiology is the representativeness of the monitoring site data, as the example described above makes clear. This chapter introduces the topic of designing, or redesigning, an environmental monitoring network. A recent handbook article provides a comprehensive overview of the topic Zidek and Zimmerman (2019).

Within this chapter, we explore issues arising and methods needed when designing environmental monitoring networks, with particular focus on ensuring that they

DOI: 10.1201/9781003352655-14

can provide the information that is required to assess the health impacts of an environmental hazard.

14.2 Design objectives?

Introductory courses on design of experiments emphasize the need to clearly articulate the objectives of the experiment as the first step in design. An example where this was done through a preliminary workshop convened by the contractor is seen in Example 12.1. There, the goal of the USA's National Oceanic and Atmospheric Agency (NOAA) was the detection of change in the concentration of trace metals in the seabed before and after the startup of exploratory drilling for oil on the north slopes of Alaska (Schumacher and Zidek, 1993). In other words, it was to test the hypothesis of no change. However, not all, possibly even very few, of the existing networks were designed in accordance with the ideal of meeting a specific objective. For those that were, the objective may have been so vague that it could not lead to a scientific approach to choosing specific locations for sampling sites. This section will give examples of important environmental monitoring networks and describe how they were established.

We begin by listing the myriad of purposes for which environmental monitoring networks have been established:

- Monitoring a process or medium such as drinking water to ensure quality or safety.
- Determining the environmental impact of an event, such as a policy-induced intervention or the closure of an emissions source.
- Detecting non-compliance with regulatory standards.
- Enabling health risk assessments to be made and to provide accurate estimates of relative risk.
- To determine how well sensitive subpopulations are protected, including all life, not only human.
- Issuing warnings of impending disaster.
- Measuring process responses at critical points, for example near a new smelter using arsenic or near an emitter of lead.

In other cases, the goals have been more technical in nature, even when the ultimate purpose concerned human health and welfare:

- Monitoring an easy-to-measure surrogate for a process or substance of real concern.
- Monitoring the extremes of a process.
- Enabling predictions of unmeasured responses.
- Enabling forecasts of future responses.
- Providing process parameter estimates for physical model parameters or stochastic model parameters, for example covariance parameters.
- Assessing temporal trends, for example assessing climate change.

As the examples that follow will show, a network's purpose may also change over time and its objectives may conflict with one another. For example, non-compliance detection suggests siting the monitors at the places where violations are seen as most likely to occur. However, an environmental epidemiologist would want to divide the sites equally between high- and low-risk areas in order to maximize contrasts and hence maximize the power of their health effects analyzes. Even objectives that seem well-defined, for example monitoring to detect extreme values of a process over a spatial domain, may lead to a multiplicity of objectives when it comes to implementation Chang, Fu, Le, and Zidek (2007).

As noted by Zidek and Zimmerman (2019), often many different variables of varying importance are to be measured at each monitoring site. To minimize cost, the network designer may elect to measure different variables at different sites. Further savings may accrue from making the measurements less frequently, forcing the designer to consider the inter-measurement times. In combination, these many choices lead to a bewildering set of objective functions to optimize simultaneously. That has led to the idea of designs based on multi-attribute theory, ones that optimize an objective function that embraces all the purposes (Zhu and Stein, 2006; Müller and Zimmerman, 1999).

However, such an approach will not be satisfactory for long-term monitoring programs when the network's future uses cannot be foreseen, as in the example described in Zidek, Sun, and Le (2000). Moreover, in some situations, the 'client' may not even be able to precisely specify the network's purposes (see for example, Ainslie, Reuten, Steyn, Le, and Zidek (2009)). As noted above, the high cost of network construction and maintenance will require the designer to select a defensible number of approaches that may provide such a justification.

Example 14.1. *The Metro Vancouver air quality network*

As with most modern urban areas in developed countries, Metro Vancouver, together with the Fraser Valley Regional District, operates an air quality monitoring network. Like many such networks, it was not planned as an integrated whole Ainslie et al. (2009) but instead grew without planned structure from a small initial nucleus of stations. Although it was seen from its inception as growing to enable monitoring air quality over the entire city and surrounding areas, there was no structure in the ways it would be expanded.

A redesign was undertaken in 2008 to develop a strategy that was consistent with the joint Air Quality Management Plan of Metro Vancouver and the Fraser Valley

The network included 27 ozone monitoring sites (stations) as well as sites for the other criteria air pollutants. Using the methods described in this chapter, the redesign analysis suggested a number of changes. One particular recommendation was that one suburban site was redundant and that it could profitably be relocated between the two most easterly sites in the Fraser Valley Ainslie et al. (2009). Overall, the redesign showed that the quality of the network could be improved at relatively low cost.

Even when an objective is prescribed for a network, meeting it may not be easy for both technical as well as conceptual reasons. For example, detecting non-compliance with regulations may be the objective of an urban network Guttorp and Sampson (2010). but interpreting that objective in a concrete, quantitative way can pose difficult conceptual challenges (Chang et al., 2007). For example, what does 'detecting non-compliance' actually mean? And what might be an optimal network design for that purpose during a three-year period might not be optimal for the next, depending on different climate regimes. How should a compromise be made between conflicting objectives?

Some networks were designed for one purpose, but developed to serve others. Some networks are a synthesis of networks that were set up at different times.

Example 14.2. *The CAPMoN Network*

During the 1980s, acid precipitation was deemed to be a serious problem worldwide because of its deleterious effects on the terrestrial as well as aquatic regions. Impacts were seen on fish and forest, for example, due to acids that were formed in the atmosphere during precipitation events and were then deposited on the earth's surface. This in turn had adverse effects on human welfare.

As a result, acid rain monitoring networks were established to monitor trends. The CAPMoN (Canadian Acid and Precipitation Monitoring Network) was one such network, however in reality it consisted of the union of three monitoring networks established at different times for various purposes Zidek et al. (2000); Ro et al. (1988); Sirois and Fricke (1992).

CAPMoN's history is particularly instructive (Zidek et al., 2000). It was established in 1978 with just three sites in remote areas but in 1983 its size increased when it was merged with the Air and Precipitation Network (APN). However, the merged network ended up with a second purpose; to trace source – receptor relationships in acid rain generation and monitoring sites were added close to urban areas. Later a third purpose was identified, that of discovering relationships between air pollution and human health (Burnett et al., 1994; Zidek et al., 1998)

This example shows us that the purpose of a network may not have been foreseen when it was established, and it may therefore not be optimal for its current purpose.

Example 14.3. *The Mercury Deposition Monitoring Network*

When ingested, mercury (Hg) is dangerous to human health. In general, it comes in three forms: elemental mercury, such as that found in thermometers and dental amalgams; organic mercury, mainly methyl mercury, found in foods such as fish; and non-elemental mercury, found in batteries and some disinfectants. The consumption of fish is a primary pathway for exposure to methyl mercury (MeHg), the most bioaccumulative form of mercury in humans and wildlife Schmeltz et al. (2011).

Mercury is a neurotoxin that can affect many areas of the brain, leading to diminished fine motor capacity and language. People exposed to mercury can develop acrodynia commonly known as pink disease whose symptoms include leg cramps, irritability, redness and the peeling of skin of the hands, nose and soles of the feet. Other symptoms include itching, fever, sweating, salivating, rashes including the 'baboon syndrome', which produces rashes in the buttocks, anal and genital regions, and sleeplessness. Mercury also has severe impacts on biota such as fish and birds.

Concern about toxicity of mercury in all its forms led to the establishment in the US Clean Air Act Amendments of 1990 (CAA) of section 112(n)(1)(B) that requires the U.S. EPA to study the impacts of mercury air pollution.

That, and the recognition of the serious human health risk associated with mercury, led to the establishment of MercNet. This is a multi-objective National US network that embraces a number of monitoring programs, notably the Mercury Deposition Network (MDN). The latter, working under the aegis of the National Atmospheric Deposition Network (NADP), consists of the monitoring site locations depicted in Figure 14.1. Data were obtained from the NADP site concerned with Atmospheric Hg is deposited on the earth's

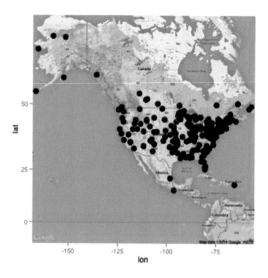

Figure 14.1: Locations of the sites maintained in the United States to monitor atmospheric deposition of mercury. The metadata containing these locations were obtained from National Atmospheric Deposition Program (NRSP-3), 2007, NADP Program Office, Illinois State Water Survey, Nation2204 Griffith Dr., Champaign, IL 61820.

surface through precipitation and is a major source of mercury in the environment. As originally conceived, MercNet would provide a comprehensive multi-objective mercury network that would amongst other things enable the development, calibration, and refinement of predictive mercury models to guide effective management Schmeltz et al. (2011).

14.3   Design paradigms

The spatial domain in which the monitors are to be sited is denoted by $\mathscr{S}$ and it can be treated as either a continuum or a discrete set, the latter commonly being chosen due to practical considerations. The potential sites $s \in D$ could be points on a regular or irregular grid. They could mark features in a geographical region, such as rivers, that could be selected for chemical assessment. (See Example 14.10 below.) They could be centroids of grid cells to be sampled. The process $Z = Z_s$ to be monitored over time and space is parametrized by those points. The network designer is required to specify a finite set of points at which monitors are to be placed. In the Le – Zidek approach Le and Zidek (2006) in a multivariate setting, each site s is equipped with a small, finite set of pseudo-site locations where individual monitors can be placed. The design problem becomes one of deciding at which pseudo-sites gauges (monitors) should be placed, and the choice to a considerable extent is subjective.

Example 14.4. *The acid deposition monitoring network*

The National Atmospheric Deposition Network, referred to above, stipulates that when siting network monitors:

'The COLLECTOR should be installed over undisturbed land on its standard 1 – meter – high aluminum base. Naturally vegetated, level areas are preferred, but grassed areas and up or down slopes up to 15% will be tolerated. Sudden changes in slope within 30 meters of the collector should also be avoided. Ground cover should surround the collector for a distance of approximately 30 meters. In farm areas, a vegetated buffer strip must surround the collector for at least 30 meters.'

Most design strategies fall into one of three categories or 'paradigms' (Le and Zidek, 2006; Müller, 2007; Dobbie, Henderson, and Stevens Jr, 2008), which we describe in the next three sections. The first are the geometry-based designs. These sites are selected from the population $\mathscr{S}$ without reference to the responses indexed by $\mathscr{S}$ that are to be measured. The second category are the probability-based designs, the domain of the survey sampler. Like the geometry-based designs, these are selected by randomly sampling from the list $\mathscr{S}$, again without reference to the process $\mathscr{S}$ or the joint distribution of those processes. Finally, we have the model-based designs, where now the joint distribution of the $\{Z_s\}$ responses over $\mathscr{S}$ is taken into account. Thus, for example, these designs will tend not to pick sites that are geographically close to one another. Here the focus may be parameters, as for example the coefficients in a model that relates covariates to the process. Or it may be on prediction, as was the case for most designs developed in geostatistics over the past half century.

14.4   Geometry-based designs

This approach seems to be based on the heuristic idea of covering a region and would have included things like corner points of a grid spread over a region as well as space-filling designs Nychka and Saltzman (1998). Müller (2007) points to their use when the purpose of the network is exploratory, while Cox, Cox, and Ensor (1997) rationalize this choice for multi-objective analysis.

Example 14.5. *Redesigning a freshwater monitoring network*

Olea (1984) performed an interesting simulation study to find an optimal geo-metric sampling plan in a geostatistical setting where prediction performance through universal kriging was the criterion for assessing network quality. Their result showed sites arranged in hexagonal patterns proved best among the twelve geometric patterns he considered. He used his result to redesign the network for monitoring the freshwater levels in the Equus Beds of Kansas. The original design, which was not the result of careful planning, proved quite unsatisfactory judged by the criteria they used.

Example 14.6. *Space-filling design*

Royle and Nychka (1998) give an algorithm for finding the optimum space-filling design. Given a set $S \subset D$ as a proposed set of monitoring points define the distance from a point $s \in D$ to S to be

$$d_p(s,D) = \left(\sum_{s' \in S} \| s - s' \|^p \right)^{1/p}$$

Then the overall coverage criterion is given by

$$C_{p,q}(S) = \left(\sum_{s \in D} d_p(s,D)^q \right)^{1/q}$$

The (sub-) optimal design is found using a point swapping algorithm: given a starting set S, visit each of S's points in successive steps; at any given step replace the point in S with one not in S and keep it if and only if it improves (reduces) the coverage criterion; go on to the next point in S and repeat the search for an improvement using points not in S including those that have been dumped in an earlier round; continue until convergence.

Royle and Nychka (1998) apply their algorithm to an ozone network in the city of Chicago. They impose a grid of 720 candidate sites over the City, excluding points in Lake Michigan but located in the convex hull of the existing sites. In their first analysis, analysis, they reduce the existing network of 21 down to 5, by picking the best space-filling subset using the coverage criterion. Notice that no ozone data are required for this analysis.

The space-filling approach to design is very appealing due to its simplicity. It is also robust, since unlike other approaches, it does not rely on data from the environmental fields and associated stochastic modeling.

14.5   Probability-based designs

This approach to design goes back at least half a century and is now widely used for such things as public opinion polling. This is the domain of the 'survey sampler'. The approach has appeal due to its apparent objectivity, since the sample is drawn purely at random from a list of the population elements, the *sampling frame*. Designers need not know anything about the population distribution to complete that process, except possibly for optimizing the sample size.

In our application, the sampling frame would consist of the elements s of the finite population $\mathscr{S}$. The responses of interest would be the $\{Z_s\}$ at a specific time (or possibly a sequence of responses over time) depending on the nature of the inquiry. However, these would not be considered random, even if they were unknown. The survey assisted approach to survey sample assumes that $\mathscr{S}$ itself is a random sample from a superpopulation and that therefore the $\{Z_s\}$ have a joint probability distribution whose unknown parameter vector θ would itself be unknown. And the unknown 'estimate' of θ would then be regarded as a population 'parameter'.

Example 14.7. *Superpopulation modeling*

Suppose $D = \{s_1, \ldots, s_N\}$ so that the population is of unknown size N. Assume the $Z_i = Z_{s_i} = (Y_i, X_i)$, $i = 1, \ldots, N$ are drawn independently of the superpopulation each element having a bivariate normal distribution with $\mu_{1\cdot2} = E(Y_i \mid X_i)\alpha + \beta X_i$ while $\sigma_{1\cdot2} = Var(Y_i \mid X_i) = \sigma_Y(1 - \rho^2)$. Then it is easily shown that the maximum likelihood estimator for β would be

$$\hat{\beta} = \frac{\Sigma_i Y_i X_i}{\Sigma_i X_i X_i} \qquad (14.1)$$

The sample $\tilde{d}$ from $\mathscr{S}$ would now yield the data needed to estimate $\hat{\beta}$ and yield $\hat{\hat{\beta}}$, an estimate of the 'estimate'.

The superpopulation helps define the relevant finite population parameters. They would commonly be linear functions of $\{Z_s\}$, such as the average pollution level for a given year, $\bar{Z} = \Sigma_{s \in S} Z_s / N_S$ where N_S denotes the number of elements in S. Or they may be combinations of linear functions, as in Equation 14.1.

However, these so-called *population parameters* are unknown and need to be estimated and hence a sample needs to be selected from $\mathscr{S}$. The probability-based sample design is specified by the probabilities of selecting a random sample say $\tilde{d} \subset D$, that is by the list $\{P(\tilde{d} = s) : d \subset D\}$. Of particular importance are the selection probabilities $\pi_s = P(s \in \tilde{d})$. Equiprobability sampling would mean $\pi_s \equiv K$ for some constant K. Note $\sum_{s \in D} \pi_s \neq 1$ in general, but they can be used to enable inference in complex sampling designs as seen in the following examples.

Example 14.8. *Simple random sampling*

In simple random sampling (SRS) n elements, $\tilde{d}$ are selected without replacement at random from the total of N elements in the sampling frame $\mathscr{S}$ in such a way that $\pi_s = n/N$. The responses Z_s would then be measured for the elements $s \in \tilde{d}$. In our applications, these elements would commonly be site locations.

Example 14.9. *Stratified random samples*

This approach can be very effective when $\mathscr{S}$ can be stratified into subsets $\mathscr{S}_j$, $j = 1, \ldots, J$ with $\mathscr{S} = \cup \mathscr{S}_j$ where the responses are thought to be quite similar within the $\mathscr{S}_j$. In an extreme case, suppose all the elements in $\mathscr{S}_j$ were identical. Then you would need to sample only one element in that strata to gain all the available information. More generally, the expectation is that only a small SRS of size n_j would need to be taken from each $\mathscr{S}_j$, with its subpopulation total N_j, to get a good picture of the population of Z responses for all of $\mathscr{S}$. Thus, in SRS sampling $\pi_\mathbf{S} = n_j/N_j$, $\mathbf{s} \in \mathscr{S}_j$, $j = 1, \ldots, J$.

To complete this discussion, we turn to inference and the Horwitz – Thompson (HT) estimator. Consider first the case of a population parameter of the form, $\hat{\theta} = \sum_{s \in \mathscr{S}} \omega_s Z_s$ where the ωs are known constants. Then the HT estimator is defined by

$$\hat{\theta}_{HT} = \sum_{s \in \tilde{d}} \omega_s Z_s / \pi_\mathbf{S} \qquad (14.2)$$

An important property of the HT estimator is its design-unbiasedness:

$$E\left[\hat{\theta}_{HT}\right] = \hat{\theta} \qquad (14.3)$$

where the expectation in Equation 14.3 is taken over all possible $\tilde{d}$ (see Exercise 14.6).

However, the population parameter may not be a linear function of the process responses Z. If it is a function of such linear combinations as in Example 14.7 then the HT estimator can be used to estimate each of the linear combinations; these will then be unbiased estimators of their population level counterparts, even if the function of

them, which defines the parameter, is not. In other words, in Example 14.7 we would
get

$$\hat{\beta} = \frac{\sum_i Y_i X_i / \pi_i}{\sum_i X_i X_i / \pi_i} \tag{14.4}$$

that is not a design unbiased estimator, unlike the numerator and denominator that
are.

Probability-based designs have been used in designing environmental sampling
plans. The US EPA's Environmental Monitoring and Assessment Program, which
ran from 1990 to 2006, was concerned with ecological risk and environmental risk.
Example 14.10 illustrates the use of probability-based design in a situation where
other approaches would be difficult to use.

Example 14.10. *The National Stream Survey*

The National Stream Survey was carried out as part of the US EPA's National
Surface Water Survey. The survey sought to characterize the water chemistry
of streams in the United States, 26 quantitative physical and chemical variables being of interest Mitch (1990). The elements of target population $\mathscr{S}$
were 'stream reaches' defined as Stehman and Overton (1994) the segment of
a stream between two confluences or, in the case of a headwaters reach, the
segment between the origin of a stream and the first confluence (with some
additional technical restrictions). A confluence is a point at which two or more
streams flow together. Sampling units were selected using a square dot grid
with a density of 1 grid point per 64 square miles, which was imposed (via
a transparent acetate sheet) on a 1:250,000 scale topographical map. A reach
was included if a grid point fell into its watershed, meaning that the selection
probability for a reach was proportional to the area of that watershed. In other
words, if we denote by X_s the area of the watershed s and $X.$ the population
total of these X's (Stehman and Overton, 1994)

$$\pi_s = n \frac{X_s}{X.} \tag{14.5}$$

Much more complex examples may be used as in multi-stage sampling where
primary units, for example urban areas, are selected at stage one, with secondary
units (e.g. dwelling units) at stage two and tertiary units (e.g. an individual within
the dwelling unit) at stage three. The selection probabilities may still be found in
such situations.

We have now seen some of the advantages of the probability-based sampling
approach. However, these can also be seen as some of the disadvantages in that some
implicit modeling will be required. For example, choosing the strata effectively will
require having enough information to be able to pick homogeneous strata. Modeling
can be seen as a good thing in that it enables the analyst to bring a body of background knowledge to the problem; knowledge whose inclusion probability sampling

would restrict or exclude altogether. Finally, while stratified sampling has the advantage of forcing the sampling sites to be spread out over an area, you could still end up in the awkward situation of having two sites right next to each other across a strata boundary. These shortcomings have led to the development of model-based alternatives.

14.6   Model-based designs

Broadly speaking, model-based designs optimize some form of inference about the process or its model parameters. This section will present a number of those approaches. There are two main categories of design theory of this type:

- Parameter estimation approaches.
- Random fields approaches.

We begin by looking at parameter estimation approaches.

14.6.1   Regression parameter estimation

This approach was developed outside the framework of spatial design, and so we focus more generally on optimizing the fitting of regression models. This topic has a long history and was developed for continuous sampling domains (Smith, 1918; Elfving et al., 1952; Kiefer, 1959). The result was an elaborate theory for design that differed greatly from the established theory of the time. That new theory was pioneered by Silvey (1980); Fedorov and Hackl (1997); Müller (2007).

Example 14.11. *An optimal design for regression*
Consider a dataset that consists of a fixed number n of vectors (x_i, y_i), $i = 1, \dots, n$ that are assumed to be independent realizations of $(x, Y) \in [a, b] \times (-\infty, \infty)$ where the x's are chosen by the experimenter while Y is generated by the model

$$Y = \alpha + \beta x + \varepsilon \qquad (14.6)$$

where α and β are unknown parameters and ε has zero mean and variance σ_ε^2. The least squares estimate of β is given by

$$\hat{\beta} = \frac{\sum_i (x_i - \bar{x})((y_i - \bar{y}))}{\sum_i (x_i - \bar{x})^2} \qquad (14.7)$$

How should the experimenter choose the x's?

The answer is to ensure that the accuracy of $\hat{\beta}$ is maximized, that is its standard error (*se*) is minimized. Conditional on the unknown parameters, that *se* is the square root of

$$Var(\hat{\beta}) = \frac{\sigma_\varepsilon^2}{\sum_i (x_i - \bar{x})^2} \qquad (14.8)$$

Obviously the optimal strategy is to put half of the x's at either end of their range $[a,b]$, a result that can be substantially generalized in spatial sampling (Schumacher and Zidek, 1993).

14.7 An entropy-based approach

So far we have described a number of approaches to designing networks where a specific objective, such as parameter estimation, can be prescribed. However, in our experience, most major networks are not planned for a single purpose. Instead, the purpose may be too ill-defined to yield a specific quantitative objective function to be maximized. There may be a multiplicity of purposes or the purpose, or purposes, may be unforeseen. The conundrum here is that despite those challenges, the designer may need to provide and justify specific monitoring site locations.

One way forward recognizes that most networks have a fairly fundamental purpose of reducing uncertainty about some aspect of the random environmental process of interest, unknown parameters or unmeasured responses, for example. This uncertainty can be reduced or eliminated by measuring the quantities of interest. An entropy-based approach provides a unified, general approach to optimizing a network's design. Chapter 3 gives the foundation needed to develop that theory, which has a long history, including general theory (Good, 1952; Lindley, 1956) and applications to network design (Shewry and Wynn, 1987; Caselton and Zidek, 1984; Caselton et al., 1992; Sebastiani and Wynn, 2002; Zidek et al., 2000).

The entropy approach is implemented within a Bayesian framework. To explain the approach in a specific case, assume the designer's interest lies in the process response vector Z one time step into the future where T denotes the present time, $T+1$ for all sites in $\mathscr{S}$, that is monitored and unmonitored (i.e. gauged and ungauged in alternate terminology).

For simplicity, let $\mathscr{D}$ denote the set of all available data upon which to condition and get posterior distributions. Entropy also requires that we specify h_1 & h_2 as baseline reference densities against which to measure uncertainty. With H denoting the entropy and θ the process parameters, define with expectation being conditional on $\mathscr{D}$ and taken over both the unknown Z and θ:

$$
\begin{aligned}
H(\mathbf{Z} \mid \theta) &= E[-\log(p(\mathbf{Z} \mid \theta, \mathscr{D})/h_1(\mathbf{Z}) \mid \mathscr{D}] \\
H(\theta) &= E[-\log(p(\theta \mid \mathscr{D})/h_2(\tilde{\theta})) \mid \mathscr{D}]
\end{aligned}
$$

Finally, we may restate the fundamental identity in Equation 3.6 as

$$
H(\mathbf{Z}, \theta) = H(\mathbf{Z} \mid \theta) + H(\theta) \tag{14.9}
$$

Example 14.12. *Elements of the entropy decomposition in the Gaussian case*

Assume that the process in Equation 14.9 has been non-dimensionalized along with its unknown distribution parameters in θ. Then we may take

$h_1 = h_2 \equiv 1$ (although there would be more judicious choices perhaps in some applications). Furthermore, assume the $\mathscr{S}$ consists of a single point $\mathscr{S} = \{1\}$. We assume the response at time t at this site, Z_{1t} is measured without error so that $Z_{1t} = Y_{1t}$. We now adopt the assumptions made in Example 5.1. Moreover, conditional on the unknown mean θ and known variance σ^2, they $Y_{1t} \sigma N(\theta, \sigma^2)$, $t = 1, \ldots, T$ are independently observed to yield the dataset $\mathscr{D} = \{y_{11}, \ldots, y_{1T}\}$ with mean $\hat{y}$. A conjugate prior is assumed so that

$$\theta \sim N(\theta_0, \sigma_0^2) \tag{14.10}$$

The posterior distribution for θ is found to be

$$\theta \sim N(\hat{\theta}_{Bayes}, \sigma_1^2) \tag{14.11}$$

where $\hat{\theta} = w\hat{y} + (1-w)\theta_0$, $\sigma_1^2 = [w\sigma^2 n^{-1}]$ and $w = \sigma_0^2(\sigma_0^2 + \sigma^2/n)$. At the same time $-\log p(Z \mid \theta, \mathscr{D} = -\log p(Y \mid \theta) = -n/[2\sigma^2](\theta - \hat{y})^2 + \ldots$ where we have ignored for now some known additive constants.

We can now compute the first term in Equation 14.9, call it T_1 for short, as

$$
\begin{aligned}
T_1 &= \frac{n}{2}\left[\frac{\sigma_1^2}{\sigma^2} + \frac{(\hat{\theta}_{Bayes} - \hat{y})^2}{\sigma^2} + \right. \\
&\quad \left. \log 2\pi\sigma^2 + \frac{s^2}{\sigma^2}\right]
\end{aligned}
\tag{14.12}
$$

where s^2 denotes the sample variance (calculated by dividing by n rather than $(n-1)$. The second term in Equation 14.9, call it, T_2 is given by

$$T_2 = \frac{1}{2}[1 + \log 2\pi\sigma_1^2] \tag{14.13}$$

Thus, Equation 14.9 reduces to,

$$T = T_1 + T_2 \tag{14.14}$$

where we denote the total uncertainty $H(Z, \theta)$ by T. A number of sources of uncertainty contribute to the total uncertainty (while recalling that we have rescaled the responses/parameters a priori to eliminate the units of measurement). First, when we look at T_1 we see that if we ignore additive constants, it is essentially the expected squared prediction error incurred were θ to be used to predict the uncertain future, Y, the log likelihood is essentially $(Y - \theta)^2$, whose expectation is being computed. However, we don't know θ, which adds to the uncertainty in T_1. The result is that our uncertainty grows if the following apply:

- The known sampling variance σ^2 is large, although that effect is relatively small since its logarithm is being taken.

- The sample variance proves much larger than the supposedly known sampling variance σ^2, almost as though that prior knowledge is being assessed.
- The posterior mean and sample mean differ a lot relative to the natural variance of the sample mean σ^2/n.
- A large component of w comes from the prior variance σ_0^2 meaning the designer is not sure of his prior opinions about the value of the predictor θ of Y, this same uncertainty will inflate T_2 as well.

In summary, even in this simple example, the uncertainty as discussed in Chapter 3 is complex, even without taking model uncertainty into consideration.

14.7.1   The design of a network

We now consider the design of a network. Assume for simplicity $Y = Z$ is measurable without error and take the network's design goal to be that of adding or subtracting sites. We focus on adding new sites to an existing network to reduce uncertainty in an optimal way at time $T + 1$. We now have all the data $\mathscr{D}$ up to the present time T and we have the sites that provided it. We will be adding new sites and these as well as current sites will provide measurements at time $T + 1$, that will help us predict the measurable but unmeasured responses at the sites that will not be gauged at that time. The question is how do we choose the sites to add.

The total future uncertainty will be the total entropy TOT by $H[\mathbf{Y}_{(T+1)}, \theta \mid \mathscr{D}]$. We can partition the response vector as follows

$$\mathbf{Y}_{(T+1)}\mathbf{Y}_{(T+1)} = (\mathbf{Y}_{(T+1)}^{(1)}, \mathbf{Y}_{(T+1)}^{(2)}) \qquad (14.15)$$

where $\mathbf{Y}_{(T+1)}^{(1)}$ and $\mathbf{Y}_{(T+1)}^{(2)}$ are respectively, the responses corresponding to the sites that are not and are currently monitored. The sites without monitors need to split into two groups, corresponding to the ones which will be gauged and those that will not. After relabeling them, this will correspond to a partition of the vector of responses $\mathbf{Y}_{(T+1)}^{(1)} = (\mathbf{Y}_{(T+1)}^{(rem)}, \mathbf{Y}_{(T+1)}^{(add)})$, $\mathbf{Y}_{(T+1)}^{(rem)}$ and $\mathbf{Y}_{(T+1)}^{(add)}$ being respectively the responses at sites that will remain ungauged and those will be added to the existing network and yield measurements at time $T + 1$.

Let's simplify notation by letting

$$\mathbf{U} = \mathbf{Y}_{(T+1)}^{(rem)}, \; \mathbf{G} = (\mathbf{Y}_{(T+1)}^{(add)}, \mathbf{Y}_{(T+1)}^{(2)}), \; \mathbf{Y}_{(T+1)} = [\mathbf{U}, \mathbf{G}] \qquad (14.16)$$

Then we get a revised version of the fundamental identity:

$$\boxed{\text{TOT} = \text{PRED} + \text{MODEL} + \text{MEAS}}$$

where

$$
\begin{aligned}
PRED &= E[-\log(f(\mathbf{U} \mid \mathbf{G}, \theta, \mathscr{D})/h_{11}(\mathbf{U})) \mid \mathscr{D}] & (14.17) \\
MODEL &= E[-\log(f(\theta \mid \mathbf{G}, \mathscr{D})/h_2(\theta)) \mid \mathscr{D}] & (14.18)
\end{aligned}
$$

and

$$MEAS = E[-\log(f(\mathbf{G} \mid \mathscr{D})/\mathbf{h_{12}}(\mathbf{G})) \mid \mathscr{D}] \qquad (14.19)$$

Here TOT denotes the total amount of uncertainty. The identity states that it has three components. The first PRED is the residual uncertainty in the field after it has been predicted. The predictor involves the uncertain process parameter vector θ, so that also is reflected in PRED. MOD represents model uncertainty due to its unknown parameters. An extended version of this identity could include model uncertainty, and given the model, for example Gaussian, the parameter uncertainty for the model. Finally, MEAS is the amount of uncertainty that would be removed from TOT simply by measuring the random field at the monitoring sites. We immediately see the remarkable result that maximizing MEAS through judicious selection of the sites will simultaneously minimize the combination of uncertainties about the unmonitored sites in the field as well as the model. Since the total uncertainty TOT is fixed, this decomposition must hold, no matter which sites we decide to monitor.

Finding entropy – optimal designs

The following material is included for completeness to briefly describe one way of creating an optimal design.The foundations of the approach are those underlying the the BSP method (Chapter 12, Section 12.5) and the EnviroStat package. The latter includes a function for finding entropy-based optimal designs whose use will be described in Example 14.14.

The BSP assumes that in an initial step, the process is transformed and prefiltered by removing regional level spatio-temporal components. These would include things like trend and periodicity, along with regional autocorrelation. These are commonly the largest source of variation. Furthermore, since a single parameter set is fitted for all sites, the standard errors of estimation for these parameters will be essentially negligible. Yet, most of the trend and autocorrelation may be taken out of the process spatio-temporal mean field, leaving the site-specific parameters much less work to do. The entropy, however, will be unaffected as it is determined by the stochastic variation in the residuals.

For completeness, we briefly describe the BSP model for the residuals process, which we denote by Y rather than Z. This is because the previous steps remove the same mean model across all sites, making the residual process observable by subtracting it from the measurements at the monitored sites.

The important result is the posterior predictive distribution for the unmeasured responses, as this is needed to find PRED above Le and Zidek (2006). We use once again the notation $\mathscr{D}$ to represent the totality of data. The notation $\mathscr{H}$ is used to represent the set of all hyperparameters, of which there are many. The latter are estimated by maximizing the marginal likelihood as an empirical Bayes step in fitting the model, in order to reduce computation times. The superscript u will refer below to an ungauged site, while the superscript g will refer to an observation at a gauged site. The general version of the BSP, which is included in EnviroStat allows a (monotone) staircase pattern in the data matrix. There the superscript g_m is attached to responses at gauged sites that go unmeasured, and these too are part of the predictive distribution. This staircase pattern is commonly seen due to the variable start or termination dates of the sites in a network (Shaddick and Zidek, 2014; Zidek, Shaddick, and Taylor, 2014). They are sometimes important due to the need to reconstruct exposure histories of subjects involved in the study of the chronic effects of exposure to environmental hazards. An example is the study of the relationship between air pollution and cancer. The latter has a long latency period, so Le and Zidek (2010) used the BSP to infer those long-term exposures of patients in a cancer register. The result did not show a significant result, although the measurement error in such a study would be large, greatly reducing the power to detect an association.

However, for instructional purposes, we are going to present the simplest version of the model – no staircase and just one response per site – not the multivariate version of the BSP. This models the random response field over the time period, $1, \ldots, (T+1)$ the last of these time points being one time step into the future. This is the model proposed by Zidek et al. (2000):

$$\mathbf{Y}^{(T+1) \times p} \mid \beta, \Sigma \sim N_p(\mathbf{X}^{(T+1) \times k} \beta^{k \times p}, I_{(T+1)} \otimes \Sigma)$$

$$\beta \mid \Sigma, \beta_0, F \sim N(\beta_0, \mathbf{F}^{-1} \otimes \Sigma) \qquad (14.20)$$

$$\Sigma \sim IW(\Phi, \delta) \text{ \# Inverted Wishart distribution}$$

where k denotes the number of covariates at each time point. Here the notation of Dawid (1981) is used for the inverted Wishart (IW) distribution, which is replaced by the generalized inverted Wishart (GIW) distribution in the general theory (Brown, Le, and Zidek, 1994) The distribution theory that is required for this can be found in Appendix A. Note that the β matrix represents the site-specific effects that the covariates have, after removing the regional version which is embedded in β_0. The model is more flexible than it appears at first glance. For example, monthly effects can be represented by eleven indicator variables in X as covariates to capture seasonality. In that case, a column of the B matrix for a site at location s can represent the impact of different months on different sites. Those near the mountain would respond differently in winter to those near the sea. The regional model would not capture that difference.

The posterior predictive distributions we need for $\mathbf{U}^{1 \times u}$ and $\mathbf{G}^{1 \times g}$ as defined above in Equation 14.16, given the data to time T $\mathscr{D}$ are (Le and Zidek, 1992; Le and Zidek, 2006)

$$\mathbf{G} \mid \mathscr{D} \quad \sim \quad t_g\left(\mu^g, \frac{c}{l}\hat{\Phi}, l\right)$$

$$\mathbf{U} \mid \mathbf{G} = \mathbf{g}, \mathscr{D} \quad \sim \quad t_u\left(\mu^u, \frac{d}{q}\Phi_{u|g}, q\right). \qquad (14.21)$$

The product of the distributions in Equation 14.21 yields the joint distribution of all responses at time $T+1$. We see in that equation, a lot of undefined symbols.

It turns out we do not need to know them. For a start it can be shown that for any multivariate normal random variable with covariance $\Sigma \sim IW(\Phi, \delta)$ must have entropy of a remarkably simple form, that of the -multivariate-t distribution (Caselton et al., 1992)

$$\frac{1}{2} \log | \Phi | + c \tag{14.22}$$

with a known constant c whose value is irrelevant. Our design goal is to add sites to the existing sites to maximize the entropy of the resulting network's response $\mathbf{G}$–that will make maximizing the uncertainty we remove by measurement at time $T + 1$. After permuting coordinates appropriately, we may partition $\mathbf{G}$ as $(\mathbf{G}^{add}, \mathbf{G}^{original})$. Elementary probability tells us that we write the joint distribution $[\mathbf{G}]$ as the product of the joint distribution $[\mathbf{G}^{original}]$ and the conditional distribution $[\mathbf{G}^{add} | \mathbf{G}^{original}]$. However, Equation 14.21 shows that each of these distributions will have a multivariate-t distribution. Moreover, taking logarithms of the product of the densities leads to the sum of their logarithms. In other words,

$$H(\mathbf{G} \mid \mathscr{D}) = H(\mathbf{G}^{add} \mid \mathbf{G}^{original}, \mathscr{D}) + H(\mathbf{G}^{original} \mid \mathscr{D}) \tag{14.23}$$

The second term in Equation 14.23 is fixed — those sites are not to be removed. Thus, to maximize MEAS, in other words, $H(\mathbf{G} \mid \mathscr{D})$ means maximizing $H(\mathbf{G}^{add} \mid \mathbf{G}^{original}, \mathscr{D})$. In other words, the responses for the add sites should be the ones that are least predictable from $\mathbf{G}^{original}$ and hence maximally uncertain. As noted above that conditional distribution must be a multivariate-t and hence its entropy must be of the form given in Equation 14.22, in other words,

$$H(\mathbf{G}^{add} \mid \mathbf{G}^{original}, \mathscr{D}) = \frac{1}{2} | \Phi_{add|original} | + c* \tag{14.24}$$

where in an obvious notation

$$\Phi_{add|original} = \Sigma_{add,add} - \Sigma_{add,original} \Sigma_{original,original}^{-1} \Sigma_{original,add}$$

the Φ being that which appears in the inverted Wishart prior as a matrix of hyperparameters.

This matrix can be specified in a variety of ways, but in line with our empirical Bayes approach, EnviroStat estimates it for the data at the original sites using a maximum likelihood approach . For a staircase data pattern, the EM algorithm needs to be employed due to the missing data (Le and Zidek, 2006). This estimate can then be extended to the entire network of sites $\mathscr{S}$ by fitting a spatial semivariogram and using this to determine the missing elements of Φ. That second step may require use of the Sampson–Guttorp method to address field non-stationarity. We will see this approach in Example 14.13.

Example 14.13. *Redesign of Metro-Vancouver's PM$_{10}$ network*

Le and Zidek (2006) present a case study which anticipates the redesign described in Example 14.1 although they had no forewarning of it. It is concerned with Metro Vancouver's air quality monitoring sites as seen in Figure 14.2. Purely as a hypothetical case study, 10 PM$_{10}$ sites scattered

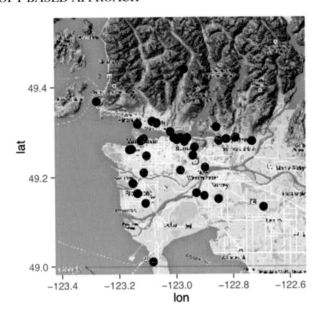

Figure 14.2: Locations of the sites maintained in the Lower Mainland of British Columbia, Canada to monitor the air quality in the region. Notice the topography of the region, which in summer combines with the prevailing wind from the west to push the pollution cloud eastward into the Fraser valley. Ten of the sites were selected in a hypothetical redesign of the PM_{10} network as described in the text.

through the region were chosen as a network, to which an additional 6 sites were to be added from 20 potential sites located in census tracts with relatively large populations. The entropy-based approach was used with an interesting result.

Their study used the approach described above and described in the vignette accompanying the EnviroStat package for network design. After transforming and prefiltering the data, a posterior predictive distributive distribution was created as described above. The Sampson–Guttorp approach Sampson and Guttorp (1992) had to be applied and the estimated hypercovariance for the field of all 30 sites estimated with its help (an exponential semi-variogram was used).

They began by ranking the 20 potential sites by the size of the posterior variance of their future PM_{10} concentrations and labelling the sites from [1] to [20], site [20] being the one with the largest variance. They then applied the greedy algorithm to find, one-by-one, the best 6 sites as far as uncertainty reduction was concerned and labelled these from (1) to (6), where (1) being the single site that reduces uncertainty the most.

The results were quite interesting. The site (1) chosen for first place was not a surprise, its posterior variance was large placing it second from the top, giving it a label of [19] according to the variance ranking and hence its measurements were quite uncertain. A lot could be gained by making measurements there. The next five best choices had variance ranks [18], [20], [10], [16] and [17]. Things went more or less as expected as sites (1) to (3) were picked, but then we see an abrupt divergence, site [10] gets selected for inclusion in the 'add' set. Why is that? The answer is that the entropy recognizes that once (1)–(3) have been included, more information could be gained from the variance ranked site [10] than from any of the sites [17]–[11]. It turned out that [10] was on the edge of the network and so able to provide information not available from other sites. Curiously, this is close to the site that was chosen in the redesign described in Example 14.1. These results show the subtlety of the entropy criterion in the way it picks its optimal sites.

14.7.2   Redesigning networks

In this subsection, we will see step-by-step how to redesign an existing network. The approach in the example follows that of the vignette for the EnviroStat package, used here since it includes a function for warping to achieve non-stationarity as well as one for entropy-based design.

Example 14.14. *Adding temperature monitoring sites in California*

This example follows Example 10.5 and concerns what may be increasingly seen as an environmental hazard, as discussed in that example. We have simplified the modeling of the field for this illustrative example. In fact, finding good spatio-temporal models is challenging and the subject of current research Kleiber, Katz, and Rajagopalan (2013).

We begin by plotting the locations of the 18 temperature monitoring sites we selected for this example. The ultimate goal is that of adding 5 additional sites to this network we have artificially created. First, we need to load the necessary libraries along with the necessary data. Then we plot the 18 sites that constitute the 'current' network.

```
### The libraries
library(EnviroStat)
library(sp)
library(rgdal)
library(ggmap)

### The data
dat <- read.csv("MaxCaliforniaTemp.csv", header=T)
crs.org <-   read.table("metadataCA.txt", header=T)
```

```
### Now we plot the sites
Cal.sp = crs.org
coordinates(Cal.sp) = ~Long+Lat
proj4string(Cal.sp) = CRS("+proj=longlat
        +ellps=WGS84")
latLongBox = bbox(Cal.sp)
location = c(-126, 32, -114, 42)
CaliforniaMap = get_map(location = location, source
        = "google", maptype = "roadmap")
CaliforniaMap = ggmap(CaliforniaMap)
CaliforniaMap = CaliforniaMap +
        geom_point(data = metadata,
        aes(x = Long, y = Lat), size = 3, col = 2)
        + xlab("Longitude") + ylab("Latitude")
```

We see the result in Figure 14.3, a set of sites selected to cover the State. The datasets consist of two files. The first (metadataCA.txt) is the metadata for the 17 sites: elevations above sea level (feet); geographic coordinates (latitude, longitude); (in the two right-hand most columns for each site) a reference point's coordinates on the west coast of California that are closest to the site to enable a calculation of its distance from the ocean. The second (MaxTempCalifornia.csv) gives the maximum daily temperatures for those sites from 1 Jan 2012 to 30 Dec 2012. For convenience, we divide 2012 into 13 'months' of 28 days each by dropping days at the end of the year. This is not necessary, but it makes life easier.

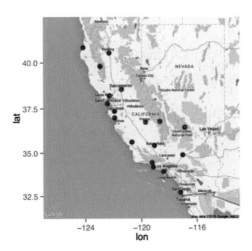

Figure 14.3: The current network of eighteen temperature monitoring sites in California to which five sites must be added.

The analysis begins with standard data analysis. The assumption of a conditional Gaussian distribution underlying EnviroStat seems valid, as a result of a site-by-site analysis using standard methods such as the qq-plot. In any case, EnviroStat is fairly robust against departures from that assumption provided that the distribution is symmetric since the marginal process model conditional on the hyperparameters is the large family of multivariate (or matric) t distributions, conditional on hyperparameters. The ultimate test of all such assumptions is the performance of the resulting spatial process model (Fu, Le, and Zidek, 2003), for example by cross validation, although that was not done for this example.

Next we compute the monthly averages of data at each site and then their grand mean for each month. This gives thirteen 28-day averages at each site and then thirteen regional averages. The latter are estimated from a lot of data, so effectively can be treated as constants. Subtract the regional averages from the site-specific monthly averages to get the site-specific deviations for each month. The regional means will capture a very large amount of temporal variation due to the movement of the sun around earth, which produces the winter to summer variation. The residuals are also important, since they represent the deviations due to such things as distance from the ocean. A plot of these 13 residuals for San Francisco is V-shaped with a minimum in the summer, which is pretty cool compared with the overall state average. That for Death Valley is the exact opposite, the desert reaches its maximum in the summer. This analysis can be captured in the EnviroStat model by setting up the design matrix which removes these major time trends along with the big site-specific deviations as follows:

```
month <- 1:13day <- 1:28
dgrid <- expand.grid(d=day, m=month)
dat <- dat[-365, ]
ZZ <-   model.matrix(~as.factor(dgrid\$m))
```

We can now fit the hyperparameters in the model using EnviroStat's <staircase.EM> function designed to handle a staircase pattern in the data matrix. In particular, this gives us estimates of the covariance parameters.

Next, we project latitude and longitude using the Lambert projection to get a flat surface on which intersite distances are measured in kilometers. Recall that the lines of longitude are not parallel like those of latitude, so for an area as large as California, Euclidean distance cannot be calculated using geographic coordinates. That job is done using EnviroStat's Flamb2 function. The code is included in the online resources.

The next check takes the fitted covariance matrix and assesses it for non-stationarity using the Sampson–Guttorp warping method. Two versions of the warping approach are shown here. The first finds the best possible fit when there is no smoothing involved, that is $\lambda = 0.0$. The result is seen in Figure 14.4, where the right panel shows a near perfect fit of an exponential

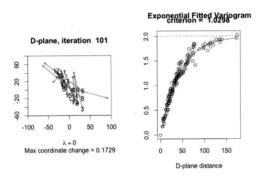

Figure 14.4: The effect of applying the Sampson–Guttorp warping method is seen in this figure, where no smoothing has been used $\lambda = 0$. The left-hand panel shows how the sites must be moved around on California's surface to achieve stationarity and a near perfect variogram.

variogram while the left-hand panel in that row shows with vectors the tremendous degree to which the sites would need to be moved to overcome the non-stationarity reflected in the covariance matrix fitted to the 18 temperature sites.

```
par(mfrow=c(1, 2))
### First approach
sg.est = Falternate3(disp, scoord, max.iter=100,
+ alter.lim=100, model=1)

### Second approach
apply(scoord, 2, range)
coords.grid = Fmgrid(range(scoord[,1]), range(scoord
    [,2]))
par(mfrow=c(1,2))
temp = setplot(scoord, ax=T)
deform  = Ftransdraw(disp=disp, Gcrds=scoord, MDScrds=
    sg.est\$ncoords, gridstr=coords.grid)

Tspline = sinterp(scoord, sg.est\$ncoords, lam = 50 )
```

The second piece of code above requires the analyst to get interactively involved by choosing increasing values of λ starting from $\lambda = 0$ until a satisfactory degree of smoothing is achieved. Thus, the first fit in the first row of Figure 14.5 shows a crumpled mess instead of the flat surface of California in the right panel. Moving to $\lambda = 20$ resolves that surface to some extent.

Most of the basic work is now done. We now move onto the new design, and here we omit a lot of the relevant code for brevity and refer the reader

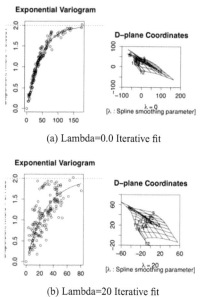

(a) Lambda=0.0 Iterative fit

(b) Lambda=20 Iterative fit

Figure 14.5: The effect of applying the Sampson–Guttorp warping method is seen in these figures beginning with the first row where we see the results for $\lambda = 0$. The analyst must then become involved and experimentally try a sequence of λs until $\lambda = 20$ is reached. The first row shows the same variogram fit, but also in the right-hand panel, that the surface of California would be a crumpled mess. To achieve some interpretability and a more recognizable surface, we must go to $\lambda = 20$ in the second row.

to the online resources for the code. The first step is that of creating potential new design points, five of which are to be selected. That we do by overlaying a regular grid based on equal latitude and longitude spacing. That grid will have points that lie outside California's boundaries, so we need to intersect the grid with those boundaries to keep the sites inside the state. Finally, we have to project the new site with the Lambert projection and extend the original estimated spatial covariance structure to cover all the points in the grid. The principal functions and steps are as follows, the last two being for the selection of the five new sites as shown in Figure 14.6.

```
Tspline.var = sinterp(allcrds[(u+1):(u+18),],matrix(
    diag(cov.est),ncol=1),lam=50)
###
varfit = seval(allcrds,Tspline.var)\$y
temp = matrix(varfit,length(varfit),length(varfit))
covfit = corr.est\$cor * sqrt(temp * t(temp))
```

```
###
hyper.est = staircase.hyper.est(emfit= em.fit,covfit=
    covfit,u =u, p=1)
###
nsel = 5
yy = ldet.eval((hyper.est\$Lambda.0+ t(hyper.est\$
    Lambda.0))/2,nsel,all =F)
```

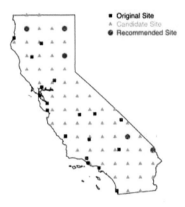

Figure 14.6: A redesigned network in California for monitoring temperatures. Here, the entropy design approach has been used to add 5 new sites to a hypothetical network of 18 sites, the latter picked from sites already existing in the State.

Applying the Sampson–Guttorp approach showed residuals of the temperature field to be highly non-stationary suggesting the need to try much more sophisticated mean models as functions of the geographic coordinates and time (e.g. months). Nevertheless, the approach does do a great job of removing the non-stationarity albeit at the price of losing some interpretability due to a heavily warped geographic space.

14.8 Implementation challenges

Finding the optimal design entails finding a best subset of sites from the entire set of possibilities, which may be infinite in the case of a continuous domain $\mathscr{S}$. In the rest of this chapter, we will continue to assume that for practical reasons $\mathscr{S}$ is finite. (The continuous case is discussed in Section 14.6.1.) Thus, the problem is one of combinatorial optimization whose solution is famously difficult. First, it is an NP-hard problem: finding an exact solution when many sites are involved is essentially impossible. Le and Zidek (2006) provide an exact branch-and-bound algorithm developed given in Ko, Lee, and Queyranne (1995). It can find optimum designs up to about the level of selecting 40 out of 80 sites when the objective function, like ours, is a monotone function of the determinant of a matrix. Many designs will involve far more sites than that. The greedy algorithm is often used when the goal is to expand the network; first add the best site and then find the second best and so on. This process would be reversed should the goal be the contraction of a network.

Deciding how many sites to include is also a practical issue that can prove difficult to solve, although the issue is mute since budget is the deciding factor in our experience. However, more formal analyzes are possible. One approach would treat this as a two criterion optimization problem: maximize the entropy but minimize the cost. That cost will entail the fixed startup costs – the equipment will be expensive and so is acquiring a site – the running costs are more modest when the equipment is automated and online, but that equipment has to be monitored and fixed or replaced when it breaks down during its long operating life. Basic multi-attribute optimization theory tells us that the optimal subset of sites $\tilde{S}^o$ given by

$$\tilde{S}^o = argmax_{\tilde{S}} entropy(\tilde{S}) - \lambda cost(\tilde{S}) \qquad (14.25)$$

in a simplified notation, where λ is the information to setup and operating cost trade-off coefficient. We have not found any systematic way of finding that coefficient. A more practical approach was suggested in personal communication by Dr Larry Phillips, maximize the 'information bang – per – sampling buck' criterion.

$$\tilde{S}^o = argmax_{\tilde{S}} \ entropy(\tilde{S})/cost(\tilde{S}) \qquad (14.26)$$

The curve of $entropy(\tilde{S}^o)/cost(\tilde{S}^o)$ as a function of the number $N_{\tilde{S}}$ of sites in $\tilde{S}$ will increase to a maximum and then decrease when one reaches the point of diminishing information returns from adding another site. We have found this works quite well.

Convincing a user of the importance of a good design can be a problem, meaning that inevitably a suboptimal plan may be chosen. For example, a survey of fresh water bodies involved sending float equipped helicopters into pristine areas to collect water samples to determine the levels of toxic substances. 'Were these samples representative?' the second author asked. 'Oh yes' came the reply, 'We took two separate samples in different spots in each lake and then combined them to ensure the result was representative before we sent it to the lab for analysis'. In another case, the second author learned that the mayor of a local area had applied unsuccessfully for years to have an air quality monitor installed in her area. She was unsuccessful every time. The reason: 'Your air pollution is too low, so you don't need a monitor'. We hope, by this stage of the book, the reader will recognize the fallacies in both of these cases.

Of course, the optimal design methods are indeed too simplistic since they overlook practical problems on the ground. Site locations thought to be optimal may be inaccessible. Costs will generally be hard to pin down since a lot of these will be soft costs, for example the administration time involved in managing a monitoring network. Then again, despite the best of intentions the process of setting up the sites will involve committees, politics, negotiations, setting up the requisite infrastructure and so on.

Even an initially optimal design can decline over time in value for various reasons, changing societal concerns being an important one where the costs are to be borne by that society. For example, the dominance of acid rain as an issue gave way to the health effect impacts of air pollution and that in turn to climate change. The purpose of the design may then change (Example 14.2) along with its suitability for its new purposes, pointing anew to the need for regular reviews of a network in terms of its current purposes.

The redesign of the Metro Vancouver air quality monitoring network (Example 14.1) is encouraging. First, administrators recognized that the network had grown somewhat haphazardly since it started and that it might therefore not be satisfactory for current uses. Secondly, they contracted out the planned redesign of the network to experts. Also, they were willing to listen to the recommendations made by the experts and act on them. This is not a unique example, but in our experience it is very rare!

14.9 Summary

In the plethora of objectives we have seen in this chapter, we see the emergence of a central purpose; to explore or reduce uncertainty about aspects of the environmental processes of interest. One form of uncertainty, aleatory, cannot be reduced by definition whereas with the other, epistemic, where uncertainty can be reduced (see Chapter 3). However, that reduction does not stop the original network from becoming suboptimal over time, pointing to the need to regularly reassess its performance. From that perspective, we see that the design criteria must allow for the possibility of 'gauging' (adding monitors to) sites that

- maximally reduce uncertainty at their space – time points (measuring their responses eliminates their uncertainty);
- best minimize uncertainty at other locations;
- best inform about process parameters;
- best detect non-compliance.

In this chapter, the reader will have gained an understanding of many of the challenges that the network designer may face. These involve the following topics:

- A multiplicity of valid design objectives;
- Unforeseen and changing objectives;
- A multiplicity of responses at each monitoring location, that is which ones should be measured;
- The need to use prior knowledge, characterize prior uncertainty
- How to formulate process models;
- The need to develop realistic designs, contending with economic and administrative demands and constraint in addition to purely scientific objectives.

14.10   Exercises

Exercise 14.1. Redo the plot in Example 14.3 but this time for just the region around the Great Lakes where a lot of industrial activity is concentrated.

Exercise 14.2. Exposure to lead is, like mercury, a serious human health risk and so is now regulated.

(i) What are the specific health risks associated with lead?

(ii) Describe pathways of human exposure to lead.

(iii) Atmospheric transportation of lead in various forms has led to the establishment of monitoring programs for it. Describe some specific features of those programs.

(iv) Plot monitoring sites for lead as found on the US EPA page
    `www.epa.gov/airdata/ad_maps.html`.

Exercise 14.3. Starting with the California temperature data, use the space – filling design-based approach as in Example 14.6 to create a new temperature monitoring network with a total of twenty-three temperature monitoring sites. This will entail some reading (Royle and Nychka, 1998) as well as downloading the `fields` package. That package has the cover.design function with an example you should be able to follow to complete this exercise.

Exercise 14.4. Returning to Example 14.7, determine an estimator based on the finite population sample $\tilde{d}$, an estimator of the superpopulation parameter σ_{12} and one for the population parameter $\hat{\sigma}_{12}$.

Exercise 14.5. Redo Exercise 14.3 but this time by using the entropy-based approach, to add five sites to the existing network. This will entail downloading the `EnviroStat` package and an investigation of the stationarity of the temperature field.

Exercise 14.6. Prove the result asserted in Equation 14.3. Also find an expression for the variance of the HT estimator.

Exercise 14.7. Carbon monoxide (CO) is called the 'silent killer' because its victims experience few symptoms (dizziness and tiredness) before they become unconscious and die, essentially by asphyxiation. The reason is that CO attaches itself to hemoglobin in the blood to form carboxyhemoglobin and blocks oxygen from being carried to the brain. (Tobacco smoking also creates carboxyhemoglobin.) For these reasons, CO has long been a criterion pollutant because of its risk to human health.

In general, incomplete burning leads to the production of CO rather than its benign cousin CO_2. Thus, indoor sources can be found in gas stoves and heaters when they go out of adjustment. So it is likely to be found in the cold days of winter in the northern climates. A probability-based survey of homes is planned to determine the average level of CO in homes on cold days using portable detectors. Briefly describe how probability-based sampling could be used to survey homes on such days and how the resulting selection probabilities could be calculated.

Exercise 14.8. Return to Example 14.11.

(i) Prove the claim that it is best to make half the observations at either end of the interval $[a, b]$.

(ii) We may extend the result to the case where the vector $\varepsilon = (\varepsilon_1, \ldots, \varepsilon_n)) \sim N_n(\mathbf{0}, \Sigma_\varepsilon)$ where $\Sigma_\varepsilon = \sigma_\varepsilon \tau$ and τ is a known positive definite matrix. Determine the maximum likelihood estimator of β and optimal design for estimating it.

Exercise 14.9. Prove the result asserted in Equation 14.3. Also find an expression for the variance of the HT estimator.

Exercise 14.10. Suppose for elements s of the spatial sampling frame $\mathscr{S}$ are listed, and their sizes X_s are known. How would you go about selecting a sample of size n from this list with selection probability proportional to size, that is so that Equation 14.5 holds.

Exercise 14.11. Chang et al. (2007) carry out simulation studies when the random field distribution follows the assumptions underlying the BSP assumptions so that the field has a marginal multivariate-t distribution. They see a smaller loss of intersite dependence when the t distribution has heavy tails compared to when it has light tails (a large number of degrees of freedom).

Try the simulation experiment yourself and confirm that heavier tails lead to increased intersite correlations.

Exercise 14.12. Return to Example 10.5 and the design of 18 temperature monitoring sites.

(i) Redo the analysis in the Example, but this time removing say 3 sites. Plot the resulting new network.

(ii) In that example, 'month' was used to capture the large variation over time. Find a more sophisticated mean temperature model that depends on the spatial coordinates as well, remembering to first use regional models for the whole State and thereby keep the number of parameters used in the model to a small number.

Exercise 14.13. DISCUSSION QUESTION. How might design criteria be arrived at in practice? Who should be responsible for setting them?

Exercise 14.14. RESEARCH QUESTION. Monitor placement should recognize such things as the geographical distribution of impacted populations (e.g. trees or fish). How can an optimal design be determined in such a context?

Exercise 14.15. RESEARCH QUESTION. Develop a design theory in a non-Gaussian context.

Chapter 15

Further topics in spatio-temporal modeling

15.1 Overview

The field of spatio-temporal epidemiology has expanded rapidly in the past 10 years due to the development of statistical techniques that can accommodate variation over both space and time and the increasing availability of high-resolution data measuring a wide variety of environmental processes. Bayesian hierarchical modeling has steadily expanded, as has the ability to handle a large number (n) of measurement vectors, which may be of high dimension (p). Conventional methods for performing Bayesian analysis may be infeasible due to their high computational demands, paving the way for approximate methods for Bayesian inference such as INLA (see Chapter 6, Section 6.7).

There are a great number of specific areas that are under current active development. They include the following:

- Uncertainty Quantification (UQ) , which is defined by Wikipedia as

  'the science of quantitative characterization and reduction of uncertainties in applications. It tries to determine how likely certain outcomes are if some aspects of the system are not exactly known'.

  This topic embraces the content of Chapter 3 along with more conventional sources of uncertainty such as unknown parameters in a mathematical, physical or numerical computer models.

- Model-based geostatistics.

- Modeling high dimensional response vectors ; the 'big p problem'.

- Handling and analyzing datasets with numerous records; the 'big n problem'.

- Multivariate extreme value theory for high dimensional data.

- Preferential sampling and network design, a topic that is discussed in Chapter 14.

- Non-stationary spatio-temporal covariance structures.

- Physical-statistical modeling.

Limitations of space in this book rule out treatment of all these topics. In this chapter, we discuss three of particular importance.

DOI: 10.1201/9781003352655-15

15.2   Non-stationary fields

The topic of non-stationarity was discussed in Chapter 10 in a spatial setting. Here we expand on this topic, describing two approaches:

Spatial deformation: The Sampson–Guttorp approach (Sampson and Guttorp, 1992) warps the geographic space into dispersion space, meaning that strongly correlated sites are moved closer together with uncorrelated ones being moved further apart.

Dimension expansion: The geographic space is kept the same, but additional dimensions are added.

15.2.1   Spatial deformation

In the methodology described so far, two major assumptions have been required, stationarity and isotropy, which are unlikely to hold in many environmental problems. One approach to dealing with non-stationarity and anisotropic processes was suggested by Sampson and Guttorp (1992). The approach begins with the idea of warping the geographical plane, the G-plane, into another latent space, the D-plane, in such a way that two points whose process values are uncorrelated are pushed apart while two that are correlated are pushed The result is a stationary and isotropic process on the D-plane. In practice, this can be challenging. To find the required 1:1 transformation, g, Sampson and Guttorp (1992) rely on dispersion rather than correlation. Dispersion is similar in concept to the distance between points. For any two sites, this is defined as $s, s' \in \mathscr{S}$ by $D(Z_s, Z_{s'}) = 2(1 - Corr(Z_s, Z_{s'})$ for a process Z, which we assume here is measured without error. Here, D is assumed to be a variogram model with a suitable parametric form (Meiring, Sampson, and Guttorp, 1998) so that

$$D(Z_s, Z_{s'}) = \Gamma_\xi[||g(s) - g(s')||] \tag{15.1}$$

The transformation, g, is selected in order to ensure a smooth transformation and the parameter ξ is estimated in the process.

We can then compute the dispersion, and hence correlation, between any two points by inserting their G-plane coordinates into Equation 15.1. Using the parametric dispersion model, we can get a covariance matrix for a process over the entire spatial domain $\mathscr{S}$.

Damian, Sampson, and Guttorp (2000) and Schmidt and O'Hagan (2003) have independently proposed Bayesian approaches for spatial deformation , which incorporate the uncertainty into the choice of a transformation function and the effect this has on subsequent estimation. Schmidt and O'Hagan (2003) use a Gaussian process prior for the deformation to D-plane, whilst Damian et al. (2000) uses a prior based on thin plate splines. Both approaches use MCMC simulation to sample from the posterior.

In considering spatial predictors we adopt the notation used in Chapter 12, Section 12.5 which links the following description to the EnviroStat package which can be used to implement the Sampson–Guttorp method. We will use the terminology used in Section 12.5 and let $U = \{u_1, \ldots, u_{N_u}\}$ and $S = G = \{s_1, \ldots, s_{N_s}\}$ denote the set of ungauged and gauged sites in $\mathscr{S}$, respectively. Thus $U \cup G = \mathscr{S}$.

The process vectors indexed by the sets of sites U and G are $\mathbf{Z}_u^{N_g \times 1}$ and, $\mathbf{Z}_g^{N_s \times 1}$ respectively. The process and its distribution over $\mathscr{S}$ are represented by

$$\begin{pmatrix} \mathbf{Z}_u \\ \mathbf{Z}_g \end{pmatrix} \sim N_{N_u + N_s} \left(\mu, \begin{bmatrix} \Sigma_{uu} & \Sigma_{ug} \\ \Sigma_{gu} & \Sigma_{gg} \end{bmatrix} \right) \tag{15.2}$$

where Σ_{gg} is the covariance between gauged sites, Σ_{uu} between ungauged sites and Σ_{gu} between gauged and ungauged sites.

The predictive distribution is then given by

$$(\mathbf{Z}_u | \mathbf{Z}_g = \mathbf{z}_g) \sim N(\Sigma_{ug} \Sigma_{gg}^{-1} (\mathbf{z}_g - \mu), \Sigma_{uu} \Sigma_{ug}' \Sigma_{gg}^{-1} \Sigma_{ug}) \tag{15.3}$$

Example 15.1. *An application of the spatial deformation approach*

We now give some further details of the application described in 14.14. In that example, the geographic surface was spatially deformed to achieve a non-stationary daily maximum temperature field. The design goal there was to add 5 sites from a grid of possible new monitoring sites. The existing grid consisted of 18 of the current monitoring sites in California. The spatial field of residuals after subtracting an estimate of the mean proved highly non-stationary, so spatial deformation was used. Although a D-plane was found on which the field of residuals seemed stationary, the deformation needed was severe. Current research of the second author revealed that this was due to a failure to include in the estimated mean field the complex three-way interaction between latitude, longitude and time. In summer unlike winter the maximum temperature field was fairly flat from one longitude to the next but only in the southern latitudes. Much less warping is needed when that interaction is accounted for.

In Chapter 14 we saw examples of how a monitoring network might be expanded; one hypothetical (Example 14.14) and one real (Example 14.1). The second of these related to the need for changes in the Metro Vancouver monitoring network. The population has grown substantially and with it the levels of air pollution. So, a study of the Metro Vancouver air pollution monitoring network was undertaken by Ainslie et al. (2009). Deficiencies in the network were found, and subsequently the network was modified. Key to the analysis was deformation of the spatial fields of each of the various air pollutants being studied. In this case, the deformation was largely in response to topography, in particular the mountains on the northern edge of the urban area.

The analysis in Example 14.13, which describes the Metro Vancouver's PM_{10} monitoring network, also required spatial deformation. This hypothetical example demonstrated how 6 sites were selected from 20 candidates locations in highly populated areas to augment the existing 10 sites PM_{10} network.

Example 15.2. *Extending a composite air pollution network*

The subject of this example was the analysis reported in Zidek et al. (2000) and described in Example 14.2. Briefly, this was a network that grew out of a combination of acid rain monitoring networks that came to be used for monitoring air pollution. Spatial deformation had a critical role to play. The application in Zidek et al. (2000) statistically integrated the disparate networks into a combined network, which was then extended in an optimal way.

At the time, the combined network consisted of 31 air pollution monitoring sites in southern Ontario. Each of these sites monitored one or more pollutants including ionic sulfate (SO_4), sulfite (SO_2), nitrite (NO_2) and ozone (O_3).

This redesign presented two major challenges: (i) the spatio-temporal process was multivariate in nature; (ii) the data being collected were misaligned in that not all sites measured the same pollutants. The redesign could therefore involve either adding monitors to an existing site and/or creating new sites. A 'quasi-site' referred to existing sites to which monitors could be added. To illustrate, a location, s, with two pollution monitors would be designated as having two quasi-sites indicating that two additional monitors could be attached. This option would be less expensive than creating a new monitoring location elsewhere due to startup costs.

Zidek et al. (2000) analyzed monthly data for ozone and sulfate, as these had previously been found to be strongly associated with hospital admissions for respiratory morbidity (Burnett et al., 1994; Zidek et al., 1998). There were $2 \times 31 = 62$ quasi-sites, of which 10 measured SO_4 and 21 O_3. This left 31 ungauged sites. Monitors were to be located at an additional 15 sites (30 quasi-sites) The spatial domain $\mathscr{S}$ was taken to contain the original 31 sites plus the additional 15 to give a total of 46 sites.

The approach generally followed that described in Chapter 12, Section 12.5) but with some novel elements. The process model assumed a temporally uncorrelated sequence of two-dimensional vectors $\tilde{s}_{st}$, $s \in \mathscr{S}$ with coordinates representing the O_3 and SO_4 concentrations. These responses could then be combined into $\tilde{s}_t$ a 46×2 process matrix. It was assumed that the within site correlation matrices were identical and equal to Ω. The hyper-covariance matrix for $\tilde{s}_t$, after adopting an inverted Wishart distribution as the prior for the spatial covariance matrix, was $\Phi = \Lambda \otimes \Omega$ where Λ represents the spatial covariance between sites. Measurement error was ignored and the available data were used to estimate Λ using the EM algorithm, which was used to impute the missing data. That provided an estimate $\hat{\Lambda}_{gg}$ for Λ_{gg} from which the intersite dispersion could be estimated. The substantial non-stationarity seen in those estimates led to use of the spatial deformation method to eliminate folds in the geographic surface of southern Ontario. This allowed an approximately stationary covariance to be found.

An exponential variogram was fit based on the spatial deformation analysis and was extrapolated over the entire domain $\mathscr{S}$ of gauged and ungauged sites to obtain a hyper-covariance for the process.

Zidek et al. (2000) then consider the problem of design using the entropy approach, where keeping the quasi-site structure was essential. Given that the posterior distribution for the process had already been characterized, this turned out to be relatively straightforward. They transformed the original process vectors as $\tilde{s}_t^* = \tilde{R}^T \tilde{s}_t$ where

$$\tilde{R} = diag\{I_{2u}, R\}$$

and R, defined in Le et al. (1997), simply permutes the coordinates of $\tilde{s}_t$ corresponding to the gauged sites, that is $\tilde{s}_{gt}$ so that responses corresponding to the quasi-sites constituted the bottom rows of the $\tilde{s}_{gt}^*$ matrix.

With this transformation and the resulting change in the hypercovariance matrix, the entropy approach could be used with the transformed version of the approximately stationary spatial covariance matrix.

In this case, the optimization needed to account for costs. This was incorporated by using a linear combination of the log determinant from the entropy approach and these costs as the optimization criteria. More precisely,

$$O(\tilde{S}^{add}) = E(\tilde{S}^{add}) - ED \cdot C(\tilde{S}^{add}) \tag{15.4}$$

where instead of S^{add}, the sites to be added, we use $\tilde{S}^{add}$ to represent the quasi-sites to be added. In Equation 15.4 $E(\tilde{S}^{add})$, ED and $C(\tilde{S}^{add})$ denote the entropy, the entropy to dollar conversion ratio and cost respectively.

The costs were based on estimates from air pollution monitoring authorities. Over a 60-month period, the monthly costs for buying, installing and operating a single gauge at a formerly ungauged site were estimated to be $1,334. For an already gauged site, that monthly cost of adding a gauge would be considerably less at $292. Not surprisingly, the optimal choice of quasi-sites to add depended on the ED ratio; for all ED in the interval considered, $0.05 \leq ED \leq 0.015$, all additions were pseudo-sites on existing sites and no new sites were added.

In developing methods for coping with non-stationary in the spatio-temporal modeling, there are a number of issues that will arise. They include the following:

- Handling multivariate data.
- Dealing with high degrees of non-stationary that even the spatial deformation approach may not be able to handle well.
- The need to provide a degree of robustness against the misspecification of the spatial mean field.
- The need to contend with monotone and misaligned data patterns in the data.

15.2.2   Dimension expansion

Dimension expansion has similarities with spatial deformation, but it differs in that the locations in the geographic space are retained, with added flexibility obtained through the extra dimensions. It addresses one of the major issues with the image warping approach, the folding of the space suggested by Bornn, Shaddick, and Zidek (2012).

This idea goes back a long way; it was described by Edwin A. Abbott in 1884 although it has been reprinted many times since (Abbott, 2009).

> 'Place a penny on one of your tables in space; and, leaning over, look down upon it. It will appear as a circle. But now, drawing back to the edge of the table, gradually lower your eye....and you will find the penny becoming more and more oval...until you have placed your eye exactly on at the edge of the table [when] ...it will become a straight line'.   Edwin A. Abbott (1884).

Example 15.3. *Gaussian spatial process on half-ellipsoid*

In this example, Abbott's flatlander lives on a two-dimensional disk, as seen in the right-hand panel of Figure 15.1. He sees a distorted version of the field in which points on opposite sides of the disk have the same concentrations, unlike those in the center which have much heavier concentrations. However, a person living in three dimensions sees a much clearer pattern, with the higher values being associated with the magnitude of the third dimension. This is often the case in measuring air pollutants or solar radiation where elevation, along with x and y coordinates will be an important factor. Ignoring such a third dimension would result in a non-stationary random field, whereas including it in a model may help in achieving stationarity.

This observation is confirmed by the empirical variogram plot in Figure 15.2 based on a random sample of sites, where we see an obvious improvement when distance is now calculated using the three-dimensional coordinate (left-hand panel) compared to the original variogram seen on the right.

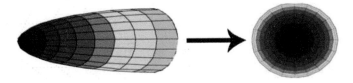

Figure 15.1: The left-hand figure shows a Gaussian process on a half-ellipsoid, with the right-hand figure showing the effect that will be seen when it is compressed to two dimensions, which results in a disk centered at the origin. The resulting field is an example of one in which Abbott's flatlander might live.

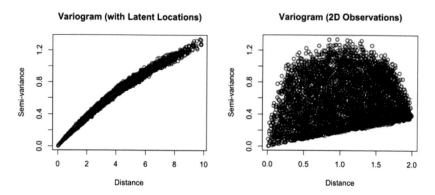

Figure 15.2: Variograms before and after dimension expansion, showing again the same effect seen in Figure 15.1. Before expansion there are obvious signs of non-stationarity which have been addressed by the dimension expansion.

The dimension expansion method starts in two-dimensional space, the disk in Figure 15.1, and seeks additional dimensions in a new domain that will resolve non-stationarity. In this example, it finds the original three-dimensional surface quite precisely without any prior specification being passed to the algorithm. In contrast, spatial deformation does not resolve the problems of non-stationarity in this example (Bornn et al., 2012).

Adding new dimensions

As seen in Example 15.3, embedding the original field in a space of higher dimension can resolve non-stationarity. This begins with the original site coordinate vectors, $s_1, \ldots, s_g \in S$ each of dimension d. These are augmented to get new site coordinate vectors $[s_1, \tilde{s}_1], \ldots, [s_g, \tilde{s}_g]$ each of dimension $d + p$. The ultimate goal is a stationary process $Z_{[s,\tilde{s}]t}$, $[s, \tilde{s}] \in S \times \tilde{S}$, $t \in T$, with variogram

$$\Gamma_\phi(d_{ij}) \tag{15.5}$$

where $d_{ij} = [s_i, \tilde{s}_i] - [s_j, \tilde{s}_j]$.

To define the search algorithm let

$$\mathbf{S} : (g \times d) = \begin{bmatrix} s_1 \\ \vdots \\ s_g \end{bmatrix}, \quad \tilde{\mathbf{S}} : (g \times p) = \begin{bmatrix} \tilde{s}_1 \\ \vdots \\ \tilde{s}_g \end{bmatrix} \tag{15.6}$$

The problem then becomes that of choosing an augmented, coordinate system denoted in shorthand in matrix notation by $[\mathbf{S}, \tilde{\mathbf{S}}]$.

There is theory in support of this approach by Perrin and Schlather (2007), which shows that (subject to moment conditions) for any Gaussian process Z on $\mathcal{R}^d$ there exists a stationary Gaussian field Z^* on $\mathcal{R}^{d+p}, p \geq 2$ such that Z on $\mathcal{R}^d$ is a realization of Z^*. However, the theory only shows existence and not how to construct Z^*.

Finding the new coordinates

One approach we could take would find the $\tilde{s}_1, \ldots, \tilde{s}_g$ such that

$$\hat{\phi}, \tilde{\mathbf{S}} = \phi, \tilde{\mathbf{S}}' \, argmin \sum_{i<j} (v_{ij}^* - \Gamma_\phi(d_{ij}([\mathbf{S}, \tilde{\mathbf{S}}'])))^2$$

where d_{ij} is defined in Equation 15.5 except that it now includes the variable coordinate system in its argument $[\mathbf{S}, \tilde{\mathbf{S}}']$. Here v_{ij}^* is an estimate of variogram (spatial dispersion between sites s_i and s_j) example with data Y,

$$v_{ij}^* = \frac{1}{|\tau|} \sum_\tau |Y_{s_i} - Y_{s_j}|^2$$

with $\tau > 1$ indexing some relevant observation pairs.

Given the matrix, $\tilde{\mathbf{S}} \in \mathcal{R}^g \times \mathcal{R}^p$ we need to construct an f with $f(\mathbf{S}) \approx \tilde{\mathbf{S}}$. Note that we could follow Sampson and Guttorp (1992) and determine thin plate splines f with a smoothing parameter λ_2. This would in turn give us f^{-1} to carry us from the manifold in $\mathcal{R}^{g+p}$ defined by $\{[\mathbf{S}, f(\mathbf{S})], \mathbf{S} \in \mathcal{R}^d\}$ back to the original space. In other words, $f^{-1}(\tilde{\mathbf{S}}) = \mathbf{S}$ and so no issues arise around the bijectivity of f.

However, this approach would not tell us the number of new coordinates that are required. This could be found using cross-validation or model selection to determine the dimension of $\tilde{S}$. However, for parsimony and to regularize in the optimization step we instead solve

$$\hat{\phi}, \tilde{\mathbf{S}} = \phi, \tilde{\mathbf{S}}' \, argmin \sum_{i<j} (v_{s_i,\tilde{s}_j}^* - \Gamma_\phi(d_{s_i,\tilde{s}_j}([\mathbf{S}, \tilde{\mathbf{S}}'])))^2 + \lambda_1 \sum_{k=1}^{p} ||\mathbf{S}'_{.,k}||_1$$

where λ_1 regularizes estimation of $\tilde{S}$ and may be estimated through cross-validation. But other model fit diagnostics or prior information could be used.

To solve the optimization problem, we could proceed as in traditional multidimensional scaling. However, this would not work since the objective function would not have unique maximum. Our optimization is more regularized, due to its penalty function, with the result that the optimization is unique (up to sign and indices of zero/non-zero dimensions). Finally, the gradient projection method of Kim, Kim, and Kim (2006) is used to carry out the optimization.

Example 15.4. *Black smoke in the United Kingdom*

In this example we consider a measure of particulate matter, black smoke, which has been measured in the United Kingdom over many decades by

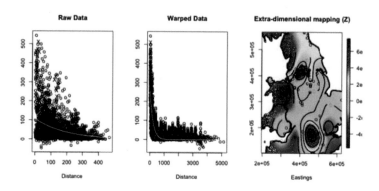

Figure 15.3: Black smoke concentrations in the United Kingdom. The covariance (against distance) of the original data appears in the left hand panel and shows clear signs of non-stationarity. The center panel shows the result of warping geographic space that shows a field much closer to being stationary. The right-hand panel shows the modeled surface after dimension expansion.

Elliott et al. (2007). This field has been shown to be highly non-stationary (Bornn et al., 2012).

The left-hand panel of Figure 15.3 shows covariance as a function of the intersite distance and gives a clear indication of non-stationarity. The spatial deformation method transforms geographic coordinates to dispersion coordinates and the result is seen in the middle panel, which shows a substantial improvement. The result of dimension expansion appears in the right-hand panel.

15.3 Physical-statistical modeling

A modern frontier in spatio-temporal modeling combines deterministic and statistical models. The former embrace scientific knowledge and are deterministic, since the future is determined by the past with certainty. Although their parameters may need to be estimated, uncertainty associated with these estimates is not reflected in the outcomes they generate. Climate models give future atmospheric temperatures (that have potential health impacts, without any expression of the uncertainty about these calculated temperatures. Statistical analysis of their outcomes has shown them to be biased (Jun, Knutti, and Nychka, 2008). Similarly, chemical transport models (CTMs) predict concentrations of air pollutants over various spatial locations without quantification of their inherent uncertainty. The outputs from such models is called 'simulated data'.

These models have a number of limitations. The numerical computer models that represent these deterministic models can take a long time to run. As a result, they are commonly simplified by avoiding microscale phenomena such as evaporation, condensation and turbulence by running them at larger spatio-temporal scales, for example the mesoscale. Climate models may generate output for grid cells of fifty kilometers squared (Kalnay, 2003). Their output may be perfectly valid at that scale of resolution but they need to be downscaled where possible, or subgrid scale processes modeled, when small spatio-temporal resolution is required. Another difficulty faced when using non-linear deterministic models, for example for weather, is their sensitivity to their initial conditions. This can lead to the so-called 'butterfly effect' where small changes in their inputs lead to large changes in their outputs. Data (observations) may therefore be required in order to periodically restart or adjust the models (data assimilation) with new inputs, although their inclusion is often somewhat ad-hoc. Also, as noted above, they are not able by their very nature to provide estimates of the uncertainty in their simulated data.

In contrast, statistical models are designed to provide just such estimates of uncertainty. However, they do not usually incorporate an extensive base of scientific knowledge, even when Bayesian methods are used. The idea of combining these two approaches seems appealing, and this is the topic of much current research. It is possible, by combining the two approaches in a hierarchical Bayesian model, to estimate the fraction of ground level ozone in Vancouver, Canada, that is transported there at a specified time from outside sources (Kalenderski and Steyn, 2011). Cressie and Wikle (2011) provide a review on the use of deterministic dynamic models in a spatio-temporal setting.

15.3.1   Dynamic processes

In this section, deterministic processes are denoted using lower case and random processes using upper case. To add clarity, we assume that the underlying processes Z are observable and are therefore represented by Y.

We begin with dynamic temporal processes which are indexed by continuous time and are characterized by

$$\frac{\partial y_t}{\partial t} = \dot{y}_t = H[y_t], \, t \geq 0 \tag{15.7}$$

In discrete time they will be characterized by

$$\nabla y_t = y_t - y_{t-1} = H[y_t], \, t \geq 0 \tag{15.8}$$

Note the formal resemblance of these equations to the state space models seen in Chapter 11, Section 11.7. As H and y_0 are specified, these equations make y a deterministic process. A non-linear H can lead to chaotic behavior in deterministic systems. In that case, small changes in y_0 can lead to huge variations in y_t, that is the butterfly effect.

A very simple linear system would be $\nabla Y_t = \theta y_t$. If Y_0 were random, we would get a stochastic system. Even a deterministic dynamic system can be subject to random environmental disturbances so that

$$\frac{dY_t}{dt} = \dot{Y}_t = H[Y_t] + v_t$$

where v is random and independent of Y. A Bayesian approach makes parameters in a deterministic system described by H random. In all these cases and others we get a random process even though we start with a conceptually deterministic one.

Example 15.5. *Dynamic growth model*

We use a simple linear dynamic model to illustrate some key ideas. After rescaling y_t so that $y_0 = 1$, it is given by

$$\frac{dy_t}{dt} = \dot{y}_t = \lambda y_t, \, t \geq 1. \tag{15.9}$$

Solving this gives the result $\ln y_t = \lambda(t-1)$, that is $y_t = \exp\{\lambda(t-1)\}$. This will become a stochastic differential equation if the value of λ is uncertain, and hence random in a Bayesian context, that is the deterministic model becomes a random process model. This model could be subject to random perturbations, and so would seem suitable for embedding in a statistical framework. One approach would be to express Equation 15.9 as a state space model by turning the differential equation into a difference equation:

$$\dot{y}_t \approx \nabla y_t \tag{15.10}$$
$$= y_t - y_{t-1} = \lambda y_{t-1} \tag{15.11}$$

Adding the random perturbation term we get $Y_t = (\lambda + 1)Y_{t-1} + v_t, \, t \geq 1$ a state space model (see Chapter 11, Section 11.7).

Example 15.6. *Infectious disease as a dynamic process*

In this example, the approach illustrated in Example 15.5, can be used for any system of partial differential equations, as long as there are not too many of them.

The left-hand panel of Figure 15.4 shows the number of cases of mumps per month in New York City during 1950–1971 (Source: Hipel and McLeod, 1994, in Times Series Data Library, file: epi/mumpsmo). A closer look at the 1970–1972 period is seen in the right-hand panel. Notice the apparent seasonal pattern. A vaccine was licensed in 1967 and led to a dramatic (99%) decline in the number of cases in the United States (van Loon et al., 1995).

One could attempt a classical temporal process modeling approach for the number of cases of mumps, however the cyclical nature of an epidemic

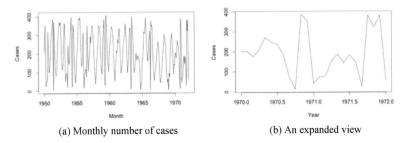

(a) Monthly number of cases   (b) An expanded view

Figure 15.4: The number of cases of mumps in New York City during the period 1950–1971. Panel (a) shows the monthly number of cases from 1950–1971, with a clear seasonal pattern in the number of cases. Panel (b) shows an expanded view for 1970–1972.

for an infectious disease is well understood, and this understanding should ideally be incorporated in a model. Attempts in that direction began at least as far back as 1927 (Kermark and Mckendrick, 1927) with the publication of the susceptibles-infected-recovered (SIR) model. Let u_t, v_t and w_t denote the numbers in the three categories of the SIR model. The sum of the numbers in the categories will be N, the population size.

The following is a dynamic process model, which describes how cases enter and exit the infective population:

$$\dot{u}_t = -\beta_N u_t v_t$$
$$\dot{v}_t = \beta_N u_t v_t - \gamma_N v_t$$
$$\dot{w}_t = \gamma_N v_t$$

This process can be turned into a stochastic model with random elements U_t, V_t, and W_t replacing their deterministic counterparts (Leduc, 2011). Since U is determined by V and W only these are stochastically modeled. They in turn can be modeled by using classical stochastic process models with their deterministic counterparts serving as model parameters as follows: U_t is a non-homogeneous pure death process with rate $\beta_N^* u_t v_t$ and W_t is a non-homogeneous Poisson (birth) process with rate γv_t.

The approaches seen above will not work in the case of complex models such as CMAQ, the Community multiscale air quality model chemical transport model for air pollutants that builds in emissions, meteorology, atmospheric chemistry and atmospheric transport. There may be as many as one hundred differential equations just to represent the chemistry alone, and hence no hope of turning the deterministic model into a stochastic one by methods like those described above. Instead, these numerical models must be treated as 'black box' simulators and their outputs used as inputs into a statistical modeling framework (Berrocal, Gelfand, and Holland, 2010b; Zidek, Le, and Liu, 2012b).

15.3.2 Dimensional analysis in scientific modeling

The results in this subsection rely heavily upon on the ArXiv report of Lee, Zidek, and Heckman (2020), hereafter referred to as LZH. Recall that two processes are involved in the quest for knowledge about a natural process of interest (see Subsection 1.9). Understanding such a process begins by defining a population of possible realizations ω generated by that process, for example a daily weather pattern. Associated with each ω is a set of p measurable attributes $Z_1, \ldots, Z_p$. These Z's are latent, that is they are not directly observable. You can sense that the 'temperature' is low, but it does not come equipped with a thermometer. Moreover, it can interact with other latent quantities like humidity.

The notation for the dimension of each Z_i customarily uses square brackets, $[Z]$, for example, $[Z] = T$ where T stands for time. The ultimate objective will usually be the imagined relationship among these latent attributes: or the predictability of one of them from the others, that is

$$0 = u(Z_1, \ldots, Z_p), \text{ or} \tag{15.12}$$
$$Z_p = u(Z_1, \ldots, Z_{p-1}). \tag{15.13}$$

15.3.3 Dimensional analysis

Dimensional analysis DA plays a key role in developing process models as well as measurement models, the latter being the subject of the next subsection. DA can reveal a hidden structure that must be considered in modeling natural processes. To illustrate this structure, we consider an instructional example.

Example 15.7. *Objects in motion*

A population of moving objects is under consideration. Each object has $p = 3$ measurable attributes of interest, that is Z_1, Z_2, Z_3. Z_1 represents the distance the object has travelled at the time it is sampled. Consulting the Directory of Standard International Units SIU , we find that 'distance' is represented by L, that is length. For Z_2 the dimension would be T, the length of time the object has travelled. Both of these attributes will be easy to measure. But Z_3 is hard to measure. It is the object's average speed of travel at the time it is measured and has dimension LT^{-1}. In summary, $[Z_1] = L$, $[Z_2] = T$ and $[Z_3] = LT^{-1}$.

Because Z_3 will be hard to measure, the modelers, using their sample, need to develop a predictor of the measured value of Z_3 based on the other two. That model could then be used in future to avoid the need to measure Z_3. We return to this example in the sequel.

As in Example 15.7, the Z's associated with a natural process will have dimensions, but not scales. You can't say, for example, that T is measured in minutes. Or that T is measured in hours. Time is just time. Nature did not equip time with a clock. But it is a natural phenomenon and it most surely passes by. Yet here Z_1 sits inside the predictor in Equation 15.12. This presents a puzzle that was solved more than a century ago using an ingenious approach to modeling natural processes. Yet scientists working outside the domain of the physical sciences, seem, by-and-large, completely unaware of this historic achievement, which we now describe.

15.3.4   Buckingham's Pi Theorem

The celebrated Buckingham Pi-theorem (Buckingham, 1914) solves the puzzle presented above. Buckingham reasoned that the solution to the problem lay in recognizing that any complete, legitimate physical model must be non-dimensionizable. It cannot depend on the dimensions of the quantities involved in specifying it! That led him to his famous Pi-theorem, which he proved rigorously through sound mathematical analysis.

Buckingham started by accepting that a natural process could be characterized by a set of p physical variables $Z_1, \ldots, Z_p$ and a relationship like that in Equation 15.12. But since ultimately these relationships could not depend on the the dimensions of these quantities, he sought a way of eliminating them. A naive solution would divide each of the Zs by some constant having the same dimension. But that would have been not only naive, but it would also create a new problem, that of finding those constants. So instead, Buckingham looked to the Z's to provide their own resolution of this dilemma. He first observed a structural redundancy amongst them in that their combined total number m of dimensions would usually be less than their total number of quantities, p. That is what pointed to a path to the problem of finding the needed resolution.

He went on to rigorously prove that if the set of quantities was 'complete', then there would exist just $q \leq p - m$ dimensionless quantities, he called π-functions, $\pi_{m+1}, \ldots, \pi_p$, which would yield a reduced non-dimensionalized U such that

$$0 \quad = \quad U(\pi_{m+1}, \ldots, \pi_p), \tag{15.14}$$

$$\text{or in predictive form}$$

$$\pi_p \quad = \quad U^*(\pi_{m+1}, \ldots, \pi_{p-1}). \tag{15.15}$$

That solution, now called Buckingham's Pi-theorem, would both govern the process and by construction, it would be invariant under changes of scale. Furthermore, it could be inverted to find how the dimensional quantities play their role in the relationship. To illustrate an application of the theorem, we turn to a famous physical model.

Example 15.8. *Newton's second law*

Newton's famous second law of motion says that for any object in motion at time $t > 0$, omitted to avoid notational clutter, $f = ma$. In other words, force equals the mass times the acceleration. This may be rewritten as $a = m^{-1}f$, when our interest lies in applying sufficient force to achieve an acceleration of a, for example the escape velocity of a rocket launched from Earth. In Newton's law, just two $m = 2$ distinct dimensions are involved. The first is mass: M. The second is more complex, the units of acceleration: L^2/T^2. The dimension of force is constructed as the product of the dimensions of mass and acceleration. In our notation, we let Z_3, Z_2 and Z_1 stand for a, m and F respectively. Then Newton's law becomes

$$Z_3 = Z_2^{-1} Z_1. \tag{15.16}$$

Note also that in the rocket application, a lot of the mass of a rocket lies in its propellant, which also diminishes in time after its launch. To escape Earth's gravitational field, a velocity of $11.186 km/s$ must be attained. Thus, the declining propellant supply must provide enough force to dominate its declining mass and accelerate the rocket to its escape velocity.

To show that Newton's law passes Buckingham's test of completeness, we first observe that only $m = 2$ distinct dimensions are involved. And the law as proposed by Newton can then be written in terms of a single *pi*-function

$$\pi_3 = Z_3 Z_2 Z_1^{-1} = 1. \tag{15.17}$$

Here we have $m = 2$ as our number of primary quantities that is variables and $q = 1$ as the number of secondary ones in a common terminology for these functions. We have used 3 as the subscript for the Pi-function, to recognize that formally, at least, there are two other unitless π functions $\pi_1 = \pi_2 = 1$ that replace Z_1 and Z_2 in the non-dimensionalized version of Newton's law.

15.3.5 *Transforming the measurements*

Assume the hard work of selecting appropriate scales of measurement along with their units has been done. Thus, we can now replace the unobserved latent variables Z with their measured values Y. But since these will be observed, we can go further in our exploration of quantity relationships. At the same time, we can carry Buckingham's principles over from the Zs to their measured surrogates Y. As a footnote, there will be complicated situations where the device for measuring the Z's to get the Y's will depend on more than one of the former. So in cases where the set of latent quantities can be vectorized as $\mathbf{Z}^{p \times 1}$, the measurement vector may then be of the form $\mathbf{Y}^{q \times 1} = H(\mathbf{Z})$.

Next comes a contemporary example that illustrates the application of Buckingham's theorem to measurements.

Table 15.1: Variables used to build that process model for disease, infection increases over time.

Number	Variable	Description	Fundamental Dimensions
1	V_p	Virus spread rate	$L\,T^{-1}$
2	P_r	Precipitation	L
3	θ	Ambient temperature	θ
4	C_a	Airflow	$L^3\,T^{-1}$
5	C_e	Seasonal changes	T
6	E_{fs}	Family & social structures	L^{-2}
7	H	Absolute humidity	$ML\,T^{-3}$
8	I_p	Pre-existing immunity	$Adimensional$

Example 15.9. *Rate in spread of infectious diseases*

This example involves a temporal process, the spread of an infectious disease. We now describe an application of Buckingham's Pi-Theorem made by Contreras, Mora, and Gómez (2020). The sampling process involves several attributes that affect the rate of growth in the infected population of individuals in a geographical region. These variables are listed in Table15.1 We see only $m = 4$ distinct dimensions in Table 15.1 from the total of $p = 8$ homogeneous variables, that is L, T, M, and θ. The redundancy implied by Buckingham's reasoning, suggests a simplified alternative to the general predictive model, after non-dimensionalizing it, when a prediction model of the form Equation (15.13) is needed. The variable of predictive interest in this natural process is Vp, which in our notation would be Y_8, that is $Y_8 = Vp$ so it cannot be taken as one of the $m = 4$ primary variables, in our terminology. Instead, for various reasons they are taken to be $Y_1 = Temperature$, $Y_2 = airflow$, $Y_3 = humidity$ and $Y_4 = precipitation$. For various reasons, these are chosen by the authors to create the π-functions, π_8 being the transformed version of Y_8 the predictand. The remaining 3 π-functions would be denoted, in our notation, as π_i, $i = 5,6,7$, the remainder being $\pi_i = 1$, $i = 1,2,3,4$ with

$$\pi_i = V_p \theta^a c_a^b H^c \dot{P}_r^d, \ i = 5,6,7,8 \tag{15.18}$$

with suitably chosen a ,b ,c ,and d .

With Buckingham's simplification, the prediction model becomes

$$\pi_8 = U^*(\pi_5, \pi_6, \pi_7), \tag{15.19}$$

with U^* yet to be chosen.

The final steps taken in the paper are fairly *ad hoc*, and in particular, rely on time series data for coronavirus infections in China. That data, in a scatter plot of the number of infected against the time in days, suggests a linear model. Then after transforming back to the original Y's, we get

$$V_p = \frac{C_a}{P_T^2}a + b\frac{C_e\,C_a^2 E_{fs}I_p}{P_r^3}. \tag{15.20}$$

Use of the linear model in Equation 15.20 could seem as objectionable since all the quantities involved lie on a ratio-scale, not interval-scale. That consideration led to the product model on page 17 in Shen's Ph.D. thesis (W. Shen, 2015).

To dig a little deeper into the domain of measurement process modeling, we revisit Example 15.7, this time in terms of the measurements.

Example 15.10. *Objects in motion – Continued*

We now find ways in which the measurements, their scales and finally their dimensions may be changed. In particular, we ultimately aim to achieve Buckingham's basic principle for process modeling, of non-dimensionalizing a process model based on the experimenter's measurements.

We start in this example, with a remarkably simple but powerful transformation, $g_{\mathbf{c}}$, of the measurements vector $\mathbf{Y} = (Y_1, Y_2, Y_3)^T$ where $\mathbf{c} = (c_1, c_2, c_3)$. More precisely,

$$g_{\mathbf{c}}(\mathbf{Y}) = (c_1 Y_1, c_2 Y_2, c_3 Y_3).^T$$

The simplest of this family might be used by an automated version of a predictive model such as that in our previous Example 15.19, only here Y_3 is the hard to measure predictand. Now we may explore hypothetical changes in the easily measured future values of Y_1 and Y_2. In this case, we would keep Y_3 as the predictive value so $c_3 = 1$. But to represent various hypothetical future values of the predictors, they would be transformed to $c_i Y_i$, $i = 1, 2$ with $c_i > 0$, $i = 1, 2$. However, the scales of the measurements such as say *km* for Y_1 would not be changed nor would the units of measurement. And the c's would be unitless – just positive real numbers. Each member of the set of all possible such transformations, say $\mathscr{G}_0$, would map $\mathbf{Y}^T$ into its set of all possible realizations. It is what is called a group in the language of mathematics. This is because:

- it has an identity mapping, with $c_i \equiv 1$, $i = 1, 2, 3$, where the cs are unitless;
- it contains an obvious inverse transformation for each $g_{\mathbf{c}}$ in $\mathscr{G}_0$;
- compositions of its transformations $g_{\mathbf{c}} \circ g_{\mathbf{d}} = g_{\mathbf{c} \times \mathbf{d}}$ remain in that same group that is $g_{\mathbf{c} \times \mathbf{d}} = (c_1 d_1, c_2 d_2, c_3 d_3)$.

We expand $\mathscr{G}_0$ to $\mathscr{G}_1$ to get a class of transformations that change the scales of one or more of the coordinates of $\mathbf{Y}$. We leave that extension as an exercise. But readers unfamiliar with quantity calculus should read Appendix C first.

Finally, we can let the c_i, $i = i, 2, 3$ depend on the measurements Y to non-dimensionalize them to get $\mathscr{G}_3$. For example, using quantity calculus, we can let $c_1 = Y_1^{-1}$, $c_2 = Y_2^{-1}$ and $c_3 = Y_2/Y_1$. We then get $g_c(Y) = \pi(Y) = (1, 1, Y_3 Y_2 / Y_1)^T$. The measurement vector has now turned into the set of Buckingham's unitless π-functions. The resulting functions are easily shown to be invariant under transformations in $\mathscr{G}_0$ and, $\mathscr{G}_1$ that is $\pi(g_c Y) = \pi(Y)$. Note that these transformations will entail a change of variables in deriving the resulting change in the probability distribution of the measurements vector $\mathbf{Y}$.

So how does this tie into sampling and measurement? The answer is that the data channel is meant to provide information to complement that provided by the knowledge channel . This is done by, amongst other things, enabling models coming out of the latter to be fitted and assessed. Pi-theory has rewritten the model in what must be an equivalent, non-dimensional form. It will have fewer quantities to be assessed in the experimental phase. So applying Newton's second law in Example 15.17 yields a model involving just a single variable. But experimental science requires reproducibility as a fundamental desideratum. Thus, repeated experiments would need to be run, and the result would change from one repetition to another. At the end of each run, an estimate of $\hat{\pi}_i$ would need to be calculated and in each case, shown to lie within the margin of error consistent with the experimental method, as to validate the process model.

15.3.6   Statistical invariance principle

A more principled approach for the analysis in the previous subsection comes from a different direction. The latter applies the statistical invariance principle in a famous unpublished paper by Hunt and Stein in the 1940s. Oddly enough, the link between the Hunt-Stein theory and Buckingham theory went unnoticed until quite recently. The link was recognized independently at around the same time by two research groups. Lee, Zidek and Heckman did so with the goal of unifying statistical and scientific approaches to what has sometimes been called phystat modeling to include other scales such as those seen in the social sciences. Their results were reported in Lee et al. (2020) who worked from Buckingham's original perspective of simplifying physical modeling by reducing the number of quantities involved (W. Shen, 2015; Shen, Lau, Kim, and Li, 2001; Lin and Shen, 2013). Both approaches recognized the Buckingham and Hunt-Stein connection.

Here is a summary of the two approaches. Each start from the measurements vector. Both eliminate the scales and the units of measurement for $\mathbf{Y}^{p \times 1}$.

Approach 1. Experimental costs are high, so cutting costs along with the number of measurements that are needed. Moreover, the -model must be non-dimensionalized as seen in both the Buckingham theory and the Hunt-Stein theory. Putting these together yields the model in Equation 15.14. The experiment can now be run by measuring just the π-functions or maximal invariants, as they were called in the Hunt-Stein theory. The experimental results can then be used to estimate the function U^* in the Equation (15.15).

Approach 1 involves two unanswered questions. First, how do you select the primary variables, that is the quantities to be used to non-dimensionalize the remainder? Second, how do you infer U^* once you have run the experiment with the reduced variable set?

The second approach of Hunt and Stein anticipates those questions. Like Buckingham, they recognize that a model for a natural process cannot depend on the units of measurement the experimenter happens to choose for an assessment of that model.

Approach 2. This approach assumes n repeated experiments have been carried out, both for selecting the primary variables and for estimating U^*. The underlying statistical invariance principle has a rich underlying theory, which can be extended to cover the case of Bayesian inference.

Despite the appeal of Approach 2, Approach 1 can still have a lot of value. Experiments such as a field trial in epidemiology can be expensive and demanding. Running them with a lot of design variables can be impractical.

We will now illustrate Approach 2 using the hypothetical Example 15.10 for instructional simplicity.

Example 15.11. *Object in motion – continued*

The quantities Y_i, $i = 1, 2, 3$ and their units are as previously defined, L, T, and LT^{-1}, respectively. Recall that the random vector $\mathbf{Y}^{3 \times 1}$ of measurements of the latent attribute vector $\mathbf{Z}^{3 \times}$ now has units of measurements attached. Recall also the transformations $\mathscr{G}_i$, $i = 0, 1, 2$ developed above with elements g_c, which transforms $\mathbf{Y}$ into $g_c(\mathbf{Y})$.

Now suppose the experiment is repeated $n = 2$ times to yield two such measurement vectors $\mathbf{Y_i}^{3 \times 2}$, $i = 1, 2$. These can be combined in a sample matrix $\tilde{\mathbf{Y}}^{3 \times 2}$. The transformation groups can be applied to each column vector in the usual way with elements to get

$$g_c(\tilde{\mathbf{Y}}) = \begin{pmatrix} c_1 Y_{11} & c_1 Y_{12} \\ c_2 Y_{21} & c_2 Y_{22} \\ c_3 Y_{21} & c_3 Y_{32} \end{pmatrix}. \tag{15.21}$$

Approach 2 forces a consideration of the entire sample in contrast to Approach 1, which presents just a single measurement vector *a priori*. But implementing Buckingham's Pi-theorem now becomes complicated. A novel approach to doing just has been described in a recent ArXiv report by Lee et al. (2020). That report chooses, in this example, the primary measurements, Y_1 and Y_2, although other choices could have been made. Then they choose a statistic, which represented the population of possible values for each of the two primary quantities, namely the sample's geometric mean based on the two samples, that is $\hat{Y}_j = (Y_{1j} Y_{2j})^{1/2}$. They then form the π-functions

$$\pi_{1j} = \frac{X_{1j}}{\hat{X}_1}, \quad \pi_{2j} = \frac{X_{2j}}{\hat{X}_2}, \quad \pi_{3j} = \frac{X_{3j} \hat{X}_2}{\hat{X}_1}, \quad j = 1, 2. \tag{15.22}$$

Each of the two samples then yields in predictive form,

$$\pi_{3j} = u^*(\pi_{1j}, \pi_{2j}), \; j = 1, 2. \tag{15.23}$$

In explicit, predictive form, we obtain

$$Y_{3j} = \frac{\hat{Y}_1}{\hat{Y}_2} u^*(\pi_{1j}, \pi_{2j}), \; j = 1, 2. \tag{15.24}$$

One might ask how this relates to this result based on Approach 2 to what might have been obtained by applying Approach 1. To see that connection, LZH take

$$u^*(\pi_{1j}, \pi_{2j}) = K \frac{\pi_{1j}}{\pi_{2j}}, \; j = 1, 2 \tag{15.25}$$

for some positive K. Then

$$Y_{3j} = \frac{\hat{Y}_1}{\hat{Y}_2} u^*(\pi_{1j}, \pi_{2j}) = \frac{\hat{Y}_1}{\hat{Y}_2} \left(K \frac{\pi_{1j}}{\pi_{2j}} \right) = K \frac{Y_{1j}}{Y_{2j}}. \tag{15.26}$$

From the last result, we obtain the model of W. Shen and Lin (2019)

$$\pi_{3j} = K, \; j = 1, 2. \tag{15.27}$$

However, the final choice for u^* could be dictated by an analysis of the data, an advantage of Approach 2.

Finally, we summarize LZH's choice of π-functions

$$M(\tilde{Y}) = \begin{pmatrix} \pi_{11} & \pi_{12} \\ \pi_{21} & \pi_{22} \\ \pi_{31} & \pi_{32} \end{pmatrix}. \tag{15.28}$$

Remarks This example shows that the LZH method can yield the same model as the method developed by the Lin group even though the latter is designed for a single 3×1 dimensional attribute vector unlike that of LZH, which starts with the entire $3 \times n$ sample matrix (with $n = 2$).

15.3.7 A theory for stochastifying deterministic models

Lee et al. (2020) presents a general theory for non-dimensionalizing models. The result embeds deterministic models in a stochastic shell, thereby quantifying uncertainty about them.

The theory admits a wide variety of dimensions and scales in the process and measurement models. Thus, it complements the work of the Lin group cited in the previous subsection. The latter takes direct Approach 1 in line with Buckingham's theory. Thus, it concerns measurements on a ratio-scale. In contrast, the former takes Approach 2. So it follows the Hunt-Stein theory and has a broader domain of application. The need for brevity limits us to a sketch of the general theory. Further detail and examples are given in Lee et al. (2020), that is LZH.

The general theory involves all the conventional elements of statistical decision theory:

- the sample space of measurements $\mathscr{Y}$;
- the sampling distribution and associated parameter space, P_λ, Λ respectively;
- the prior distribution and associated hyperparameter space, ρ_β and Beta, respectively.

To this framework, we add the building blocks of statistical invariance theory:

- a group of transformations of the sample space, that is G;
- a group of transformations of the parameter space, that is $\bar{G}$;
- a group of transformations of the hyperparameter space, that is $\hat{G}$.

The groups need to be homomorphically linked to each other. In general, two groups G and H are said to be homomorphic if there exists a mapping w between them such that:

- $w(g_1 \circ g_2) = w(g_1) \cdot w(g_2)$;
- $w(g)^{-1} = w(g^{-1})$;
- $w(e_G) = e_H$.

The novel ingredient added by LZH lies in the restriction on G imposed by the dimensions, scales and measurements. The key consequence of that structure is the maximal invariants that ultimately yield what Buckingham called π-functions. Note that for each of the groups above, a maximal invariant M is like that in Equation 15.28 for the sample space. It has the property that if two sample matrices have the property $M(\tilde{\mathbf{Y}}) = M(\tilde{\mathbf{Y}}^*)$, then these matrices are related to each other by a member $g \in \mathscr{G}_1$ of the transformation group.

LZH shows that the constraints imposed by the structure limit the set of models available for statistical inference, for example, in multivariate regression. Remarkably, this restriction seems to have gone unnoticed by statistical scientists for more than a century.

Finally, a deterministic model, for example, Newton's second law of motion, becomes the conditional expectation of the maximal invariant into which the predictand is transformed, conditional on the maximal invariants into which the other secondary variables are embedded.

15.3.8 The problem of extreme values

A major component of risk analyzes is the modeling of extreme values. Reliability theory classifies events by their return periods. A 1000-year return period for the event of a failure of a nuclear power generating facility, such as Chernobyl, indicates the period in which one failure is expected.

Although the statistical study of extremes spans at least a century (Fisher and Tippett, 1928), new frontiers present themselves due to advances in technology. One developing field is that of multivariate extreme value theory with process response vectors whose dimensions can be in the hundreds of thousands. Conceptual issues may arise where there are differences in the size of the dimensions of the responses. One approach is suggested by Heffernan and Tawn (2004), who propose a conditional approach based on the assumption that the asymptotic form of the joint distribution has an extreme component.

We now describe some specific ways in which extremes arise in environmental epidemiology along with issues arising in network design, especially that of preferentially selecting locations in order to detect non-attainment of regulatory standards.

The inevitable lack of data at extreme values makes modeling the tails of a distribution difficult or even impossible. This lead to a search for distribution theory that could be justified by weak but plausible assumptions. Fisher and Tippett (1928) developed a trinity of distributions that make up the entire family of possibilities for an extreme value distribution for a single data record, for example the sequence of monthly maxima of a pollution series at a single site.

The Fisher–Tippett trinity is reached by assuming a sequence of independently and identically distributed process values observed without error Y_t, $t = 1, \ldots, T$ with a common CDF F_Y. Then $M_T = \max\{Y_1, Y_2, \ldots, Y_T\}$ must converge to one of three distributions as $T \to \infty$, the Gumbel distribution, the Fréchet distribution or the Weibull distribution, Later it was recognized that all three could be combined in a single parametric family of distributions now called the generalized extreme value distribution (GEV): More precisely for a sequence of normalizing constants a_T and b_T that keep the following limit from being degenerate,

$$P\left(\frac{M_T - b_T}{a_T} \leq m\right) \to G(m) \qquad (15.29)$$

as $T \to \infty$ where G must be of the form

$$G(m) = \begin{cases} exp\left[-\left\{1 + \xi\left(\frac{(m-\mu)}{\sigma}\right)\right\}^{-1/\xi}\right], & 1 + \xi(m-\mu)/\sigma > 0,\ \xi \neq 0 \\ exp\left\{-exp\left[-\frac{(x-\mu)}{\sigma}\right]\right\} & \xi = 0 \end{cases}.$$

$$(15.30)$$

For diagnostic analysis, a qqplot is useful. This can be constructed by letting $q_{tT} = (t - 1/2)/T$ and $e_{tT} = \hat{G}^{-1}(q_{tT})$ and plotting q against e. Notice that the q's are just the quantiles of the empirical distribution function.

Further developments have led to a rich theory for the case of a single series (Gumbel, 2012; Leadbetter, 1983; Coles, Bawa, Trenner, and Dorazio, 2001; Embrechts, Klüppelberg, and Mikosch, 1997). An alternative approach is the class of peak over threshold (POT) models that look at exceedances over high thresholds. The number of such exceedances can then be modeled using a non-homogeneous Poisson process. The response can also be modeled conditional on it's exceeding a specified threshold. Its conditional distribution will be the generalized Pareto distribution (Pickands III, 1975; Davison and Smith, 1990) with right-hand tail,

$$G(m) = 1 - \lambda\left\{1 + \frac{\xi(m-u)}{\sigma}\right\}_+^{-1/\xi}, \qquad m > u \qquad (15.31)$$

for parameters $\lambda > 0$, $\sigma > 0$, and $\xi \in (-\infty, \infty)$. Note that as $\xi \to 0$ in Equation 15.31, $G(m) \to 1 - \exp[-(m-u)/\sigma]$, $m > u$, in words to an exponential distribution, a surprisingly simple result. If you delete the residuals above u in the series, the sequences of heights of the series above u will have an approximately exponential distribution.

Example 15.12. *Hourly ozone extreme values*

Smith (1989) presented what was one of the first analyzes of the extreme values of air pollutants from the perspective of regulatory policy, where both their extreme values and their exceedances of a specified threshold are important. Amongst other things, the paper investigates the fit of the GEV model to 61 day maxima of hourly O_3 concentrations based on 199,905 observations and found the GEV provides a good fit.

Our illustrative example is much more modest in scope in that we fit the GEV distribution to the daily, one week and two week block maxima for an hourly series of O_3 measurements recorded at a site in Illinois for 2004 to 2014. The data were obtained from the EPA?s AQS database.

Here we show a selection of the code that was used. The full code is included in the online resources. We compute block maxima for four periods; daily, weekly, two weekly and four weekly. Figure 15.5 shows the series of daily maxima which shows the high degree of variability (volatility) of an extreme value compared to say the sample average.

```
library(fExtremes)
illinoiso04_14.dat <-read.table("illinois_
    aqs03data2004_2014.txt", sep="",header=FALSE)

### blockMaxima computes the block maxima for blocks
    of a specified number
### of hours Daily, Weekly Two Weekly and Four weekly
    maxima
```

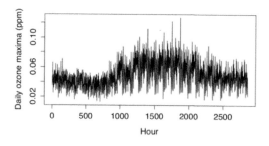

Figure 15.5: Daily ozone maxima (ppm) at a site in Illinois over the period 2004 to 2014. Notice the volatility of this series. Data source: US EPA Air Data Site

```
bm24<-blockMaxima(illinoiso04_14.dat\$V1, block = 24,
   doplot=FALSE)
bm168<-blockMaxima(illinoiso04_14.dat\$V1, block =
   168,doplot=FALSE)
bm336<-blockMaxima(illinoiso04_14.dat\$V1, block =
   336,doplot=FALSE)
bm672<-blockMaxima(illinoiso04_14.dat\$V1, block =
   672,doplot=FALSE)
```

Next, we fit a GEV distribution and plot the fit using a histogram. This can be seen in Figure 15.6 and indicates a good fit.

```
fit24<-gevFit(illinoiso04_14.dat\$V1, block = 24, type
   = "mle")

######## Results: Estimated Parameters:
########   xi          mu          beta
######## -0.10574035  0.04434469  0.01323267

hist(bm24, nclass = NULL, freq = FALSE,, xlim = c
   (0,0.12), ylim=c(0,30),xlab = "O3 daily maxima (
   ppm)", ylab="density", main = "")
x = seq(0,0.12, by = 0.001)
lines(x, dgev(x, xi = -0.09164308, mu = 0.04218148,
   beta = 0.01400470), col = "black")
```

Remember the upper tail is particularly important and so further diagnostics are important and to assess this we construct a qqplot. This can be seen in Figure 15.7.

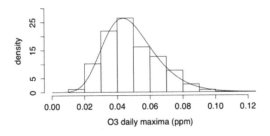

Figure 15.6: A comparison of the fitted generalized extreme value distribution with the raw data for daily ozone maxima (ppm) at a site in Illinois over the period 2004 to 2014. The fit seems reasonably good but note that it's the right tail that counts most. Data source: US EPA Air Data Site

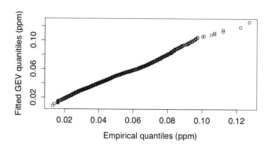

Figure 15.7: A comparison of the fitted generalized extreme value distribution with the raw data through a diagnostic qqplot. Again the fit looks good except for the all important right tail where it droops a little. Data source: US EPA Air Data Site

```
e<-(1:length(bm24)-1/2)/length(bm24)
empq<-sort(bm24)
fitq<-qgev(e,xi = -0.09164308, mu = 0.04218148, beta =
    0.01400470)
plot(empq,fitq,xlab='empirical quantiles (ppm)',ylab='
    Fitted GEV quantiles (ppm)')
```

Again the result looks good except for the all important right tail. On the right-hand side, we see that the fitted quantiles are too high relative to their empirical quantiles, as seen by the empirical demonstration shown in Figure 15.7.

```
#Interpreting the plot.
length(e)-length(e[e>=0.99])
### Result: 2827
bigq<-cbind(empq[2828:2856],fitq[2828:2856])
bigq
```

The calculations above show that the first empirical quantile above the 0.99 level in empq is 0.091 ppm while for the fitted GEV distribution it is 0.095 ppm. That result shows the fit to be unsatisfactory, as it shows the 99th percentile of the fitted distribution is too high. To emphasize this, suppose if it had been 0.400 ppm instead of 0.095 ppm. In this case, the model would indicate that the population living near that monitor would experience O_3 concentrations in excess of 400 ppb about 3 or 4 days a year.

Example 15.13. *Air quality criteria and non-attainment*

This example shows how problems of extreme values arise in relation to health impact analysis. The National Ambient Air Quality Standards are exemplary; the US Clean Air Act (1970) requires that they be set and regularly reviewed to protect human health and welfare while allowing for a margin of safety. Specifically Section 109(b)i states:

'National primary ambient air quality standards, prescribed, under subsection (a) shall be ambient air quality standards the attainment and maintenance of which in the judgment of the Administrator, based on such criteria and allowing an adequate margin of safety, are requisite to protect the public health. Such primary standards may be revised in the same manner as promulgated'.

Regions found to be in non-attainment of the NAAQS are required to submit a plan for getting back into attainment. Specifically Section 172(a)(2) states:

'(2) ATTAINMENT DATES FOR NONATTAINMENT AREAS (A) The attainment date for an area designated nonattainment with respect to a national primary ambient air quality standard shall be the date by which attainment can be achieved as expeditiously as practicable, but no later than 5 years from the date such area was designated nonattainment under section 107(d), except that the Administrator may extend the attainment date to the extent the Administrator determines appropriate, for a period no greater than 10 years from the date of designation as nonattainment, considering the severity of nonattainment and the availability and feasibility of pollution control measures'.

In other words, areas in non-attainment must get back into attainment within ten years at most. Severe financial penalties are imposed for non-attainment, so the impact of a change in the standards can cost states with areas not in attainment a small fortune.

The criteria vary for different air pollutants. The eight-hour standards made by a US EPA Clean Air Scientific Advisory Committee for Ozone (on which the second author served) are based on daily maximum 8-hour averages over the entire year. The standard states that the 'Annual fourth-highest daily maximum 8-hour concentration, averaged over 3 years, shall not exceed 0.075ppm'. It is understood that this will be computed for each site in an urban area, with network design standards stipulating a minimum number of sites for such an area based on population size. The area will be in non-attainment if any site is in non-attainment.

This complicated standard was reached after much risk analysis using concentration response functions (CRFs) that had been published by environmental epidemiologists. Other averaging times were considered along with other quantiles. The standards had to make a compromise between competing targets. They had to be relatively stable over time, for example weather conditions influence the production of ozone and three-year averaging was deemed to be sufficiently long as to make the metric sensitive to a structural change in ozone production, while insensitive to changes in weather. On the other hand, the primary goal of the standards was to protect human health and too much smoothing of the series might result in important changes, which may be important with regard to human health, being overlooked.

Of course, underlying all of this analysis were the raw data, and these will to a large extent depend on the siting of the monitors. Preferential siting was conclusively demonstrated in the UK as the black smoke monitoring network changed over time (Shaddick and Zidek, 2014; Zidek, Shaddick, and Taylor, 2014) although to the knowledge of the authors no such analysis has been performed for the networks in the US.

Example 15.13 shows that where environmental risk is concerned, it's the extreme values, however measured, that matter. Networks should therefore be designed with this in mind. It shows that the extremes can be calculated from complex metrics whose distributions would not have simple analytic forms. This points to the need for spatial predictive distributions that can be used to realistically simulate these metrics over a spatial region of interest. Such predictive distributions would allow calculation of the metric at locations where there are no monitoring sites However, the spatial prediction of extremes is much more difficult than predicting central values. Finally, the example points to the need for an optimal design theory and with it clearly stated objectives. Should the network be designed to optimally detect non-attainment? Or to protect human health by monitoring areas with susceptible populations? How many sites are needed to do that effectively? Recall that each site in an area must be in attainment of the air quality standards that are deemed to protect human health, but what would happen if a location that was currently unmonitored was predicted to be in non-attainment?

Chang et al. (2007) explore the problem of finding designs for regulating and controlling air pollution in urban regions. Their findings using a combination of empirical analysis and simulation studies include the following:

1. Current networks may provide data that can characterize the environmental hazard field relatively well, but are less able to characterize extremes. That is in part because extremes, for example using the metric in Example 15.13, tend to lose spatial correlation.

2. Even if the objective is to find areas in non-attainment, the interpretation of that goal may be difficult. Presumably it would be based on the probability of detecting non-attainment, but should locations be chosen to give the highest probability of detecting non-attainment, that is where levels might be expected to be highest, or where non-attainment is least likely to occur? These two approaches give different networks!

3. In the absence of a clear criterion, the entropy-based criterion has been shown to give reasonable results as long as the multivariate – marginal distribution for the environmental field is appropriate.

15.4 Summary

In this chapter, the reader will have been introduced to a selection of advanced topics in spatio-temporal modeling, including a number of topics currently under active development. These include:

- Two modern approaches to addressing the problem of non-stationarity in random spatio-temporal fields; warping and dimension expansion.

- How dimension expansion can be used to reduce non-stationarity and suggest possible causes (for non-stationarity).

- The Buckingham Pi-Theorem and how it may be applied to simplify a deterministic model for the spread of infectious diseases.

- How the statistical invariance principle can be used to quantify model uncertainty.

- An approach to combining both physical and statistical modeling within a single framework.

15.5 Exercises

Exercise 15.1. Return to Example 15.12 and

(i) plot the times series for weekly, two weekly and four weekly blocks. Comment on the differences you see between them and the 24-hour version in Example 15.12.

(ii) fit the generalized extreme value distribution for each of the cases in part (i). Comment on the quality of the fits.

Exercise 15.2. Return to Example 15.12, but this time use the peak over threshold approach with various thresholds including the 0.075 *ppm* which is currently the US Air Quality Standard.

(i) Plot a histogram of the exceedances of your thresholds and comment on its shape in respect to any resemblance that might be expected for an exponential distribution.

(ii) Plot a generalized Pareto distribution's PDF over your histogram in Part (i).

Exercise 15.3. Repeat Exercise 15.1 for $PM_{2.5}$.

Exercise 15.4. Show that the set of transformations $\mathcal{G}_1$ in Subsection 1.12 is a transformation group acting on the range of $\mathbf{Y}$.

Exercise 15.5. Return to Example 15.9 and derive another model for the spread of infectious diseases by choosing different primary variables. Which model seems preferential.

Exercise 15.6. Return to Example 15.9 and develop a transformation group model theory for the process involved. After selecting the primary and secondary variables, apply the statistical invariance theory and find the maximal invariants into which the secondary variables are transformed. Finally, build a stochastic model that would quantify the uncertainty in the deterministic model derived by the authors of the paper cited in the Example.

Appendix A: Distribution theory

A.1 Overview

This appendix provides some normal and related probability distribution theory. Much more detail about this theory and its application can be found in Le and Zidek (2006) and Brown (2002)

A.2 The multivariate and matric normal distributions

The random vector $\mathbf{Z}^{p \times 1}$ is said to have a multivariate normal distribution, $\mathbf{Z} : p \times 1 \sim N_p(\mu, \Sigma)$, if for any $\mathbf{a} : p \times 1$,

$$\mathbf{a}^T \mathbf{Z} \sim N(a'\mu, \mathbf{a}^T \Sigma \mathbf{a}) \tag{A.1}$$

where $N(\mu, \sigma^2)$ denotes the univariate normal distribution with expectation and variance, respectively, μ and σ^2. If $\Sigma : p \times p > 0$ (i.e. is positive definite and hence invertible) Equation A.1 implies that $\mathbf{Z}$ has the pdf

$$f_{\mathbf{Z}}(\mathbf{z}) = (2\pi)^{-p/2} |\Sigma|^{-1/2} \exp \left\{ -(\mathbf{z} - \mu)^T \Sigma^{-1} (\mathbf{z} - \mu)/2 \right\}$$

Moreover it implies the following properties:

- $E(\mathbf{Z}) = \mu$
- $Cov(\mathbf{Z}) = \Sigma = (\Sigma_{ij})$, $\Sigma_{ij} = E[(Z_i - \mu_i)(Z_j - \mu_j)]$.

For a Gaussian spatial field $\Sigma_{ij} = Cov(Z_i, Z_j)$ is the covariance between process responses at sites i and j.

The multivariate normal distribution is a special case of the matric normal distribution $\mathbf{Z} : n \times m \sim N(\mu, \mathbf{A} \otimes \mathbf{B})$ meaning

$$f_{\mathbf{Z}}(\mathbf{z}) = \frac{1}{(2\pi)^{nm/2}} |\mathbf{A}|^{-m/2} |\mathbf{B}|^{-n/2} \operatorname{etr} \left\{ -\frac{1}{2} [\mathbf{A}^{-1}(\mathbf{z} - \mu)][(\mathbf{z} - \mu)\mathbf{B}^{-1}]^T \right\} \tag{A.2}$$

where $\mathbf{A} = (a_{ij}) : n \times n > 0$ and $\mathbf{B} = (b_{ij}) : m \times m > 0$, and $etr = \exp tr()$ and $tr(\mathbf{A}) = trace(\mathbf{A}) = \sum a_{ii}$ for any matrix $\mathbf{A}$.

Let *vec* denote an operator that converts a matrix to a vector by stacking its transposed rows into a tall column vector. Then the matric-normal distribution defined by Equation A.2 has the following properties:

- $E(\mathbf{Z}) = \mu$.
- $\operatorname{var}[vec(\mathbf{Z})] = \mathbf{A} \otimes \mathbf{B}$ and $\operatorname{var}[vec(\mathbf{Z}^T)] = \mathbf{B} \otimes \mathbf{A}$.

DOI: 10.1201/9781003352655-A

- $\mathbf{Z} \sim N(\mu, \mathbf{A} \otimes \mathbf{B})$ if and only if $\mathbf{Z}^T \sim N(\mu^T, \mathbf{B} \otimes \mathbf{A})$.
- $\mathrm{cov}(\mathbf{Z}_i, \mathbf{Z}_j) = a_{ij}\mathbf{B}, \mathrm{cov}(\mathbf{Z}^{(i)}, \mathbf{Z}^{(j)}) = b_{ij}\mathbf{A}$.

  For any matrices $\mathbf{C} : c \times n$, $\mathbf{D} : m \times d$, $\mathbf{F} : m \times m$ and $\mathbf{G} : n \times n$:
- $\mathbf{CZD} \sim N(\mathbf{C}\mu\mathbf{D}, \mathbf{CAC}^T \otimes \mathbf{D}^T\mathbf{BD})$
- $E[\mathbf{ZFZ}^T] = \mu\mathbf{E}\mu^T + \mathbf{A}\mathrm{tr}(\mathbf{FB})$ and
- $E[\mathbf{Z}^T\mathbf{GZ}] = \mu\mathbf{D}\mu^T + \mathrm{tr}(\mathbf{AG})\mathbf{B}$.

Thus

$$E[\mathbf{ZB}^{-1}\mathbf{Z}^T] = \mu\mathbf{B}^{-1}\mu^T + m\mathbf{A}$$

and

$$E[\mathbf{Z}^T\mathbf{A}^{-1}\mathbf{Z}] = \mu^T\mathbf{A}^{-1}\mu + n\mathbf{B}$$

Multivariate and matric t-distribution

The multivariate t-distribution is related to the multivariate normal distribution in much the same way as in the univariate case. We designate it by $\mathbf{Z} : p \times 1 \sim t_p(\mu, \mathbf{A}, \nu)$ which means

$$f_{\mathbf{Z}}(\mathbf{z}) = \frac{\Gamma\left(\frac{p+\nu}{2}\right)\sqrt{|\mathbf{A}|}}{\Gamma(\nu/2)\sqrt{2\pi p}} \times \left[1 + \frac{1}{\nu}(\mathbf{z}-\mu)^T\mathbf{A}(\mathbf{z}-\mu)\right]^{-(p+\mu)/2}$$

where $\mathbf{A} > 0$ represents the precision matrix, $E(\mathbf{Z}) = \mu$ and $Cov(\mathbf{Z}) = \frac{\nu}{\nu-2}\mathbf{A}^{-1}$.

Likewise for the matric t-distribution $Z : n \times m \sim t_{n \times m}(\mu, \mathbf{A} \otimes \mathbf{B}, \delta)$, δ being the degrees of freedom means

$$f_{\mathbf{Z}}(\mathbf{z}) \propto |\mathbf{A}|^{-m/2}|\mathbf{B}|^{-n/2}|I_n + \delta^{-1}[\mathbf{A}^{-1}(\mathbf{z}-\mu)][(\mathbf{z}-\mu)\mathbf{B}^{-1}]^T|^{-\frac{\delta+n+m-1}{2}}$$

for matrices $\mathbf{A} : n \times n > 0$, $\mathbf{B} : m \times m > 0$ and $\mu : n \times m$. The normalizing constant is

$$K = (\delta\pi^2)^{-\frac{nm}{2}} \frac{\Gamma_{n+m}[(\delta+n+m-1)/2]}{\Gamma_n[(\delta+n-1)/2]\Gamma_m[(\delta+m-1)/2]}$$

$$\Gamma_p(t) = \pi^{\frac{p(p-1)}{4}} \prod_{i=1}^{p} \Gamma[t-(i-1)/2]$$

We now summarize the properties of the matric t-distribution:

- $\mathbf{Z} \sim t_{n \times m}(\mu, \mathbf{A} \otimes \mathbf{B}, \delta)$, if and only if $\mathbf{Z}^T \sim t_{m \times n}(\mu^T, \mathbf{B} \otimes \mathbf{A}, \delta)$.
- If $n = 1$ and $\mathbf{A} = 1$, $\mathbf{Z}$ has an m-variate t-distribution, that is,

$$\mathbf{Z} \sim t_m(\mu, \mathbf{B}, \delta)$$

- If $m = 1$ and $\mathbf{B} = 1$, $\mathbf{Z}$ has an n-variate t-distribution, that is,

$$\mathbf{Z} \sim t_n(\mu, \mathbf{A}, \delta)$$

- If $\mathbf{Z} \sim t_{n \times m}(\mu, \, \mathbf{A} \otimes \mathbf{B}, \, \delta)$, and $\mathbf{C}_{c \times n}$ and $\mathbf{D}_{m \times d}$ are of full rank (ie. rank c and d respectively), then

$$\mathbf{Y} = \mathbf{CZD} \sim t_{c \times d}(\mathbf{C}\mu\mathbf{D}, \mathbf{CAC}^T \otimes \mathbf{D}^T \mathbf{BD}, \, \delta)$$

- $E(\mathbf{Z}) = \mu$.
- When $\delta > 2$,

$$\text{var}[vec(\mathbf{Z})] = \delta(\delta - 2)^{-1} \mathbf{A} \otimes \mathbf{B}$$

and

$$\text{cov}(\mathbf{Z}_i, \mathbf{Z}_j) = \delta(\delta - 2)^{-1} a_{ij} B, \quad \text{cov}(\mathbf{Z}^{(i)}, \mathbf{Z}^{(j)}) = \delta(\delta - 2)^{-1} b_{ij} A$$

The Wishart distribution

Recall that the chi-squared random variable with p degrees of freedom can be defined by $\chi_p^2 = \sum_{i=1}^{p} Z_i^2$ where the $Z_i \sim N(0,1)$, $i = 1, \ldots p$ are independently distributed. The Wishart random variable generalizes the chi-squared—the one with p degrees of freedom replaces the $\{Z_i\}$ by independent vectors $\mathbf{Z}_i : m \times 1 \sim N_m(\mathbf{0}, \mathbf{I}_m)$, $i = 1, \ldots p$ to get

$$\mathbf{S}_p = \sum_{i=1}^{p} \mathbf{Z}_i \mathbf{Z}_i^T \tag{A.3}$$

This may be extended by replacing $\mathbf{Z}_i$ by $\mathbf{A}^{1/2}\mathbf{Z}$ in Equation A.3 where $\mathbf{A} > 0$. We denote the resulting random variable's distribution by $\mathbf{S}_p : p \times p \sim W_p(\mathbf{A}, m)$. It can be shown that the pdf of $\mathbf{S}_p$ is

$$f_{S_p}(\mathbf{s}) = \left[2^{mp/2} \Gamma_p(m/2) \right]^{-1} |\mathbf{A}|^{-m/2} |\mathbf{s}|^{(m-p-1)/2} \exp^{-\frac{1}{2} tr(\mathbf{A}^{-1}\mathbf{S})} \tag{A.4}$$

for any $\mathbf{A} > 0$.

Many of the properties of the Wishart are easiest to derive with the help of the representation A.3. For example its expectation is given by $E(\mathbf{S}_p) = n\mathbf{A}$.

Inverted Wishart distribution

This important distribution is simply obtained by inverting the Wishart random variable. In other words, $\mathbf{Z}_p \sim W_p^{-1}(\Psi, \delta)$ if and only if $\mathbf{S}_p = \mathbf{Z}^{-1} \sim W_p(\Psi^{-1}, \delta)$. It may be shown that

$$f_{Z_p}(\mathbf{z}) = 2^{mp/2} \Gamma_p(m/2) |\Psi|^{-\frac{1}{2}(\delta+p+1)} \exp^{\{ -\frac{1}{2} \mathbf{z}^{-1}\Psi \}} \tag{A.5}$$

for some $\Psi > 0$. This distribution generalizes the inverse gamma distribution.

Properties

- If $\mathbf{Z} \sim W_p(\Sigma, \delta)$ then $E(\mathbf{Z}) = \delta\Sigma$ and $E(\mathbf{Z}^{-1}) = \Sigma^{-1}/(\delta - p - 1)$ provided $\delta - p - 1 > 0$.
- If $\mathbf{Y} \sim W_p^{-1}(\Psi, \delta)$, then $E(\mathbf{Y}) = \Psi/(\delta - p - 1)$ and $E(\mathbf{Y}^{-1}) = \delta\Psi^{-1}$.
- If $\mathbf{Y} \sim W_p^{-1}(\Psi, \delta)$, then

$$E \log|\mathbf{Y}| = -p\log 2 - \sum_{i=1}^{p} \eta\left[\frac{1}{2}(\delta - i + 1)\right] + \log|\Psi|$$

where $\eta = $ digamma function $= d[\log\Gamma(x)]/dx$.

Bartlett decomposition

Let

$$\Sigma = \begin{pmatrix} \Sigma_{11} & \Sigma_{12} \\ \Sigma_{21} & \Sigma_{22} \end{pmatrix}$$

$$\Delta = \begin{pmatrix} \Sigma_{1|2} & 0 \\ 0 & \Sigma_{22} \end{pmatrix} \text{ and}$$

$$T = \begin{pmatrix} I & \tau \\ 0 & I \end{pmatrix}$$

where $\Sigma_{1|2} \equiv \Sigma_{11} - \Sigma_{12}\Sigma_{22}^{-1}\Sigma_{21}, \tau \equiv \Sigma_{12}\Sigma_{22}^{-1}$. Then

$$\Sigma = T\Delta T^T \tag{A.6}$$

Hence

$$\Sigma = \begin{pmatrix} \Sigma_{1|2} + \tau\Sigma_{22}\tau^T & \tau\Sigma_{22} \\ \Sigma_{22}\tau^T & \Sigma_{22} \end{pmatrix} \tag{A.7}$$

A problem with the Wishart distribution is that only a single degree of freedom is available to characterize uncertainty about all the parameters in the distribution. This deficiency leads us to the distribution in Subsection A.2.

Generalized Inverted Wishart

The two block version of the inverted Wishart above can be easily be extended to k blocks as follows. First apply the Bartlett decomposition to

$$\Sigma = \begin{pmatrix} \Sigma_{11} & \Sigma_{12} \\ \Sigma_{21} & \Sigma_{22} \end{pmatrix}$$

Then $\mathbf{Z} \sim GIW(\Psi, \delta)$ would mean that

$$\Sigma_{22} \sim IW(\Psi_{22}, \delta_2)$$
$$\Sigma_{1|2} \sim IW(\Psi_{1|2}, \delta_1), \text{ and}$$
$$\tau \mid \Sigma_{1|2} \sim N(\tau_{01}, H_1 \otimes \Sigma_{1|2})$$

where

$$\Psi_{1|2} = \Psi_{11} - \Psi_{12}(\Psi_{22})^{-1}\Psi_{21}$$

In the next step we would partition $(\Psi_{1|2}$ and so on leaving a sequence of degrees of freedom to represent the uncertainties that go with the different blocks in the decomposition.

Appendix B: Entropy decomposition

B.1 Overview

This appendix provides details of the entropy decomposition for the multivariate t-distribution.

Assume for the $p \times 1$ vector $\mathbf{Z}$

$$
\begin{aligned}
\mathbf{T} \mid \Sigma &\sim N_p(0, \Sigma) \\
\Sigma \mid \Psi, \delta &\sim W_p^{-1}(\Psi, \delta)
\end{aligned}
$$

Then

$$\mathbf{T} \mid \Psi, \delta \sim t_p(0, \delta^{*-1}\Psi, \delta^*)$$

with $\delta^* = \delta - p + 1$.

It can be shown that

$$\Sigma \mid \mathbf{T}, \Psi, \delta \sim W_p^{-1}(\Psi + \mathbf{TT}', \delta + 1)$$

Conditional on Ψ & δ

$$
\begin{aligned}
H(\mathbf{T}, \Sigma) &= H(\mathbf{T} \mid \Sigma) + H(\Sigma) \\
H(\mathbf{T}, \Sigma) &= H(\Sigma \mid \mathbf{T}) + H(\mathbf{T})
\end{aligned}
$$

Hence

$$H(\mathbf{T}) = H(\mathbf{T} \mid \Sigma) + H(\Sigma) - H(\Sigma \mid \mathbf{T})$$

with

$$
\begin{aligned}
H(\mathbf{T} \mid \Sigma) &= \frac{1}{2} E(\log|\Sigma| \mid \Psi) + \frac{p}{2}(\log(2\pi) + 1) \\
&= \frac{1}{2} E(\log|\Psi|) + \frac{1}{2} E(\log|\Sigma\Psi^{-1}|) + \frac{p}{2}(\log(2\pi) + 1) \\
&= \frac{1}{2} E(\log|\Psi|) + c(p, \delta)
\end{aligned}
$$

the constant $c(g, \delta)$ depending on g and δ and noting that $\Psi\Sigma^{-1} \sim W_p(I_p, \delta)$.

DOI: 10.1201/9781003352655-B

Using $h(\mathbf{T},\Sigma) = h(\mathbf{T})h(\Sigma) = |\Sigma|^{-(g+1)/2}$ we obtain

$$
\begin{aligned}
H(\Sigma) &= E[\log f(\Sigma)/h(\Sigma)] \\
&= \frac{1}{2}\delta \log|\Psi| - \frac{1}{2}\delta E(\log|\Sigma|) \\
&\quad - \frac{1}{2}E(tr\Psi\Sigma^{-1}) + c_1(p,\delta) \\
&= -\frac{1}{2}\delta E(\log|\Sigma\Psi^{-1}|) - \frac{1}{2}E(tr\Psi\Sigma^{-1}) + c_1(p,\delta) \\
&= \frac{1}{2}\delta E(\log|\Sigma^{-1}\Psi|) - \frac{1}{2}E(tr\Psi\Sigma^{-1}) + c_1(p,\delta) \\
&= c_2(p,\delta)
\end{aligned}
$$

Similarly

$$
\begin{aligned}
H(\Sigma \mid \mathbf{T}) &= \frac{1}{2}(\delta+1)\log|\Psi| - \frac{1}{2}(\delta+1)E(\log|\Psi+\mathbf{T}\mathbf{T}^T)|) \\
&\quad + c_3(p,\delta) \\
&= -\frac{1}{2}(\delta+1)E(\log|1+\mathbf{T}'\Psi^{-1}\mathbf{Z})|) + c_3(p,\delta) \\
&= c_4(p,\delta)
\end{aligned}
$$

Note $|\Psi|(1+\mathbf{Z}^T\Psi^{-1}\mathbf{Z}) = |\Psi+\mathbf{Z}\mathbf{Z}^T)|$ and $\mathbf{Z}^T\Psi^{-1}\mathbf{Z} \sim F$ with degrees of freedom depending only on g, δ and thus $H(\mathbf{Z}) = \frac{1}{2}\log|\Psi| + c_5(p,\delta)$.

Appendix C: Quantity calculus

C.1 Overview

The topic of this appendix belongs in the domain of dimensional analysis (Lee et al., 2020). Quantity calculus underlies a discussion of these key ideas. That calculus needs notation: $u = \{u\}[u]$ for any measurement u, where $\{u\}$ and $[u]$ stand respectively for the numerical part of u and its units. It tells us, for example, that $a + b$ is meaningless unless $[a] = [b]$, while a/b is a valid calculation whatever their units. Powers a^b are OK provided that b is a rational number, that is a ratio of two integers.

Quantity calculus also tells us that models that involve the measurable attributes Z can only be meaningful if they involve algebraic functions $h(\mathbf{Z})$ or ratios of such functions. These functions are defined by algebraic equations that is solutions of polynomial equations

$$p_r(\mathbf{Z})h^r + \ldots p_0(\mathbf{Z})h^0 = 0[0]. \tag{C.8}$$

Here r is an integer, $\{p_i(\mathbf{Z})\}$ is a polynomial in $\mathbf{Z}$ of order $i = 1, \ldots, r$, Equation (C.8) is dimensionally consistent, and finally $[0]$ has the same as the units on the left-hand side of that equation. An example would be $h(Z) = Z^{1/2}$, which is the solution of $y = h^2 - Z = 0[X]$. Functions that are not algebraic, are called transcendental. indexFunctions!algebraic

When Y has units of measurement assigned, $h(Y)$ can only be meaningful in a measurement or process model if it is an algebraic function. That rules out $\ln Y$. To apply transcendental functions like $\ln Y$ requires that Y be rescaled to Y/Y_0 where Y_0 is a known reference level.

What about the regression model, which is valid in principle when Y_1 is on an interval scale,

$$y(Y_1) = \beta_0 + \beta_1 Y_1? \tag{C.9}$$

Here we have an algebraic function and the units of Y_1 can be absorbed in β_1. However, even in that case, non-dimensionalizing Y_1 is desirable. If we do so, we get

$$Y(Y_1) = \beta_0^* + \beta_1^*(Y_1/Y_0). \tag{C.10}$$

Now the two β^*s are on the same scale and so are directly comparable-their relative sizes now matter and indicate the relative importance of the two factors, intercept and slope in model variation. This same idea is proposed in (Faraway, 2015).

However, the conventional regression model like that seen in Equation C.9, would not be appropriate if attributes were being measured on a ratio-scale, that is one that has a true zero on its measurement scale 0. In, such a case, to be meaningful, change must be measured by ratios, not differences. As an example, changes in stock prices change are measured in percentages. Strictly speaking, it also rules out the use of the bell curve as a potential approximation for the model of X's sampling distribution, although the distribution is extensively used as an approximation. Rather than a linear model, For regression analysis on the ratio-scale, the product model rather than a linear model would be more appropriate.

C.2   Exercises

Exercise C.2.7. Is $Y(Y_1) = (Y_1^2 + 1mm)/(Y_1^5 + (3mm)\,Y_1^2 + 2\,(mm)^5)$ a polynomial function? What units of measurement should be attached?

Exercise C.2.8. Under what conditions is the Box-Cox transformation in Equation (10.10) an algebraic function?

References

Abbott, E. (2009). *Flatland*. Broadview Press.

Adar, S., D'Souza, J., Shaddick, G., Langa, K., Bloom, D., Arokiasamy, P., ... others (2019). Ambient air pollution and cognition in india. *Environmental Epidemiology*, *3*, 105.

Ainslie, B., Reuten, C., Steyn, D. G., Le, N. D., and Zidek, J. V. (2009). Application of an entropy-based Bayesian optimization technique to the redesign of an existing monitoring network for single air pollutants. *Journal of Environmental Management*, *90*(8), 2715–2729.

Alves, M. B., Gamerman, D., and Ferreira, M. A. (2010). Transfer functions in dynamic generalized linear models. *Statistical Modelling*, *10*(1), 03-40.

Ashagrie, A., De Laat, P., De Wit, M., Tu, M., and Uhlenbrook, S. (2006). Detecting the influence of land use changes on floods in the Meuse River basin? the predictive power of a ninety-year rainfall-runoff relation? *Hydrology and Earth System Sciences Discussions*, *3*(2), 529–559.

Austen, P. B. (2012). *1812: Napoleon in Moscow*. Frontline Books.

Aven, T. (2013). On Funtowicz and Ravetz's "Decision stake–system uncertainties" structure and recently developed risk perspectives. *Risk Analysis*, *33*(2), 270–280.

Bakka, H., Rue, H., Fuglstad, G.-A., Riebler, A., Bolin, D., Illian, J., ... Lindgren, F. (2018). Spatial modeling with r-inla: A review. *Wiley Interdisciplinary Reviews: Computational Statistics*, *10*(6), e1443.

Bandeen-Roche, K., Hall, C. B., Stewart, W. F., and Zeger, S. L. (1999). Modelling disease progression in terms of exposure history. *Statistics in Medicine*, *18*, 2899–2916.

Banerjee, S., Carlin, B. P., and Gelfand, A. E. (2015). *Hierarchical Modeling and Analysis for Spatial Data. Second edition*. CRC Press.

Bartlett, M. S. (1935). Contingency table interactions. *Supplement to the Journal of the Royal Statistical Society*, *2*(2), 248–252.

Basu, D. (1975). Statistical information and likelihood [with discussion]. *Sankhyā: The Indian Journal of Statistics, Series A*, 1–71.

Baxter, P. J., Ing, R., Falk, H., French, J., Stein, G., Bernstein, R., ... Allard, J. (1981). Mount St Helens eruptions, May 18 to June 12, 1980: An overview of the acute health impact. *Journal of the American Medical Association*, *246*(22), 2585–2589.

Bayarri, M., and Berger, J. O. (1999). Quantifying surprise in the data and model verification. *Bayesian Statistics*, *6*, 53–82.

Bayarri, M., and Berger, J. O. (2000). P values for composite null models. *Journal of the American Statistical Association*, *95*(452), 1127–1142.

Bergdahl, M., Ehling, M., Elvers, E., Földesi, E., Korner, T., Kron, A., ... Sæbø, H. (2007). *Handbook on Data Quality Assessment Methods and Tools.* Ehling, Manfred Körner, Thomas.

Berger, J. (2012). Reproducibility of science: P-values and multiplicity. SBSS Webinar, Oct, 4.

Berger, J. O., and Wolpert, R. L. (1988). The likelihood principle. IMS. In S. Kotz and N. Johnson, "Encyclopedia of Statistical Sciences," John Wiley and Sons, Inc., New York, 1982.

Berhane, K., Gauderman, W. J., Stram, D. O., and Thomas, D. C. (2004). Statistical issues in studies of the long-term effects of air pollution: The Southern California Children's Health Study. *Statistical Science*, *19*(3), 414–449.

Berliner, L. M. (1996). Hierarchical Bayesian time series models. In *Maximum entropy and bayesian methods* (pp. 15–22). Springer.

Bernardo, J. M., and Smith, A. F. M. (2009). *Bayesian Theory*. John Wiley & Sons.

Bernoulli, J. (1713). Ars conjectandi: Usum & applicationem praecedentis doctrinae in civilibus, moralibus & oeconomicis. *Translated into English by Oscar Sheynin. Basel: Turneysen Brothers,. Chap.*

Berrocal, V., Gelfand, A., and Holland, D. (2010b). A bivariate space-time downscaler under space and time misalignment. *Annals of Applied Statistics.*

Berrocal, V., Gelfand, A. E., and Holland, D. M. (2010a). A spatio-temporal downscaler for output from numerical models. *Journal of Agricultural, Biological, and Environmental Statistics*, *15*(2), 176–197.

Berry, G., Gilson, J., Holmes, S., Lewinshon, H., and Roach, S. (1979). Asbestosis: A study of dose-response relationship in an asbestos textile factory. *British Journal of Industrial Medicine*, *36*, 98–112.

Berry, S. M., Carroll, R. J., and Ruppert, D. (2002). Bayesian smoothing and regression splines for measurement error problems. *Journal of the American Statistical Association*, *97*(457), 160–169.

Besag, J. (1974). Spatial interaction and the statistical analysis of lattice systems. *Journal of the Royal Statistical Socety, Series B*, *36*, 192–236.

Besag, J., York, J., and Mollié, A. (1991). Bayesian image restoration, with two applications on spatial statistics. *Annals of the Institute of Statistical Mathematics*, *43*, 1-59.

Bishop, Y., Feinburg, S., and Holland, P. (1975). *Discrete Multivariate Analysis: Theory and Practice*. MIT Press.

Blangiardo, M., and Cameletti, M. (2015). *Spatial and Spatio-Temporal Bayesian Models with R-INLA*. John Wiley & Sons.

Blyth, C. R. (1972). On Simpson's paradox and the sure-thing principle. *Journal of the American Statistical Association*, *67*(338), 364–366.

Bodnar, O., and Schmid, W. (2010). Nonlinear locally weighted kriging prediction for spatio-temporal environmental processes. *Environmetrics*, *21*, 365–381.

Bornn, L., Shaddick, G., and Zidek, J. V. (2012). Modeling nonstationary processes through dimension expansion. *Journal of the American Statistical Association*, *107*(497), 281–289.

Bowman, A. W., Giannitrapani, M., and Scott, E. M. (2009). Spatiotemporal smoothing and sulphur dioxide trends over Europe. *Journal of the Royal Statistical Society: Series C (Applied Statistics)*, *58*(5), 737–752.

Box, G. E., and Draper, N. R. (1987). *Empirical Model–Building and Response Surfaces*. John Wiley & Sons.

Breslow, N., and Clayton, D. (1993). Approximate inference in Generalized Linear Mixed Models. *Journal of the American Statistical Association*, *88*(421), 9–25.

Breslow, N., and Day, N. (1980). *Statistical Methods in Cancer Research, Volume 2 — The Analysis of Cohort Studies*. Scientific Publications No. 82. Lyon: International Agency for Research on Cancer.

Breslow, N., Lubin, J. H., Marek, P., and Langholz, B. (1983). Multiplicative models and cohort analysis. *Journal of the American Statistical Association*, *78*(381), 1–12.

Briggs, D. J., Sabel, C. E., and Lee, K. (2009). Uncertainty in epidemiology and health risk and impact assessment. *Environmental Geochemistry and Health*, *31*(2), 189–203.

Brook, D. (1964). On the distinction between the conditional probability and the joint probability approaches in the specification of nearest-neighbour systems. *Biometrika*, *51*(3/4), 481–483.

Brown, P. E., Diggle, P. J., Lord, M. E., and Young, P. C. (2001). Space-time calibration of radar-rainfall data. *Journal of the Royal Statistical Society: Series C (Applied Statistics)*, *50*(2), 221–241.

Brown, P. E., Karesen, K. F., Roberts, G. O., and Tonellato, S. (2000). Blur-generated non-separable space-time models. *Journal of the Royal Statistical Society: Series B (Statistical Methodology)*, *62*, 847–860.

Brown, P. J. (2002). *Measurement, Regression, and Calibration*. Oxford University Press.

Brown, P. J., Le, N. D., and Zidek, J. V. (1994). Inference for a covariance matrix. In A. F. M. Smith and P. R. Freeman (Eds.), *Aspects of Uncertainty: A Tribute to DV Lindley*. Wiley.

Brumback, B. A. (2021). *Fundamentals of Causal Inference: With R*. CRC Press.

Buckingham, E. (1914). On physically similar systems; illustrations of the use of dimensional equations. *Physical Review*, *4*(4), 345–376.

Burke, J. M., Zufall, M. J., and Ozkaynak, H. (2001). A population exposure model for particulate matter: case study results for PM2. 5 in Philadelphia, PA. *Journal of Exposure Analysis and Environmental Epidemiology*, *11*(6), 470–489.

Burnett, R. T., Dales, R. E., Raizenne, M. E., Krewski, D., Summers, P. W., Roberts, G. R., ... Brook, J. (1994). Effects of low ambient levels of ozone and sulfates on the frequency of respiratory admissions to ontario hospitals. *Environmental Research*, *65*(2), 172–194.

Burton, P., Gurrin, L., and Sly, P. (1998). Extending the simple linear regression model to account for correlated responses: An introduction to generalized estimating equations and multi-level modelling. *Statistics in Medicine, 11*, 1825–1839.

Calder, C. A., and Cressie, N. (2007). Some topics in convolution-based spatial modeling. *Proceedings of the 56th Session of the International Statistics Institute*, 22–29.

Cameletti, M., Lindgren, F., Simpson, D., and Rue, H. (2011). Spatio-temporal modeling of particulate matter concentration through the spde approach. *AStA Advances in Statistical Analysis*, 1–23.

Carlin, B. P., and Louis, T. A. (2000). *Bayes and Empirical Bayes Methods for Data Analysis*. Chapman and Hall/CRC.

Carlin, B. P., Xia, H., Devine, O., Tolbert, P., and Mulholland, J. (1999). Spatio-temporal hierarchical models for analyzing Atlanta pediatric asthma ER visit rates. In *Case studies in Bayesian Statistics* (pp. 303–320). Springer.

Carroll, R., Chen, R., George, E., Li, T., Newton, H., Schmiediche, H., and Wang, N. (1997). Ozone exposure and population density in harris county, texas. *Journal of the American Statistical Association, 92*(438), 392–404.

Carroll, R. J., Chen, R., Li, T. H., Newton, H. J., Schmiediche, H., Wang, H., and George, E. I. (1997). Ozone exposure and population density in Harris County, Texas. *Journal of the American Statistical Association, 92*, 392-413.

Carroll, R. J., Ruppert, D., and Stefanski, L. A. (1995). *Measurement Error in Nonlinear Models*. Chapman and Hall, London.

Carstairs, V., and Morris, R. (1989). Deprivation: Explaining differences between mortality between Scotland and England. *British Medical Journal, 299*, 886-889.

Carter, C. K., and Kohn, R. (1994). On Gibbs sampling for state space models. *Biometrika, 81*, 541–553.

Carvalho, C. M., Polson, N. G., and Scott, J. G. (2010, 04). The horseshoe estimator for sparse signals. *Biometrika, 97*(2), 465-480.

Caselton, W. F., Kan, L., and Zidek, J. V. (1992). Quality data networks that minimize entropy. *Statistics in the Environmental and Earth Sciences*, 10–38.

Caselton, W. F., and Zidek, J. V. (1984). Optimal monitoring network designs. *Statistics & Probability Letters, 2*(4), 223–227.

Chang, H., Fu, A., Le, N., and Zidek, J. (2007). Designing environmental monitoring networks to measure extremes. *Environmental and Ecological Statistics, 14*(3), 301–321.

Chang, H. H., Peng, R. D., and Dominici, F. (2011). Estimating the acute health effects of coarse particulate matter accounting for exposure measurement error. *Biostatistics, 12*(4), 637–652.

Chatfield, C. (1995). Model uncertainty, data mining and statistical inference. *Journal of the Royal Statistical Society, Series A, 158*, 419-466.

Chatfield, C. (2000). *Time–Series Forecasting*. Chapman and Hall/CRC.

Chatfield, C. (2013). *The Analysis of Time Series: An Introduction*. CRC press.

Chatfield, C., and Collins, A. (1980). *Introduction to Multivariate Analysis*. Chapman and Hall.

Chen, J. (2013). A partial order on uncertainty and information. *Journal of Theoretical Probability*, *26*, 349–359.

Chen, J., van Eeden, C., and Zidek, J. (2010). Uncertainty and the conditional variance. *Statistics & Probability Letters*, *80*(23–24), 1764–1770.

Clayton, D., and Hills, M. (1993). *Statistical Models in Epidemiology*. Oxford Scientific Publications.

Coles, S., Bawa, J., Trenner, L., and Dorazio, P. (2001). *An Introduction to Statistical Modeling of Extreme Values*. Springer.

Contreras, G. S., Mora, M. R., and Gómez, P. J. (2020). Speed of virus infection by classical dimensional analysis. *Contemporary Engineering Sciences*, *13*(1), 131–147.

Copernicus Atmosphere Monitoring Service. (2018). *CAMS: Hourly Reanalysis – One Year Data for NO_2, O_3, $PM_{2.5}$ and PM_{10} for 2010–2016 in Europe*. Retrieved 2018-10-10, from `http://www.regional.atmosphere.copernicus.eu`

Cox, D. D., Cox, L. H., and Ensor, K. B. (1997). Spatial sampling and the environment: some issues and directions. *Environmental and Ecological Statistics*, *4*(3), 219–233.

Craigmile, P. F., Guttorp, P., and Percival, D. B. (2005). Wavelet-based parameter estimation for polynomial contaminated fractionally differenced processes. *Signal Processing, IEEE Transactions on*, *53*(8), 3151–3161.

Cressie, N. (1985). Fitting variogram models by weighted least squares. *Journal of the International Association for Mathematical Geology*, *17*(5), 563–586.

Cressie, N. (1986). Kriging nonstationary data. *Journal of the American Statistical Association*, *81*(395), 625-634.

Cressie, N. (1990). The origins of kriging. *Mathematical Geology*, *22*(3), 239–252.

Cressie, N. (1993). *Statistics for Spatial Data, revised edition*. John Wiley, New York.

Cressie, N. (1997). Discussion of Carroll, R.J. et al. 'Modeling ozone exposure in Harris county, Texas'. *Journal of the American Statistical Association*, *92*, 392–413.

Cressie, N., and Hawkins, D. M. (1980). Robust estimation of the variogram: I. *Mathematical Geology*, *12*(2), 115–125.

Cressie, N., and Johannesson, G. (2008). Fixed rank kriging for very large spatial data sets. *Journal of the Royal Statistical Society: Series B (Statistical Methodology)*, *70*(1), 209–226.

Cressie, N., and Wikle, C. K. (1998). Discussion of Mardia *at al.*, the kriged Kalman filter. *Test*, *7*, 257–263.

Cressie, N., and Wikle, C. K. (2011). *Statistics for Spatio-Temporal Data*. Wiley.

Cressie, N. A. C. (1993). *Statistics for Spatial Data*. Wiley.

Cullen, A. C., and Frey, H. C. (1999). *Probabilistic Techniques in Exposure Assessment: A Handbook for Dealing with Variability and Uncertainty in Models and Inputs*. Springer.

Damian, D., Sampson, P. D., and Guttorp, P. (2000). Bayesian estimation of semi-parametric non-stationary spatial covariance structures. *Environmetrics, 12*(2), 161–178.

Daniels, M. J., Dominici, F., Zeger, S. L., and Samet, J. M. (2004). The National Morbidity, Mortality, and Air Pollution Study Part III: Concentration-Response Curves and Thresholds for the 20 Largest US Cities. *HEI Project, 96–97*, 1-21.

Davison, A. C., and Smith, R. L. (1990). Models for exceedances over high thresholds. *Journal of the Royal Statistical Society. Series B (Methodology)*, 393–442.

Dawid, A. P. (1981). Some matrix-variate distribution theory: Notational considerations and a bayesian application. *Biometrika, 68*(1), 265–274.

de Valpine, P., Paciorek, C., Turek, D., Michaud, N., Anderson-Bergman, C., Obermeyer, F., ... Paganin, S. (2022). NIMBLE: MCMC, particle filtering, and programmable hierarchical modeling [Computer software manual]. Retrieved from https://cran.r-project.org/package=nimble (R package version 0.12.2) doi: 10.5281/zenodo.1211190

de Valpine, P., Turek, D., Paciorek, C., Anderson-Bergman, C., Temple Lang, D., and Bodik, R. (2017). Programming with models: writing statistical algorithms for general model structures with NIMBLE. *Journal of Computational and Graphical Statistics, 26*, 403–417.

DeGroot, M. H., and Schervish, M. J. (2010). *Probability and Statistics.* Addison Wesley.

de Hoogh, K., Gulliver, J., van Donkelaar, A., Martin, R. V., Marshall, J. D., Bechle, M. J., ... Hoek, G. (2016). Development of West-European $PM_{2.5}$ and NO_2 land use regression models incorporating satellite-derived and chemical transport modelling data. *Environmental Research, 151*, 1–10.

Dellaportas, P., and Smith, A. F. (1993). Bayesian inference for generalized linear and proportional hazards models via gibbs sampling. *Journal of the Royal Statistical Society Series C: Applied Statistics, 42*(3), 443–459.

Denison, D. G. T., Mallick, B. K., and Smith, A. F. M. (1998). Automatic Bayesian curve fitting. *Journal of the Royal Statistical Society, Series B, 60*(2), 333–350.

De Oliveira, V. (2012). Bayesian analysis of conditional autoregressive models. *Annals of the Institute of Statistical Mathematics, 64*(1), 107–133.

DETR. (1998). *Review and Assessment: Monitoring Air Quality.* Department of the Environment, Transport and the Regions. LAQM.TGI.

Dewanji, A., Goddard, M. J., Krewski, D., and Moolgavkar, S. H. (1999). Two stage model for carcinogenesis: number and size distributions of premalignant clones in longitudinal studies. *Mathematical Bioscience, 155*, 1–12.

Diggle, P., Moyeed, R., Rowlingson, B., and Thomson, M. (2002). Childhood malaria in the gambia: A case-study in model-based geostatistics. *Journal of the Royal Statistical Society. Series C (Applied Statistics), 51*(4), 493–506.

Diggle, P. J. (1991). *Time Series, a Biostatistical Introduction.* Oxford University Press.

Diggle, P. J. (1993). Point process modelling in environmental epidemiology. *Statistics for the Environment*.

Diggle, P. J. (2013). *Statistical Analysis of Spatial and Spatio-Temporal Point Patterns*. CRC Press.

Diggle, P. J., Heagerty, P., Liang, K.-Y., and Zeger, S. L. (2002). *Analysis of Longitudinal Data*. Oxford University Press.

Diggle, P. J., Menezes, R., and Su, T. (2010). Geostatistical inference under preferential sampling. *Journal of the Royal Statistical Society: Series C (Applied Statistics)*, *59*(2), 191–232.

Diggle, P. J., and Ribeiro, P. J. (2007). *Model–Based Geostatistics*. Springer.

Diggle, P. J., Tawn, J. A., and Moyeed, R. A. (1998). Model-based geostatistics (with discussion). *Journal of the Royal Statistical Society (C)*, *47*, 299–350.

Director, H., and Bornn, L. (2015). Connecting point-level and gridded moments in the analysis of climate data. *Journal of Climate*, *28*(9), 3496–3510.

Dobbie, M., Henderson, B., and Stevens Jr, D. (2008). Sparse sampling: Spatial design for aquatic monitoring. *Statistics Surveys*, *2*, 113–153.

Dockery, D., and Spengler, J. (1981). Personal exposure to respirable particulates and sulfates. *Journal of Air Pollution Control Association*, *31*, 153–159.

Dominici, F., Samet, J. M., and Zeger, S. L. (2000). Combining evidence on air pollution and daily mortality from the 20 largest US cities: a hierarchical modelling strategy. *Journal of the Royal Statistical Society: Series A (Statistics in Society)*, *163*(3), 263–302.

Dominici, F., and Zeger, S. L. (2000). A measurement error model for time series studies of air pollution and mortality. *Biostatistics*, *1*, 157-175.

Dou, Y. (2007). *Dynamic Linear and Multivariate Bayesian Models for Modelling Environmental Space–Time Fields* (Unpublished doctoral dissertation). University of British Columbia, Department of Statistics.

Dou, Y., Le, N., and Zidek, J. (2010). Modeling hourly ozone concentration fields. *Ann Applied Statistics*, *4*(3), 1183-1213.

Dou, Y., Le, N. D., and Zidek, J. V. (2007). *A Dynamic Linear Model for Hourly Ozone Concentrations* (Tech. Rep. No. TR228). UBC.

Dou, Y., Le, N. D., and Zidek, J. V. (2012). Temporal forecasting with a Bayesian spatial predictor: Application to ozone. *Advances in Meteorology, Article ID 191575*.

Draper, N. R., Guttman, I., and Lapczak, L. (1979). Actual rejection levels in a certain stepwise test. *Communications in Statistics*, *A8*, 99–105.

Eaton, M. L., and George, E. I. (2021). Charles stein and invariance: Beginning with the Hunt–Stein theorem. *The Annals of Statistics*, *49*(4), 1815–1822.

Elfving, G., et al. (1952). Optimum allocation in linear regression theory. *The Annals of Mathematical Statistics*, *23*(2), 255–262.

Elliott, P., Shaddick, G., Kleinschmidt, I., Jolley, D., Walls, P., Beresford, J., and Grundy, C. (1996). Cancer incidence near municipal solid waste incinerators in Great Britain. *British Journal of Cancer*, *73*(5), 702.

Elliott, P., Shaddick, G., Wakefield, J. C., de Hoogh, C., and Briggs, D. J. (2007). Long-term associations of outdoor air pollution with mortality in great britain. *Thorax*, *62*(12), 1088–1094.

Elliott, P., Wakefield, J. C., Best, N. G., and Briggs, D. J. (2000). *Spatial Epidemiology: Methods and Applications.* Oxford University Press.

Elliott, P., and Wartenberg, D. (2004). Spatial epidemiology: Current approaches and future challenges. *Environmental Health Perspectives*, 998–1006.

Embrechts, P., Klüppelberg, C., and Mikosch, T. (1997). *Modelling Extremal Events: for Insurance and Finance.* Springer.

EPA. (2002). *Health and environmental effects of particulate matter.* Retrieved from `https://www.epa.gov/pm-pollution/health-and-environmental-effects-particulate-matter-pm`

EPA. (2004). *Air Quality Criteria for Particulate Matter.* U.S. Environmental Protection Agency.

EPA. (2005). (Final Report, 2006). U.S. Environmental Protection Agency, Washington, DC, EPA/600/R-05/004aF-cF, 2006.

ETC-LC Land Cover (CLC2000). (2013). *Raster Database (version 12/2009).* Retrieved 2013-10-30, from `https://www.eea.europa.eu/data-and-maps/data/corine-land-cover-2000-clc2000-100-m-version-12-2009`

ETC-LC Land Cover (CLC2006). (2014). *Raster Database (version 12/2013).* Retrieved from `https://www.eea.europa.eu/data-and-maps/data/clc-2006-raster-3`

European Commision. (1980). Council directive 80/779/eec of 15 july 1980 on air quality limit values and guide values for sulphur dioxide and suspended particulates.

European Environment Agency. (2018). *Air Quality e-Reporting (AQ e-Reporting) – European Environment Agency.* Retrieved 2018-08-01, from `https://www.eea.europa.eu/data-and-maps/data/aqereporting-8`

EUROSTAT. (2016). *GEOSTAT 1km^2 population grid for Europe in 2011.* Retrieved 2018-10-10, from `https://ec.europa.eu/eurostat/web/gisco/geodata/reference-data/population-distribution-demography/geostat`

Eynon, B., and Switzer, P. (1983). The variability of rainfall acidity. *Canadian Journal of Statistics*, *11*(1), 11–23.

Fanshawe, T. R., Diggle, P. J., Rushton, S., Sanderson, R., Lurz, P. W. W., Glinianaia, S. V., ... Pless-Mulloli, T. (2008). Modelling spatio-temporal variation in exposure to particulate matter: A two-stage approach. *Environmetrics*, *19*(6), 549–566.

Faraway, J. J. (2015). *Linear models with R: Second Edition.* Chapman and Hall/CRC.

Fedorov, V. V., and Hackl, P. (1997). *Model-Oriented Design of Experiments* (Vol. 125). Springer Science & Business Media.

Ferreira, G. S., and Schmidt, A. M. (2006). Spatial modelling of the relative risk of dengue fever in Rio de Janeiro for the epidemic period between 2001 and 2002. *Brazilian Journal of Probability and Statistics*, *20*, 47–63.

Finazzi, F., Scott, E. M., and Fassò, A. (2013). A model-based framework for air quality indices and population risk evaluation, with an application to the analysis of scottish air quality data. *Journal of the Royal Statistical Society: Series C (Applied Statistics)*, *62*(2), 287–308.

Fisher, R. A., and Tippett, L. H. C. (1928). Limiting forms of the frequency distribution of the largest or smallest member of a sample. In *Mathematical Proceedings of the Cambridge Philosophical society* (Vol. 24, pp. 180–190).

Freitas, L., Schmidt, A., Cossich, W., Cruz, O., and Carvalho, M. (2021). Spatio-temporal modelling of the first chikungunya epidemic in an intra-urban setting: The role of socioeconomic status, environment and temperature. *PLoS Negl Trop Dis.*, *15*(6), e0009537.

Frey, H. C., and Rhodes, D. S. (1996). Characterizing, simulating, and analyzing variability and uncertainty: an illustration of methods using an air toxics emissions example. *Human and Ecological Risk Assessment*, *2*(4), 762–797.

Frühwirth-Schnatter, S. (1994). Data augmentation and dynamic linear models. *Journal of Time Series Analysis*, *15*(2), 183–202.

Fu, A., Le, N. D., and Zidek, J. V. (2003). *A statistical characterization of a simulated Canadian annual maximum rainfall field* (Vol. TR 2003-17; Tech. Rep.). Statistical and Mathematical Sciences Institute, RTP, NC.

Fuentes, M. (2002a). Interpolation of nonstationary air pollution processes: a spatial spectral approach. *Statistical Modelling*, *2*(4), 281–298.

Fuentes, M. (2002b). Spectral methods for nonstationary spatial processes. *Biometrika*, *89*(1), 197–210.

Fuentes, M., Chen, L., and Davis, J. M. (2008). A class of nonseparable and non-stationary spatial temporal covariance functions. *Environmetrics*, *19*(5), 487–507.

Fuentes, M., Song, H. R., Ghosh, S. K., Holland, D. M., and Davis, J. M. (2006). Spatial association between speciated fine particles and mortality. *Biometrics*, *62*(3), 855–863.

Fuglstad, G.-A., Simpson, D., Lindgren, F., and Rue, H. (2018). Constructing Priors that Penalize the Complexity of Gaussian Random Fields. *Journal of the American Statistical Association*, *114*(525), 445-452.

Fuller, G., and Connolly, E. (2012). *Reorganisation of the UK Black Carbon network*. Department for Environment, Food and Rural Affairs.

Fuller, W. A. (1987). *Measurement Error Models*. Wiley and Sons.

Funtowicz, S. O., and Ravetz, J. R. (1990). *Uncertainty and Quality in Science for Policy* (Vol. 15). Springer.

Funtowicz, S. O., and Ravetz, J. R. (1993). Science for the post-normal age. *Futures*, *25*(7), 739–755.

Gamerman, D., and Lopes, H. (2006). *Markov Chain Monte Carlo: Stochastic Simulation for Bayesian Inference*. Chapman and Hall/CRC.

Gatrell, A. C., Bailey, T. C., Diggle, P. J., and Rowlingson, B. S. (1996). Spatial point pattern analysis and its application in geographical epidemiology. *Transactions of the Institute of British Geographers*, 256–274.

Gelfand, A. E., Banerjee, S., and Gamerman, D. (2005). Spatial process modelling for univariate and multivariate dynamic spatial data. *Environmetrics*, *16*(5), 465–479.

Gelfand, A. E., Kim, H. J., Sirmans, C. F., and Banerjee, S. (2003). Spatial modeling with spatially varying coefficient processes. *Journal of the American Statistical Association*, *98*(462), 387–396.

Gelfand, A. E., and Sahu, S. K. (1999). Identifiability, improper priors, and Gibbs sampling for generalized linear models. *Journal of the American Statistical Association*, *94*, 247–253.

Gelfand, A. E., Sahu, S. K., and Holland, D. M. (2012). On the effect of preferential sampling in spatial prediction. *Environmetrics*, *23*(7), 565–578.

Gelfand, A. E., Zhu, L., and Carlin, B. P. (2001). On the change of support problem for spatio-temporal data. *Biostatistics*, *2*(1), 31–45.

Gelman, A., Carlin, J. B., Stern, H. S., Dunson, D. B., Vehtari, A., and Rubin, D. B. (2013). *Bayesian Data Analysis* (3rd ed.). Chapman & Hall / CRC.

Geman, S., and Geman, D. (1984). Stochastic relaxation, gibbs distributions, and the bayesian restoration of images. *Pattern Analysis and Machine Intelligence, IEEE Transactions on*(6), 721–741.

Geyer, C. J., and Thompson, E. A. (1992). Constrained monte carlo maximum likelihood for dependent data. *Journal of the Royal Statistical Society: Series B (Methodological)*, *54*(3), 657–683.

Giannitrapani, M., Bowman, A., Scott, E. M., and Smith, R. (2007). Temporal analysis of spatial covariance of SO_2 in Europe from 1990 to 2001. *Environmetrics*, *1*, 1–12.

Gilks, W. R., Richardson, S., and Spiegelhalter, D. J. (1996). *Markov Chain Monte Carlo in Practice*. Chapman and Hall.

Givens, G. H., and Hoeting, J. A. (2013). *Computational Statistics* (2nd ed.). Hoboken, NJ, USA: John Wiley & Sons.

Gneiting, T., Genton, M., and Guttorp, P. (2006). Geostatistical space-time models, stationarity, separability, and full symmetry. *Monographs on Statistics and Applied Probability*, *107*, 151.

Goldstein, H. (1987). *Multilevel Models in Educational and Social Research*. Charles Griffin.

Golub, G. H., and Loan, C. F. V. (1996). *Matrix Computations* (Third ed.). The Johns Hopkins University Press.

Good, I. J. (1952). Rational decisions. *Journal of the Royal Statistical Society. Series B (Methodological)*, 107–114.

Gotway, C. A., and Young, L. J. (2002). Combining incompatible spatial data. *Journal of the American Statistical Association*, *97*(458), 632–648.

Green, P. J., and Silverman, B. W. (1994). *Nonparametric Regression and Generalized Linear Models: A Roughness Penalty Approach*. Chapman & Hall/CRC.

Greenland, S., and Morgenstern, H. (1989). Ecological bias, confounding, and effect modification. *International Journal of Epidemiology*, *18*(1), 269–274.

Gryparis, A., Paciorek, C. J., Zeka, A., Schwartz, J., and Coull, B. A. (2009). Measurement error caused by spatial misalignment in environmental epidemiology. *Biostatistics*, *10*(2), 258–274.

Gu, C. (2002). *Smoothing Spline ANOVA Models*. Springer.

Guan, Y., and Afshartous, D. R. (2007). Test for independence between marks and points of marked point processes: a subsampling approach. *Environmental and Ecological Statistics*, *14*, 101–111.

Gumbel, E. J. (2012). *Statistics of Extremes*. Courier Dover Publications.

Guttorp, P., Meiring, W., and Sampson, P. D. (1994). A space-time analysis of ground-level ozone data. *Environmetrics*, *5*(3), 241–254.

Guttorp, P., and Sampson, P. D. (2010). Discussion of Geostatistical inference under preferential sampling by Diggle, P. J., Menezes, R. and Su, T. *Journal of the Royal Statistical Society: Series C (Applied Statistics)*, *59*(2), 191–232.

Haas, T. C. (1990). Lognormal and moving window methods of estimating acid deposition. *Journal of the American Statistical Association*, *85*(412), 950–963.

Hadley, W. (2014). Tidy data. *Journal of Statistical Software*, *59*(10), 1–23.

Hamilton, J. (1994). *Time Series Analysis*. Princeton University Press.

Handcock, M., and Wallis, J. (1994). An approach to statistical spatial-temporal modelling of meteorological fields (with discussion). *Journal of the American Statistical Association*, *89*, 368-390.

Harris, B. (1982). Entropy. In S. Kotz and N. Johnson, "Encyclopedia of Statistical Sciences," John Wiley and Sons, Inc., New York, 1982.

Harrison, J. (1999). *Bayesian Forecasting & Dynamic Models*. Springer.

Harrison, P. J., and Stevens, C. F. (1971). A Bayesian approach to short-term forecasting. *Operational Research Quarterly*, 341–362.

Harvey, A. (1993). *Time Series Models* (2nd ed.). MIT Press.

Haslett, J., and Raftery, A. E. (1989). Space-time modelling with long-memory dependence: assessing Ireland's wind power. *Applied Statistics*, *38*, 1–50.

Hassler, B., Petropavlovskikh, I., Staehelin, J., August, T., Bhartia, P. K., Clerbaux, C., ... Dufour, G. (2014). Past changes in the vertical distribution of ozone–part 1: Measurement techniques, uncertainties and availability. *Atmospheric Measurement Techniques*, *7*(5), 1395–1427.

Hastie, T., and Tibshirani, R. (1990). *Generalized Additive Models*. Chapman and Hall, London.

Hastings, W. (1970). Monte Carlo sampling methods using Markov chains and their applications. *Biometrika*, *57*(1), 97.

Hauptmann, M., Berhane, K., Langholz, B., and Lubin, J. H. (2001). Using splines to analyse latency in the Colorado Plateau uranium miners cohort. *Journal of Epidemiology and Biostatistics*, *6*(6), 417–424.

Heaton, M. J., Datta, A., Finley, A. O., Furrer, R., Guhaniyogi, R., Gerber, F., ... Zammit-Mangion, A. (2018). A Case Study among Methods for Analyzing Large Spatial Data. *arXiv preprint arXiv:1710.05013*.

Heffernan, J. E., and Tawn, J. A. (2004). A conditional approach for multivariate extreme values (with discussion). *Journal of the Royal Statistical Society: Series B (Statistical Methodology)*, 66(3), 497–546.

Helton, J. C. (1997). Uncertainty and sensitivity analysis in the presence of stochastic and subjective uncertainty. *Journal of Statistical Computation and Simulation*, 57(1–4), 3–76.

Hempel, S. (2014). *The Medical Detective: John Snow, Cholera and the Mystery of the Broad Street Pump*. Granta Books.

Hickling, J., Clements, M., Weinstein, P., and Woodward, A. (1999). Acute health effects of the Mount Ruapehu (New Zealand) volcanic eruption of June 1996. *International Journal of Environmental Health Research*, 9(2), 97–107.

Higdon, D. (1998). A process-convolution approach to modelling temperatures in the North Atlantic Ocean. *Environmental and Ecological Statistics*, 5(2), 173–190.

Higdon, D. (2002). Space and space-time modeling using process convolutions. In *Quantitative Methods for Current Environmental Issues* (pp. 37–56). Springer.

Higdon, D., Swall, J., and Kern, J. (1999). Non-stationary spatial modeling. In *Bayesian statistics 6 – proceedings of the sixth valencia meeting* (p. 761-768). J.M. Bernardo, J.O. Berger, A.P. Dawid, and A.F.M. Smith, (editors). Clarendon Press, Oxford.

Hill, A. B. (1965). The environment and disease: association or causation? *Proceedings of the Royal Society of Medicine*, 58(5), 295.

Hjelle, Ø., and Dæhlen, M. (2006). *Triangulations and Applications*. Springer Science & Business Media.

Hoek, G., Brunekreef, B., Goldbohm, S., Fischer, P., and van den Brandt, P. A. (2002). Associations between mortality and indicators of traffic-related air pollution in the Netherlands: A cohort study. *Lancet*, 360, 1203–1209.

Hosseini, R., Le, N. D., and Zidek, J. V. (2011). A characterization of categorical Markov chains. *Journal of Statistical Theory and Practice*, 5(2), 261–284.

Huerta, G., Sansó, B., and Stroud, J. (2004). A spatiotemporal model for Mexico city ozone levels. *Journal of the Royal Statistical Society: Series C (Applied Statistics)*, 53(2), 231–248.

Hume, D. (2011). *An Enquiry Concerning Human Understanding*. Broadview Press.

Iman, R. L., and Conover, W. (1982). A distribution-free approach to inducing rank correlation among input variables. *Communications in Statistics-Simulation and Computation*, 11(3), 311–334.

Inness, A., Baier, F., Benedetti, A., Bouarar, I., Chabrillat, S., Clark, H., … the MACC team (2013). The MACC reanalysis: An 8 yr data set of atmospheric composition. *Atmospheric Chemistry and Physics*, 13, 4073–4109.

Ioannidis, J. P. (2005). Contradicted and initially stronger effects in highly cited clinical research. *Journal of the American Medical Association*, 294(2), 218–228.

Jacob, P. E., Murray, L. M., Holmes, C. C., and Robert, C. P. (2017). Better together? statistical learning in models made of modules. *arXiv preprint arXiv:1708.08719*.

Jarvis, A., Reuter, H. I., Nelson, A., and Guevara, E. (2008). Hole-filled srtm for the globe version 4. *available from the CGIAR-CSI SRTM 90m Database (http://srtm.csi.cgiar.org)*, *15*(25-54), 5.

Jaynes, E. T. (1963). Information theory and statistical mechanics (notes by the lecturer). In *Statistical Physics 3* (Vol. 1, p. 181).

Jones, A., Zidek, J. V., and Watson, J. (2023). Preferential monitoring site location in the Southern California Air Quality Basin. *arXiv preprint arXiv:2304.10006*.

Journel, A., and Huijbregts, C. (1978). Mining geostatistics. *New York*.

Jun, M., Knutti, R., and Nychka, D. W. (2008). Spatial analysis to quantify numerical model bias and dependence: How many climate models are there? *Journal of the American Statistical Association*, *103*(483), 934–947.

Kaiser, M. S., and Cressie, N. (2000). The construction of multivariate distributions from Markov random fields. *Journal of Multivariate Analysis*, *73*(2), 199–220.

Kalenderski, S., and Steyn, D. G. (2011). Mixed deterministic statistical modelling of regional ozone air pollution. *Environmetrics*, *22*(4), 572–586.

Kalnay, E. (2003). *Atmospheric Modeling, Data assimilation, and Predictability*. Cambridge University Press.

Kass, E., and Wasserman, L. (1995). A reference Bayesian test for nested hypothesis and its relationship to the Schwarz criterion. *Journal of the American Statistical Association*, *90*(431), 928-934.

Kass, R. E., and Raftery, A. E. (1995). Bayes factors. *Journal of the American Statistical Association*, *90*, 773-795.

Katsouyanni, K., Schwartz, J., Spix, C., Touloumi, G., Zmirou, D., Zanobetti, A., ... Anderson, H. (1995). Short term effects of air pollution on health: A European approach using epidemiologic time series data: the APHEA protocol. *Journal of Epidemiology and Public Health*, *50 (Suppl 1)*, S12–S18.

Katzfuss, M. (2017). A Multi-Resolution Approximation for Massive Spatial Datasets. *Journal of the American Statistical Association*, *112*(517), 201–214.

Kelsall, J. E., Zeger, S. L., and Samet, J. M. (1999). Frequency domain log-linear models; air pollution and mortality. *Journal of the Royal Statistical Society: Series C (Applied Statistics)*, *48*(3), 331–344.

Kermark, M., and Mckendrick, A. (1927). Contributions to the mathematical theory of epidemics. Part I. *Proc. R. Soc. A*, *115*(5), 700–721.

Kiefer, J. (1959). Optimum experimental designs. *Journal of the Royal Statistical Society. Series B (Methodological)*, 272–319.

Kim, Y., Kim, J., and Kim, Y. (2006). Blockwise sparse regression. *Statistica Sinica*, *16*(2), 375.

Kinney, P., and Ozkaynak, H. (1991). Associations of daily mortality and air pollution in Los Angeles County. *Environmental Research*, *54*, 99–120.

Kleiber, W., Katz, R. W., and Rajagopalan, B. (2013). Daily minimum and maximum temperature simulation over complex terrain. *The Annals of Applied Statistics*, *7*(1), 588–612.

Kleinschmidt, I., Hills, M., and Elliott, P. (1995). Smoking behaviour can be predicted by neighbourhood deprivation measures. *Journal of Epidemiology and Community Health*, *49 (Suppl 2)*, S72-7.

Kloog, I., Chudnovsky, A. A., Just, A. C., Nordio, F., Koutrakis, P., Coull, B. A., ... Schwartz, J. (2014). A new hybrid spatio-temporal model for estimating daily multi-year $PM_{2.5}$ concentrations across northeastern USA using high resolution aerosol optical depth data. *Atmospheric Environment*, *95*, 581–590.

Knorr-Held, L. (1999). Conditional Prior Proposals in Dynamic Models. *Scandinavian Journal of Statistics*, *26*, 129-144.

Ko, C.-W., Lee, J., and Queyranne, M. (1995). An exact algorithm for maximum entropy sampling. *Operations Research*, *43*(4), 684–691.

Kolmogorov, A. (1941). Interpolated and extrapolated stationary random sequences. *Izvestia an SSSR, Seriya Mathematicheskaya*, *5*(2), 85–95.

Krainski, E. T., Gómez-Rubio, V., Bakka, H., Lenzi, A., Castro-Camilo, D., Simpson, D., ... Rue, H. (2018). *Advanced Spatial Modeling with Stochastic Partial Differential Equations Using R and INLA*. CRC Press.

Krige, D. (1951). *A Statistical Approach to Some Mine Valuation and Allied Problems on the Witwatersrand* (Unpublished doctoral dissertation). University of the Witwatersrand.

Laird, N., and Ware, J. (1982). Random-effects models for longitudinal data. *Biometrics*, *38*, 963-974.

Law, P., Zelenka, M., Huber, A., and McCurdy, T. (1997). Evaluation of a probabilistic exposure model applied. *Journal of the Air & Waste Management Association*, *47*(3), 491–500.

Lawson, A. B. (2013). *Statistical Methods in Spatial Epidemiology*. John Wiley & Sons.

Le, N. D., Sun, W., and Zidek, J. V. (1997). Bayesian multivariate spatial interpolation with data missing by design. *Journal of the Royal Statistical Society: Series B (Statistical Methodology)*, *59*(2), 501–510.

Le, N. D., and Zidek, J. V. (1992). Interpolation with uncertain spatial covariances: a bayesian alternative to kriging. *Journal of Multivariate Analysis*, *43*(2), 351–374.

Le, N. D., and Zidek, J. V. (1994). Network designs for monitoring multivariate random spatial fields. *Recent Advances in Statistics and Probability*, 191–206.

Le, N. D., and Zidek, J. V. (2006). *Statistical Analysis of Environmental Space–Time Processes*. Springer Verlag.

Le, N. D., and Zidek, J. V. (2010). Air pollution and cancer. *Chronic Diseases in Canada*, *29, Supplement 2*(144–163).

Leadbetter, M. (1983). Extremes and local dependence in stationary sequences. *Probability Theory and Related Fields*, *65*(2), 291–306.

Leduc, H. (2011). *Estimation de Paramètres dans des Modéles d'Épidémies* (Unpublished master's thesis). Département de mathématiques, University of Quebec.

Lee, D. (2013). CARBayes: an R package for Bayesian spatial modeling with conditional autoregressive priors. *Journal of Statistical Software*, *55*(13), 1–24.

Lee, D., Ferguson, C., and Scott, E. M. (2011). Constructing representative air quality indicators with measures of uncertainty. *Journal of the Royal Statistical Society: Series A (Statistics in Society)*, *174*(1), 109–126.

Lee, D., and Shaddick, G. (2010). Spatial modeling of air pollution in studies of its short-term health effects. *Biometrics*, *66*, 1238-1246.

Lee, J.-T., Kim, H., Hong, Y.-C., Kwon, H.-J., Schwartz, J., and Christiani, D. C. (2000). Air pollution and daily mortality in seven major cities of Korea, 1991–1997. *Environmental Research*, *84*(3), 247–254.

Lee, T. Y., Zidek, J. V., and Heckman, N. (2020). Dimensional analysis in statistical modelling. *arXiv preprint arXiv:2002.11259*.

Leroux, B. G., Lei, X., and Breslow, N. (1999). Estimation of disease rates in small areas: A new mixed model for spatial dependence. In D. B. M. E. Halloran (Ed.), *Statistical Models in Epidemiology, the Environment, and Clinical Trials* (pp. 135–178). Springer-Verlag, New York.

Li, K., Le, N. D., Sun, L., and Zidek, J. V. (1999). Spatial-temporal models for ambient hourly PM10 in Vancouver. *Environmetrics*, *10*, 321-338.

Lin, D. K., and Shen, W. (2013). Comment: Some statistical concerns on dimensional analysis. *Technometrics*, *55*(3), 281–285.

Lindgren, F., Rue, H., and Lindström, J. (2011). An explicit link between Gaussian fields and Gaussian Markov random fields: The stochastic partial differential equation approach. *Journal of the Royal Statistical Society: Series B (Statistical Methodology)*, *73*(4), 423–498.

Lindley, D. V. (1956). On a measure of the information provided by an experiment. *The Annals of Mathematical Statistics*, *27*(4), 986–1005.

Lioy, P., Waldman, J., Buckley, Butler, J., and Pietarinen, C. (1990). The personal, indoor and outdoor concentrations of pm-10 measured in an industrial community during the winter. *Atmospheric Environment. Part B. Urban Atmosphere*, *24*(1), 57–66.

Little, R. J. A., and Rubin, D. B. (2014). *Statistical Analysis with Missing Data*. John Wiley & Sons.

Liu, F., Bayarri, M. J., and Berger, J. O. (2009). Modularization in Bayesian analysis, with emphasis on analysis of computer models. *Bayesian Analysis*, *4*(1), 119-150.

Livingstone, A. E., Shaddick, G., Grundy, C., and Elliott, P. (1996). Do people living near inner city main roads have more asthma needing treatment? Case-control study. *British Medical Journal*, *312*(7032), 676–677.

Lubin, J. H., Boice, J. D., Edling, C., Hornung, R. W., Howe, G. R., Kunz, E., ... Samet, J. M. (1995). Lung cancer in radon-exposed miners and estimation of risk from indoor exposure. *Journal of the National Cancer Institute*, *87*(11), 817–827.

Lumley, T., and Sheppard, L. (2000). Assessing seasonal confounding and model selection bias in air pollution epidemiology using positive and negative control analyses. *Environmetrics*, *11*(6), 705–717.

Lunn, D., Jackson, C., Best, N., Thomas, A., and Spiegelhalter, D. (2012). *The BUGS Book: A Practical Introduction to Bayesian Analysis.* CRC press.

Lunn, D., Thomas, A., Best, N., and Spiegelhalter, D. (2000). WinBUGS – a Bayesian modelling framework: Concepts, structure, and extensibility. *Statistics and Computing, 10*(4), 325–337.

MacIntosh, D., Xue, J., Ozkaynak, H., Spengler, J., and Ryan, P. (1994). A population-based exposure model for benzene. *Journal of Exposure Analysis and Environmental Epidemiology, 5*(3), 375–403.

MacLeod, M., Fraser, A. J., and Mackay, D. (2002). Evaluating and expressing the propagation of uncertainty in chemical fate and bioaccumulation models. *Environmental Toxicology and Chemistry, 21*(4), 700–709.

Magnello, M. E. (2012). Victorian statistical graphics and the iconography of florence nightingale's polar area graph. *BSHM Bulletin: Journal of the British Society for the History of Mathematics, 27*(1), 13–37.

Mar, T. F., Norris, G. A., Koenig, J. Q., and Larson, T. V. (2000). Associations between air pollution and mortality in Phoenix, 1995–1997. *Environmental Health Perspectives, 108*(4), 347.

Mardia, K., Goodall, C., Redfern, E., and Alonso, F. (1998). The kriged Kalman filter. *Test, 7*, 217–276.

Martins, T. G., Simpson, D., Lindgren, F., and Rue, H. (2013). Bayesian computing with INLA: New features. *Computational Statistics and Data Analysis, 67*, 68–83.

Matérn, B. (1986). *Spatial Variation.* Springer Verlag.

Matheron, G. (1963). Principles of geostatistics. *Economic Geology, 58*, 1246–1266.

Miyasato, M. and Low, J. (2019). *Annual air quality monitoring network plan.* South Coast AQMD.

Mazumdar, S., Schimmel, H., and Higgins, I. (1982). Relation of daily mortality to air pollution: an analysis of 14 London winters, 1958/59-1971/72. *Archives of Environmental Health, 37*, 213-20.

McCullagh, P., and Nelder, J. (1989). *Generalized Linear Models* (2nd ed.). Chapman and Hall.

McKay, M., Beckman, R., and Conover, W. (2000). A comparison of three methods for selecting values of input variables in the analysis of output from a computer code. *Technometrics, 42*(1), 55–61.

McMillan, N. J., Holland, D. M., Morara, M., and Feng, J. (2010). Combining numerical model output and particulate data using Bayesian space–time modeling. *Environmetrics, 21*(1), 48–65.

Meiring, W., Sampson, P. D., and Guttorp, P. (1998). Space-time estimation of grid-cell hourly ozone levels for assessment of a deterministic model. *Environmental and Ecological Statistics, 5*(3), 197–222.

Metropolis, N., Rosenbluth, A. W., Rosenbluth, M. N., Teller, A. H., and Teller, E. (1953). Equation of state calculations by fast computing machines. *The Journal of Chemical Physics, 21*(6), 1087.

Metropolis, N., and Ulam, S. (1949). The Monte Carlo method. *Journal of the American Statistical Association, 44*(247), 335–341.

Ministry of Health. (1954). *Mortality and Morbidity during the London Fog of December, 1962.* H.M.S.O. London.

Mitch, M. E. (1990). *National Stream Survey Database Guide.* US Environmental Protection Agency, Office of Research and Development.

Moolgavkar, S. H. (2000). Air pollution and daily mortality in three US counties. *Environmental Health Perspectives, 108*(8), 777.

Moraga, P. (2019). *Geospatial Health Data: Modeling and Visualization with R-INLA and shiny.* CRC Press.

Morgan, M. G., and Small, M. (1992). *Uncertainty: A Guide to Dealing with Uncertainty in Quantitative Risk and Policy Analysis.* Cambridge University Press.

Müller, W. G. (2007). *Collecting Spatial Data: Optimum Design of Experiments for Random Fields* (3rd ed.). Heidelberg: Physica-Verlag.

Müller, W. G., and Zimmerman, D. L. (1999). Optimal design for variogram estimation. *Environmetrics*, 23-27.

Neas, L., Schwartz, J., and Dockery, D. (1999). A case-crossover analysis of air pollution and mortality in Philadelphia. *Environmental Health Perspectives, 107*, 629–631.

Nuzzo, R. (2014). Scientific method: Statistical errors. *Nature, 506*, 150–152.

Nychka, D., and Saltzman, N. (1998). Design of air-quality monitoring networks. In *Case Studies in Environmental Statistics* (pp. 51–76). Springer.

Oden, N. L., and Benkovitz, C. M. (1990). Statistical implications of the dependence between the parameters used for calculations of large scale emissions inventories. *Atmospheric Environment. Part A. General Topics, 24*(3), 449–456.

Oh, H., and Li, T. (2004). Estimation of global temperature fields from scattered observations by a spherical-wavelet-based spatially adaptive method. *Journal of the Royal Statistical Society: Series B (Statistical Methodology), 66*(1), 221–238.

O'Hagan, A. (1995). Fractional Bayes factors for model comparison. *Journal of the Royal Statistical Society. Series B (Methodology)*, 99–138.

Olea, R. A. (1984). Sampling design optimization for spatial functions. *Journal of the International Association for Mathematical Geology, 16*(4), 369–392.

Omre, H. (1984). The variogram and its estimation. *Geostatistics for Natural Resources Characterization, 1*, 107–125.

Ott, W., Thomas, J., Mage, D., and Wallace, L. (1988). Validation of the simulation of human activity and pollutant exposure (shape) model using paired days from the Denver, CO, carbon monoxide field study. *Atmospheric Environment (1967), 22*(10), 2101–2113.

Ozkaynak, H., Xue, J., Spengler, J., Wallace, L., Pellizzari, E., and Jenkins, P. (1996). Personal exposure to airborne particles and metals: Results from the particle team study in Riverside California. *Journal of Exposure Analysis and Environmental Epidemiology, 6*, 57–78.

Paciorek, C. J., and Schervish, M. J. (2006). Spatial modelling using a new class of nonstationary covariance functions. *Environmetrics, 17*(5), 483–506.

Paciorek, C. J., Yanosky, J. D., Puett, R. C., Laden, F., and Suh, H. (2009). Practical large-scale spatio-temporal modeling of particulate matter concentrations. *Annals of Applied Statistics*, *3*(1), 370–397.

Pati, D., Reich, B. J., and Dunson, D. B. (2011). Bayesian geostatistical modelling with informative sampling locations. *Biometrika*, *98*(1), 35–48.

Pebesma, E. J., and Heuvelink, G. B. (1999). Latin hypercube sampling of Gaussian random fields. *Technometrics*, *41*(4), 303–312.

Peng, R. D., and Bell, M. L. (2010). Spatial misalignment in time series studies of air pollution and health data. *Biostatistics*, *11*, 720–740.

Peng, R. D., and Dominici, F. (2008). Statistical methods for environmental epidemiology with R. In *R: A Case Study in Air Pollution and Health*. Springer.

Perrin, O., and Schlather, M. (2007). Can any multivariate Gaussian vector be interpreted as a sample from a stationary random process? *Statist. Prob. Lett.*, *77*, 881–4.

Peters, A., Skorkovsky, J., Kotesovec, F., Brynda, J., Spix, C., Wichmann, H. E., and Heinrich, J. (2000). Associations between mortality and air pollution in central Europe. *Environmental Health Perspectives*, *108*(4), 283.

Petris, G., Petrone, S., and Campagnoli, P. (2009). *Dynamic Linear Models*. Springer.

Pickands III, J. (1975). Statistical inference using extreme order statistics. *The Annals of Statistics*, 119–131.

Plummer, M. (2014). Cuts in Bayesian graphical models. *Statistics and Computing*, 1–7.

Plummer, M., and Clayton, D. (1996). Estimation of population exposure in ecological studies. *Journal of the Royal Statistical Society. Series B (Statistical Methodology)*, 113–126.

Porwal, A., and Raftery, A. E. (2022). Comparing methods for statistical inference with model uncertainty. *Proc Natl Acad Sci U S A*, *119*(16), e2120737119.

Post, E., Maier, A., and Mahoney, H. (2007). *Users Guide for TRIM.RiskHuman Health-Probabilistic Application for the Ozone NAAQS Risk Assessment*. U.S. Environmental Protection Agency.

Prentice, R., and Sheppard, L. (1995). Aggregate data studies of disease risk factors. *Biometrika*, *82*, 113–125.

Raftery, A. E., and Richardson, S. (1996). Model selection for generalised linear models via glib: Application to nutrition and breast cancer. In *Bayesian Biostatistics*. Marcel-Dekker, New York.

Rao, T. (1999). Mahalanobis' contributions to sample surveys: The origins of sampling in india. *Resonance*, *4*(6), 27–33.

Reinsel, G., Tiao, G. C., Wang, M. N., Lewis, R., and Nychka, D. (1981). Statistical analysis of stratospheric ozone data for the detection of trends. *Atmospheric Environment*, *15*(9), 1569–1577.

Rényi, A. (1961, January). On measures of entropy and information. In *Proceedings of the Fourth Berkeley Symposium on Mathematical Statistics and Probability, Volume 1: Contributions to the Theory of Statistics* (Vol. 4, pp. 547–562). University of California Press.

Richardson, S., and Gilks, W. R. (1993). Conditional independence models for epidemiological studies with covariate measurement error. *Statistics in Medicine*, *12*, 1703–1722.

Richardson, S., Leblond, L., Jaussent, I., and Green, P. J. (2002). Mixture models in measurement error problems, with reference to epidemiological studies. *Journal of the Royal Statistical Society: Series A (Statistics in Society)*, *165*(3), 549–566.

Richardson, S., Stücker, I., and Hémon, D. (1987). Comparison of relative risks obtained in ecological and individual studies: some methodological considerations. *International Journal of Epidemiology*, *16*(1), 111–120.

Riebler, A., Sørbye, S. H., Simpson, D., and Rue, H. (2016). An intuitive Bayesian spatial model for disease mapping that accounts for scaling. *Statistical Methods in Medical Research*, *25*(4), 1145–1165.

Ripley, B., and Corporation, E. (1987). *Stochastic Simulation*. Wiley Online Library.

Ro, C., Tang, A., Chan, W., Kirk, R., Reid, N., and Lusis, M. (1988). Wet and dry deposition of sulfur and nitrogen compounds in Ontario. *Atmospheric Environment (1967)*, *22*(12), 2763–2772.

Robins, J. (1986). A new approach to causal inference in mortality studies with a sustained exposure period – application to control of the healthy worker survivor effect. *Mathematical Modelling*, *7*(9–12), 1393–1512.

Robins, J., and Greenland, S. (1989). The probability of causation under a stochastic model for individual risk. *Biometrics*, *45*(4), 1125–1138.

Rothman, K. J., and Greenland, S. (1998). *Modern Epidemiology*. Lippencott-Raven.

Royle, J., and Nychka, D. (1998). An algorithm for the construction of spatial coverage designs with implementation in SPLUS. *Computers & Geosciences*, *24*(5), 479–488.

Rubinstein, R. Y., and Kroese, D. P. (2011). *Simulation and the Monte Carlo Method* (Vol. 707). John Wiley & Sons.

Rue, H., and Held, L. (2005). *Gaussian Markov Random Fields: Theory and Applications*. CRC Press.

Rue, H., Martino, S., and Chopin, N. (2009). Approximate Bayesian inference for latent Gaussian models by using integrated nested Laplace approximations. *Journal of the Royal Statistical Society: Series B (Statistical Methodology)*, *71*(2), 319–392.

Rue, H., Martino, S., and Lindgren, F. (2012). The R-INLA Project. *R-INLA* *http://www.r-inla.org*.

Ruppert, D., Wand, M. P., and Carroll, R. J. (2003). *Semiparametric Regression*. Cambridge University Press.

Sahu, S. K., Gelfand, A. E., and Holland, D. M. (2006). Spatio-temporal modeling of fine particulate matter. *Journal of Agricultural, Biological, and Environmental Statistics*, *11*(1), 61–86.

Sahu, S. K., Gelfand, A. E., and Holland, D. M. (2007). High-resolution space-time ozone modeling for assessing trends. *Journal of the American Statistical Association*, *102*(480), 1221–1234.

Sahu, S. K., and Mardia, K. (2005). A Bayesian kriged Kalman model for short-term forecasting of air pollution levels. *Journal of the Royal Statistical Society: Series C (Applied Statistics)*, *54*(1), 223–244.

Sampson, P. D., and Guttorp, P. (1992). Nonparametric estimation of nonstationary spatial covariance structure. *Journal of the American Statistical Association*, *87*, 108–119.

Schabenberger, O., and Gotway, C. A. (2000). *Statistical Methods for Spatial Data Analysis*. Chapman and Hall/CRC.

Schafer, D. W. (2001). Semiparametric maximum likelihood for measurement error model regression. *Biometrics*, *57*(1), 53–61.

Schafer, J. (1997). *Analysis of Incomplete Multivariate Data*. Chapman & Hall.

Schlather, M., Ribeiro Jr, P. J., and Diggle, P. J. (2004). Detecting dependence between marks and locations of marked point processes. *Journal of the Royal Statistical Society: Series B (Statistical Methodology)*, *66*(1), 79–93.

Schmeltz, D., Evers, D. C., Driscoll, C. T., Artz, R., Cohen, M., Gay, D., ... Morris, K. *et al.*. (2011). MercNet: a national monitoring network to assess responses to changing mercury emissions in the United States. *Ecotoxicology*, *20*(7), 1713–1725.

Schmidt, A. M., and Lopes, H. F. (2019). Dynamic models. In A. E. Gelfand, M. Fuentes, J. Hoeting, and R. Smith (Eds.), *Handbook of Environmental and Ecological Statistics* (pp. 57–80). Chapman and Hall/CRC.

Schmidt, A. M., and O'Hagan, A. (2003). Bayesian inference for non-stationary spatial covariance structure via spatial deformations. *Journal of the Royal Statistical Society: Series B (Statistical Methodology)*, *65*(3), 743–758.

Schumacher, P., Zidek, J. V. (1993). Using prior information in designing intervention detection experiments, *21*(1), 447–463.

Schwartz, J. (1994a). Nonparamteric smoothing in the analysis of air pollution and respiratory health. *Canadian Journal of Statistics*, *22*(4), 471-487.

Schwartz, J. (1994b). Total suspended particulate matter and daily mortality in Cincinnati, Ohio. *Environmental Health Perspectives*, *102*, 186–189.

Schwartz, J. (1995). Short term flucuations in air pollution and hospital admissions of the eldery for respiratory disease. *Thorax*, *50*, 531-538.

Schwartz, J. (1997). Air pollution and hospital admissions. *Epidemiology*, *8*(4), 371–377.

Schwartz, J. (2000). The distributed lag between air pollution and daily deaths. *Epidemiology*, *11*, 320–326.

Schwartz, J. (2001). Air pollution and blood markers of cardiovascular risk. *Environmental Health Perspectives*, *109*(Suppl 3), 405.

Schwartz, J., and Marcus, A. (1990). Mortality and air pollution in London: A time series analysis. *American Journal of Epidemiology*, *131*, 185-194.

Schwartz, J., Slater, D., Larson, T. V., Pierson, W. E., and Koenig, J. Q. (1993). Particulate air pollution and hospital emergency room visits for asthma in Seattle. *American Review of Respiratory Disease*, *147*(4), 826–831.

Scientific Advisory Panel. (2002). Stochastic Human Exposure and Dose Simulation Model (SHEDS): System Operation Review of a Scenario Specific Model (SHEDSWood) to Estimate Children's Exposure and Dose to Wood Preservatives from Treated Playsets and Residential Decks Using EPA's SHEDS.

Scott, A., and Wild, C. (2001). Maximum likelihood for generalised case-control studies. *Journal of Statistical Planning and Inference, 96*(1), 3–27.

Scott, A., and Wild, C. (2011). Fitting binary regression models with response-biased samples. *Canadian Journal of Statistics, 39*(3), 519–536.

Sebastiani, P., and Wynn, H. P. (2002). Maximum entropy sampling and optimal bayesian experimental design. *Journal of the Royal Statistical Society: Series B (Statistical Methodology), 62*(1), 145–157.

Sellke, T., Bayarri, M., and Berger, J. (1999). Calibration of p-values for precise null hypotheses. *The American Statistician, 55*(1).

Shaddick, G., Lee, D., and Wakefield, J. (2013). Ecological bias in studies of the short-term effects of air pollution on health. *International Journal of Applied Earth Observation and Geoinformation, 22*, 65–74.

Shaddick, G., Lee, D., Zidek, J. V., and Salway, R. (2008). Estimating exposure response functions using ambient pollution concentrations. *The Annals of Applied Statistics, 2*(4), 1249–1270.

Shaddick, G., Thomas, M. L., Green, A., Brauer, M., van Donkelaar, A., Burnett, R., ... Prüss-Ustün, A. (2018). Data integration model for air quality: a hierarchical approach to the global estimation of exposures to ambient air pollution. *Journal of the Royal Statistical Society: Series C (Applied Statistics), 67*(1), 231–253.

Shaddick, G., and Wakefield, J. (2002). Modelling daily multivariate pollutant data at multiple sites. *Journal of the Royal Statistical Society: Series C (Applied Statistics), 51*(3), 351–372.

Shaddick, G., Yan, H., Salway, R., Vienneau, D., Kounali, D., and Briggs, D. (2013). Large-scale Bayesian spatial modelling of air pollution for policy support. *Journal of Applied Statistics, 40*(4), 777–794.

Shaddick, G., and Zidek, J. V. (2014). A case study in preferential sampling: Long term monitoring of air pollution in the UK. *Spatial Statistics, 9*, 51–65.

Shannon, C. E. (2001). A mathematical theory of communication. *ACM SIGMOBILE Mobile Computing and Communications Review, 5*(1), 3–55.

Shen, S., Lau, W., Kim, K., and Li, G. (2001). A canonical ensemble correlation prediction model for seasonal precipitation anomaly. *NASA Technical Memorandum, NASA-TM-2001-209989.*

Shen, W. (2015). *Dimensional analysis in statistics: theories, methodologies and applications* (Unpublished doctoral dissertation). The Pennsylvania State University.

Shen, W., and Lin, D. K. (2019). Statistical theories for dimensional analysis. *Statistica Sinica, 29*(2), 527–550.

Sheppard, L., and Damian, D. (2000). Estimating short-term PM effects accounting for surrogate exposure measurements from ambient monitors. *Environmetrics, 11*(6), 675–687.

Shewry, M. C., and Wynn, H. P. (1987). Maximum entropy sampling. *Journal of Applied Statistics*, *14*(2), 165–170.

Silverman, B. W. (1986). *Density Estimation*. London: Chapman and Hall.

Silvey, S. D. (1980). *Optimal Design*. Springer.

Simpson, D., Rue, H., Riebler, A., Martins, T. G., and Sørbye, S. H. (2017). Penalising Model Component Complexity: A Principled, Practical Approach to Constructing Priors. *Statistical Science*, *32*(1), 1–28.

Simpson, D., Rue, H., Riebler, A., Martins, T. G., Sørbye, S. H., et al. (2017). Penalising model component complexity: A principled, practical approach to constructing priors. *Statistical Science*, *32*(1), 1–28.

Simpson, E. H. (1951). The interpretation of interaction in contingency tables. *Journal of the Royal Statistical Society: Series B (Methodological)*, *13*(2), 238–241.

Sirois, A., and Fricke, W. (1992). Regionally representative daily air concentrations of acid-related substances in canada; 1983–1987. *Atmospheric Environment. Part A. General Topics*, *26*(4), 593–607.

Smith, A. F. M., and Roberts, G. O. (1993). Bayesian computation via the Gibbs sampler and other related Markov Chain Monte Carlo methods. *Journal of the Royal Statistical Society, Series B (Statistical Methodology)*, *55*, 3–23.

Smith, K. (1918). On the standard deviations of adjusted and interpolated values of an observed polynomial function and its constants and the guidance they give towards a proper choice of the distribution of observations. *Biometrika*, *12*(1/2), 1–85.

Smith, R. L. (1989). Extreme value analysis of environmental time series: an application to trend detection in ground-level ozone. *Statistical Science*, *4*(4), 367–377.

Sobol, I. M. (1994). *A Primer for the Monte Carlo Method*. CRC press.

Spiegelhalter, D. J., Best, N. G., Carlin, B. P., and van der Linde, A. (2014). The deviance information criterion: 12 years on. *Journal of the Royal Statistical Society. Series B (Statistical Methodology)*, *76*(3), 485–493.

Spiegelhalter, D. J., Best, N. G., Carlin, B. P., and Van Der Linde, A. (2002). Bayesian measures of model complexity and fit. *Journal of the Royal Statistical Society: Series B (Statistical Methodology)*, *64*(4), 583–639.

Spix, C., Heinrich, J., Dockery, D., Schwartz, J., Völksch, G., Schwinkowski, K., . . . Wichmann, H. E. (1993). Air pollution and daily mortality in Erfurt, East Germany, 1980–1989. *Environmental Health Perspectives*, *101*(6), 518.

Stan Development Team. (2023). *RStan: the R interface to Stan*. Retrieved from https://mc-stan.org/ (R package version 2.21.8)

Stehman, S. V., and Overton, W. S. (1994). Comparison of variance estimators of the Horvitz–Thompson estimator for randomized variable probability systematic sampling. *Journal of the American Statistical Association*, *89*(425), 30–43.

Stein, M. (1987). Large sample properties of simulations using latin hypercube sampling. *Technometrics*, *29*(2), 143–151.

Stein, M. (1999). *Interpolation of Spatial Data: Some Theory for Kriging*. Springer Verlag.

Sullivan, L., Dukes, K., and Losina, E. (1999). An introduction to heirarchical linear modelling. *Statistics in Medicine, 18*, 855–888.

Sun, L., Zidek, J. V., Le, N. D., and Ozkaynak, H. (2000). Interpolating Vancouver's daily ambient PM_{10} field. *Environmetrics, 11*, 651–663.

Sun, W. (1998). Comparison of a cokriging method with a Bayesian alternative. *Environmetrics, 9*(4), 445–457.

Tadesse, M. G., and Vannucci, M. (2021). *Handbook of Bayesian Variable Selection.* Chapman and Hall/CRC.

Tibshrani, R. (1996). Regression shrinkage and selection via the LASSO. *Journal of the Royal Statistical Society. Series B (Statistical Methodology), 58*(1), 267–288.

Timbers, T., Campbell, T., and Lee, M. (2022). *Data Science: A First Introduction.* CRC Press.

Tufte, E. (1942). *The Visual Display of Quantitative Information.* Graphics Press.

van de Kassteele, J., Koelemeijer, R. B. A., Dekkers, A. L. M., Schaap, M., Homan, C. D., and Stein, A. (2006). Statistical mapping of PM_{10} concentrations over Western Europe using secondary information from dispersion modeling and MODIS satellite observations. *Stochastic Environmental Research and Risk Assessment, 21*(2), 183–194.

van der Sluijs, J. P., Craye, M., Funtowicz, S., Kloprogge, P., Ravetz, J., and Risbey, J. (2005). Combining quantitative and qualitative measures of uncertainty in model-based environmental assessment: the nusap system. *Risk Analysis, 25*(2), 481–492.

VanderWeele, T. J., and Robins, J. M. (2012). Stochastic counterfactuals and stochastic sufficient causes. *Statistica Sinica, 22*(1), 379.

van Donkelaar, A., Martin, R. V., Brauer, M., Hsu, N. C., Kahn, R. A., Levy, R. C., ... Winker, D. M. (2016). Global estimates of fine particulate matter using a combined geophysical-statistical method with information from satellites, models, and monitors. *Environmental Science & Technology, 50*(7), 3762–3772.

van Loon, F. P. L., Holmes, S. J., Sirotkin, B. I., Williams, W. W., Cochi, S. L., Hadler, S. C., and Lindegren, M. L. (1995). Mumps surveillance – United States, 1988–1993. *CDC Surveillance Summaries: Morbidity and Mortality Weekly Report, 44*(3), 1–14.

Vedal, S., Brauer, M., White, R., and Petkau, J. (2003). Air pollution and daily mortality in a city with low levels of pollution. *Environmental health perspectives, 111*(1), 45–52.

Verhoeff, A. P., Hoek, G., Schwartz, J., and van Wijnen, J. H. (1996). Air pollution and daily mortality in Amsterdam. *Epidemiology, 7*(3), 225–230.

Vianna-Neto, J. H., Schmidt, A. M., and Guttorp, P. (2014). Accounting for spatially varying directional effects in spatial covariance structures. *Journal of the Royal Statistical Society. Series C (Applied Statistics), 63*(1), 103–122.

von Kügelgen, J., Gresele, L., and Schölkopf, B. (2021). Simpson's paradox in Covid-19 case fatality rates: A mediation analysis of age-related causal effects. *IEEE Transactions on Artificial Intelligence, 2*(1), 18–27.

Wackernagel, H. (2003). *Multivariate Geostatistics: An Introduction with Applications*. Springer Verlag.

Wahba, G. (1990). *Spline Models for Observational Data* (Vol. 59). Siam.

Wakefield, J., and Salway, R. (2001). A statistical framework for ecological and aggregate studies. *Journal of the Royal Statistical Society, Series A (Statistics in Society)*, *164*, 119-137.

Wakefield, J., and Shaddick, G. (2006). Health-exposure modeling and the ecological fallacy. *Biostatistics*, *7*(3), 438–455.

Wakefield, J. C., Best, N. G., and Waller, L. A. (2000). Bayesian approaches to disease mapping. In P. Elliott, J. C. Wakefield, N. G. Best, and D. J. Briggs (Eds.), *Spatial Epidemiology: Methods and Applications*. Oxford: Oxford University Press.

Walker, W. E., Harremoës, P., Rotmans, J., van der Sluijs, J. P., van Asselt, M. B., Janssen, P., and Krayer von Krauss, M. P. (2003). Defining uncertainty: a conceptual basis for uncertainty management in model-based decision support. *Integrated assessment*, *4*(1), 5–17.

Waller, L. A., and Gotway, C. A. (2004). *Applied Spatial Statistics for Public Health Data* (Vol. 368). Wiley-Interscience.

Wang, M., Aaron, C. P., Madrigano, J., Hoffman, E. A., Angelini, E., Yang, J., ... others (2019). Association between long-term exposure to ambient air pollution and change in quantitatively assessed emphysema and lung function. *Journal of the American Medical Association*, *322*(6), 546–556.

Wasserstein, R. L., and Lazar, N. A. (2016). The asa statement on p-values: context, process, and purpose. *The American Statistician*, *70*(2), 129–133.

Watanabe, S. (2010). Asymptotic equivalence of bayes cross validation and widely applicable information criterion in singular learning theory. *Journal of Machine Learning Research*, *11*(12), 3571–3594.

Waternaux, C., Laird, N., and Ware, J. (1989). Methods for analysis of longitudinal data: blood lead concentrations and cognitive development. *Journal of the American Statistical Association*, *84*, 33–41.

Watson, J. (2021). A perceptron for detecting the preferential sampling of locations and times chosen to monitor a spatio-temporal process. *Spatial Statistics*, *43*, 100500.

Watson, J., Zidek, J. V., and Shaddick, G. (2019). A general theory for preferential sampling in environmental networks. *The Annals of Applied Statistics*, *13*(4), 2662 – 2700.

Webster, R., and Oliver, M. A. (2007). *Geostatistics for Environmental Scientists*. John Wiley & Sons.

West, M., and Harrison, J. (1997). *Bayesian Forecasting and Dynamic Models; 2 edition*. Springer.

West, M., Harrison, J., and Migon, H. S. (1985). Dynamic generalized linear models and Bayesian forecasting. *Journal of the American Statistical Association*, *80*(389), 73–83.

Whittle, P. (1954). On stationary processes in the plane. *Biometrika*, *41*(3/4), 434–449.

Wikle, C. K., Berliner, L. M., and Cressie, N. (1998). Hierarchical Bayesian space-time models. *Environmental and Ecological Statistics*, *5*, 117–154.

Wikle, C. K., and Cressie, N. (1999). A dimension reduction approach to space-time Kalman filtering. *Biometrika*, *86*, 815–829.

Wikle, C. K., Zammit-Mangion, A., and Cressie, N. (2019). *Spatio-temporal Statistics with R*. Chapman and Hall/CRC.

Wood, S. (2006). *Generalized Additive Models: An Introduction with R*. Chapman and Hall/CRC.

Yu, O., Sheppard, L., Lumley, T., Koenig, J. Q., and Shapiro, G. G. (2000). Effects of ambient air pollution on symptoms of asthma in seattle-area children enrolled in the CAMP Study. *Environmental Health Perspectives*, *108*, 1209–1214.

Zannetti, P. (1990). *Air Pollution Modeling: Theories, Computational Methods, and Available Software*. Computational Mechanics Southampton.

Zanobetti, A., Wand, M. P., Schwartz, J., and Ryan, L. M. (2000). Generalized additive distributed lag models: quantifying mortality displacement. *Biostatistics*, *1*(3), 279–292.

Zapata-Marin, S., Schmidt, A. M., Crouse, D., Ho, F., V. Labrèche, Lavigne, E., Parent, M.-E., and Goldberg, M. S. (2022). Spatial modeling of ambient concentrations of volatile organic compounds in montreal, canada. *Environmental Epidemiology*, *6*(5), e226.

Zeger, S. L., Thomas, D. C., Dominici, F., Samet, J. M., Schwartz, J., Dockery, D., and Cohen, A. (2000). Exposure measurement error in time–series studies of air pollution: Concepts and consequences. *Environmental Health Perspectives*, *108*(5), 419.

Zhang, H. (2004). Inconsistent estimation and asymptotically equal interpolations in model-based geostatistics. *Journal of the American Statistical Association*, *99*(465), 250–261.

Zhu, L., Carlin, B. P., and Gelfand, A. E. (2003). Hierarchical regression with misaligned spatial data: relating ambient ozone and pediatric asthma ER visits in atlanta. *Environmetrics*, *14*(5), 537–557.

Zhu, Z., and Stein, M. L. (2006). Spatial sampling design for prediction with estimated parameters. *Journal of Agricultural, Biological, and Environmental Statistics*, *11*(1), 24–44.

Zidek, J. (1984). Maximal simpson-disaggregations of 2×2 tables. *Biometrika*, *71*(1), 187–190.

Zidek, J., White, R., Sun, W., Burnett, R., and Le, N. (1998). Imputing unmeasured explanatory variables in environmental epidemiology with application to health impact analysis of air pollution. *Environmental and Ecological Statistics*, *5*(2), 99–105.

Zidek, J. V., Le, N. D., and Liu, Z. (2012a). Combining data and simulated data for space–time fields: application to ozone. *Environmental and Ecological Statistics*, *19*(1), 37–56.

Zidek, J. V., Le, N. D., and Liu, Z. (2012b). Combining data and simulated data for space–time fields: application to ozone. *Environmental and ecological statistics*, *19*, 37–56.

Zidek, J. V., Meloche, J., Shaddick, G., Chatfield, C., and White, R. (2003). A computational model for estimating personal exposure to air pollutants with application to London's PM10 in 1997. *2003 Technical Report of the Statistical and Applied Mathematical Sciences Institute.*

Zidek, J. V., Shaddick, G., Meloche, J., Chatfield, C., and White, R. (2007). A framework for predicting personal exposures to environmental hazards. *Environmental and Ecological Statistics*, *14*(4), 411–431.

Zidek, J. V., Shaddick, G., and Taylor, C. G. (2014). Reducing estimation bias in adaptively changing monitoring networks with preferential site selection. *The Annals of Applied Statistics*, *8*(3), 1640–1670.

Zidek, J. V., Shaddick, G., Taylor, C. G., et al. (2014). Reducing estimation bias in adaptively changing monitoring networks with preferential site selection. *The Annals of Applied Statistics*, *8*(3), 1640–1670.

Zidek, J. V., Shaddick, G., White, R., Meloche, J., and Chatfield, C. (2005). Using a probabilistic model (pCNEM) to estimate personal exposure to air pollution. *Environmetrics*, *16*(5), 481–493.

Zidek, J. V., Sun, W., and Le, N. D. (2000). Designing and integrating composite networks for monitoring multivariate gaussian pollution fields. *Journal of the Royal Statistical Society: Series C (Applied Statistics)*, *49*(1), 63–79.

Zidek, J. V., and van Eeden, C. (2003). Uncertainty, entropy, variance and the effect of partial information. *Lecture Notes-Monograph Series*, 155–167.

Zidek, J. V., Wong, H., Le, N. D., and Burnett, R. (1996). Causality, measurement error and multicollinearity in epidemiology. *Environmetrics*, *7*(4), 441–451.

Zidek, J. V., and Zimmerman, D. L. (2019). Monitoring network design. In *Handbook of Environmental and Ecological Statistics* (pp. 499–522). Chapman and Hall/CRC.

Index

413